Responsible Conduct of Research

RESPONSIBLE CONDUCT OF RESEARCH

THIRD EDITION

Adil E. Shamoo and David B. Resnik

OXFORD
UNIVERSITY PRESS

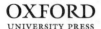

OXFORD
UNIVERSITY PRESS

Oxford University Press is a department of the University of Oxford.
It furthers the University's objective of excellence in research, scholarship,
and education by publishing worldwide.

Oxford New York
Auckland Cape Town Dar es Salaam Hong Kong Karachi
Kuala Lumpur Madrid Melbourne Mexico City Nairobi
New Delhi Shanghai Taipei Toronto

With offices in
Argentina Austria Brazil Chile Czech Republic France Greece
Guatemala Hungary Italy Japan Poland Portugal Singapore
South Korea Switzerland Thailand Turkey Ukraine Vietnam

Oxford is a registered trade mark of Oxford University Press
in the UK and certain other countries.

Published in the United States of America by
Oxford University Press
198 Madison Avenue, New York, NY 10016

Library of Congress Cataloging-in-Publication Data
Shamoo, Adil E.
  Responsible conduct of research / Adil E. Shamoo and David B. Resnik. — Third edition.
    p. cm.
  Includes bibliographical references and index.
  ISBN 978–0–19–937602–5 (alk. paper)
1. Medical ethics. 2. Bioethics. 3. Medicine—Research—Moral and ethical aspects.
4. Scientists—Professional ethics. 5. Human experimentation in medicine—Moral
and ethical aspects. I. Title.
  R724.S4545 2015
  174.2—dc23
                                        2014023963

9 8 7 6 5 4 3 2

Printed in Canada on acid-free paper

CONTENTS

PREFACE TO THE THIRD EDITION

When the first edition of this textbook went to press in 2002, the field of responsible conduct of research (RCR) was in its infancy. Since then, there has been a great deal of change at many different levels—governmental, institutional, and individual. The Office of Research Integrity (ORI), part of the U.S. government, has funded empirical research, conferences, and course development on RCR. At the institutional level, universities have developed RCR policies and implemented RCR training programs; professional societies have drafted or revised ethics codes and guidelines; and scientific journals have developed rules and policies. At the individual level, researchers have published numerous books and articles on RCR and created RCR courses, class materials, and training modules. Researchers, institutions, and government agencies have also participated in several international conferences on research integrity.

Although much has been accomplished in the last decade or so, many serious ethical challenges remain. Misconduct continues to be a serious problem in research, as illustrated by highly publicized fraud cases involving research on stem cells, nanotechnology, women's health, oncology, and animal behavior. Researchers and institutional leaders continue to wrestle with ethical issues related to collaborations with industry and the commercialization of research, such as conflicts of interest and intellectual property rights. Perennial ethical issues, such as research involving animals or human subjects, as well as new and emerging concerns in fields such as genetics/genomics, synthetic biology, neuroscience, pharmacogenomics, nutrition research, microbiology, and virology, have drawn the attention of the media, the public, and politicians.

Since 1989, the Public Health Service (PHS), which funds National Institutes of Health (NIH) research, has required trainees (such as graduate students and postdoctoral fellows) to receive RCR instruction. In 2009, the National Science Foundation (NSF) began requiring that all recipients of NSF funding have an RCR education plan for all their students on those grants. Many universities have adopted RCR training requirements that go beyond the federal conditions. Some require all doctoral students or all graduate students to receive RCR instruction. Many countries outside the United States have also begun to consider implementing RCR training requirements.

We published a second edition of the book in 2009 to take into account new developments in RCR, but the field continues to evolve rapidly, so we have decided to publish a third edition, which includes updated references, case studies, policies, and other material useful to students and scholars alike. The book presents a comprehensive introduction to RCR, with 13 chapters ranging in scope from the broad issues relating to social responsibility, research funding, and freedom of inquiry, to more narrow topics such as the ethical aspects of entering data into lab notebooks, designing experiments, citing published works, and deciding authorship matters.

We apologize for any errors or oversights in this third edition. Please feel free to send your comments and suggestions to Adil E. Shamoo, PhD, Department of Biochemistry and Molecular Biology, University of Maryland School of Medicine, 108 North Greene Street, Baltimore, Maryland 21201–1503; e-mail: ashamoo@som.umaryland.edu.

ACKNOWLEDGMENTS

Dr. Shamoo is grateful for all of the guest lecturers for his course since 1994, among them Jousef Giffels, Jack Schwartz, and Leslie Katzel. Dr. Shamoo also thanks the students in his Responsible Conduct of Research classes since 1994 for their input and discussions. For useful discussions and insight about ethics in research, Dr. Resnik is especially grateful to Dr. Loretta Kopelman, Dr. Kenneth De Ville, Dr. Thomas Feldbush, Dr. John Bradfield, Dr. Jeremy Sugarman, Frank Grassner, John Doll, and the students and co-instructors in his research ethics classes taught in 1999 and 2001 at the Brody School of Medicine. Finally, we thank the many anonymous reviewers of the prospectus during the publisher's review process for their considerable and valued suggestions for improving the textbook in content and style. Moreover, we thank Patrick L. Taylor, Children's Hospital Boston, Harvard Medical School, for his thorough review of the second edition. Research for the third edition of *Responsible Conduct of Research* was supported, in part, by the Intramural Program of the National Institute of Environmental Health Sciences, National Institutes of Health. It does not represent the views of the National Institute of Environmental Health Sciences or the National Institutes of Health.

Responsible Conduct of Research

CHAPTER 1
Scientific Research and Ethics

There is a growing recognition among scientists, government officials, research institutions, and the public that ethical conduct is essential to scientific research. Ethical conduct in research is essential to the foundation and advancement of science. It is also important to foster trust among scientists and the public's support for research. This chapter discusses the importance of ethics in research, the nature of scientific professionalism, and ethical decision making.

Ethical (or moral) problems, issues, and dilemmas occur for most people on a daily basis. Whenever we ask the question "What should I do?" there is a good chance that an ethical issue or concern lurks in the background. In everyday life, such questions frequently arise as we make choices among different interests and commitments, such as career, family, community, church, society, prestige, and money. Professional researchers—scientists, engineers, and scholars—also frequently face ethical problems, issues, and dilemmas. Consider the following cases:

CASE 1

You are a graduate student in pharmacology at a large university working under the direction of a senior researcher. After reading a paper on a new serotonin reuptake inhibitor published by the researcher, you notice that there is a problem with a diagram representing the dose-response curve. You cannot reconcile the diagram with the published data. You are a coauthor on the paper with a postdoctoral fellow, a technician, and your senior researcher (your supervisor). You approach your supervisor with this problem, and he shrugs it off, saying that you do not understand the research well enough to make a judgment about it. What should you do?

CASE 2

You are a graduate student in psychology working on a dissertation about college students' attitudes toward drug and alcohol use. When you start compiling surveys, you notice some problems with your data. It appears that about 20% of the students misunderstood the Likert-scale questions, because they answered "1" when it appears they meant "5," based on their written comments that accompanied these questions. If you exclude these data from your analysis on the grounds that they are erroneous, this could affect the statistical significance of your results and the analysis and interpretation of the data. How should you deal with this issue?

CASE 3

You are a postdoctoral fellow in epidemiology at a university, and you are collaborating with a senior researcher. You have just read an important paper in your field and contacted the author about it. The paper is one of several the author has published from a large, publicly funded database. You ask the author if you can have access to the database to confirm your own work. The author says he will share data with you only if you agree to a formal collaboration with him and name him as a coauthor in publications that use the database. What should you do?

CASE 4

You are a professor of veterinary medicine and chair of your institution's animal care and use committee, which oversees animal research. The group People for the Ethical Treatment of Animals (PETA) has staged some protests against animal research recently at your institution. A local reporter calls you on the phone and wants to do an interview with you about animal research and animal rights. How should you handle this situation?

These cases illustrate some of the complex ethical dilemmas that can arise in the conduct of research. The purpose of this book is to help enhance science students' and scientists' understanding of the ethical, legal, and social dimensions of research, so that they can act appropriately and make responsible choices.

In recent years, scientists have come to realize that ethical conduct is an essential part of basic, applied, and clinical research. A few decades ago, many scientists would not have accepted this idea. According to a view that has held sway among scientists, humanists, and the general public for centuries, science is objective (Bronowski 1956; Snow 1964) and ethics are subjective, so scientists need not deal with ethical issues and concerns when conducting research. Ethical and social questions, according to this view, occur in the applications of science, but not in the conduct of science. Humanists, politicians, and the public can grapple with the ethical (or moral) aspects of research; the main task of the scientist is to do research for its own sake (Rescher 1965).

While it is important for scientists to strive for objectivity, this does not mean that ethical questions, problems, and concerns have no place in research conduct. Indeed, ethical behavior plays a key role in promoting objectivity, since ethical transgressions, such as data fabrication or falsification, and ethical concerns, such as conflicts of interest, can lead to biased or erroneous research.

Scientists need to pay special attention to research ethics in their own work and in teaching students about how to conduct research for several reasons (Shamoo 1989; Shamoo and Dunigan 2000; Sigma Xi 1986). First, modern science is a social activity in which researchers, students, and staff work together to achieve common goals (Merton 1973; Ziman 1984). Many different aspects of science, including mentoring, education, collaborative research, data sharing, peer review, and publication depend on cooperation based on shared expectations and understandings. Unethical behavior in science can destroy the trust that holds together the social fabric of research (Committee on Science 2009; Hull 1988; Macrina 2013; Resnik 1998a; Steneck 2006).

Second, most scientists receive considerable public support, such as funding and access to resources and facilities. Even those researchers who are not funded by government contracts or grants most likely received their education at a university that benefited from public support. Public support for research is based on trust and accountability. The public trusts that scientists will perform ethical research that has the potential to benefit society, and the public may hold scientists accountable for their conduct. Over the years, political leaders have held dozens of hearings on the integrity of scientific research and have enacted laws and regulations to ensure that scientists act responsibly. Unethical and illegal conduct in science can compromise the integrity of research and lead to scandals and negative political fallout that erode public trust and support for research (Resnik 2011).

Third, all members of society, including scientists, have some basic ethical obligations and duties (Resnik 1998a). Everyone has an obligation not to lie, cheat, or steal, for example. In science, the obligation not to lie, cheat, or steal implies duties not to fabricate or falsify data or plagiarize research. Everyone also has an obligation not to harm or dehumanize other people. In science, this obligation implies duties to protect the rights and welfare of human research subjects, as well as a duty to not publish research results that could be used by others to cause significant harm to society.

For these reasons and many others, universities, funding agencies, research institutions, professional societies, and scientists are now very much aware of the importance of ethics in research (Committee on Science 2009). Responses to these ethical concerns include the development of laws and regulations, institutional policies, journal policies, and professional guidelines pertaining to research ethics; investigations of research misconduct by institutions and the government; government hearings on research integrity and oversight; research on research ethics issues, including the publication of articles and books; workshops and international conferences on research ethics; and mentoring and formal education in research ethics (or the responsible conduct of research, RCR).

SCIENCE AS A PROFESSION

Research ethics can be understood according to the professional model (Resnik 1998a; Shrader-Frechette 1994; Steneck 2006). Each profession has its own ethical standards, which govern the practices in the profession. In medicine, physicians abide by rules such as "do no harm," "promote the patient's health," "maintain confidentiality," and "honor the patient's right to make decisions" (Beauchamp and Childress 2001). Science also has its own standards, which we discuss below. Professions usually adopt codes of ethics to signal to members of the profession and the public the type of behavior that is expected in the profession (Bayles 1988). Since the 1980s, many different scientific organizations, such as the American Anthropological Association (2012), the American Physical Society (2002), the American Society for Microbiology (2005), and the American Statistical Association (1999), have adopted ethics codes and guidelines. In 2010, over 340 researchers and government and institutional officials from 51 countries adopted the Singapore Statement on Research Integrity at the 2nd World Conference on Research Integrity (Singapore Statement 2010).

In addition to adopting ethical guidelines, scientific disciplines share several other characteristics with recognized professions. First, a profession is more than an occupation; it is a career or vocation (Davis 1995a). The first people to be recognized as professionals were physicians and ministers, who viewed themselves as being "called" to serve and devoted their lives to serving society. Most scientists view their work as a career and not just an occupation. Second, professionals have social responsibilities and can be held publicly accountable (Davis 1995a). Physicians, for example, have professional duties to promote the health of not only their patients but also the public. As noted above, scientists also have social responsibilities and can be held publicly accountable. Third, professionals are allowed to be self-regulating: Professionals can make their own standards and rules, provided that they obey the law and fulfill their public responsibilities (Bayles 1988). Physicians, for example, set their own standard of care and determine what it takes to become a qualified member of the profession. Scientists are also self-regulating: Scientists make their own rules for designing experiments, drawing inferences from data, publishing results, and so on. Scientists determine what counts as "good scientific practice." Finally, professionals are recognized as having expertise. Physicians, for example, have expertise when it comes to diagnosing, treating, and preventing diseases (Bayles 1988). Scientists are recognized as experts within their domain of knowledge and professional practice.

Prior to the Scientific Revolution (ca. 1500–1700 A.D.), science was more of an avocation than a vocation. Scientists often worked in isolation and financed their own research. They did not publish very frequently— the printing press was not invented until the mid-1400s—and when they did, their works were not peer reviewed. There were no professional scientific societies or journals until the mid-1600s. Universities taught only a small number of scientific subjects, and many scientists could master several different subjects. For example, Newton made major contributions to mechanics, astronomy, optics, and mathematics (Newton 1687 [1995]). Private businesses and governments saw little reason to invest in research. Science also did not have a great deal of social status or impact—the church and the state battled for social influence and political power (Burke 1995; Ziman 1984).

Science has changed dramatically in the last 500 years. Today, there are thousands of scientific societies and professional journals. Peer review plays a key role in funding and publications decisions. Scientists now work in research groups, which may include laboratory assistants and data analysts as well as postdoctoral, graduate, and undergraduate students. Universities now offer study in hundreds of different scientific subjects, and it is virtually impossible to achieve scientific expertise without specialization. Governments and private corporations now invest billions of dollars each year in science. Science has become one of the most influential social institutions in society (Ziman 1984). Most of the technologies and many of the ideas in our modern world are the direct or indirect result of scientific research. Scientists now publish millions of articles a year, and the information boom continues to increase. Scientists give expert testimony to congressional committees and government agencies, and they provide advice to presidents, governors, generals, and corporate executives. Children learn about science in school, and most professional careers require some type of scientific and technical knowledge.

Science is now also a sizable part of the world's economy: Total (private and public) research and development (R&D) investments account for at least 2.5% of the gross domestic product (GDP) in developed countries such as the United States, United Kingdom, and Germany. Economic activity directly related to scientific research is estimated to be about 6% of the U.S. GDP (Resnik 2007). The indirect impacts of research are much larger than the direct impacts, because R&D investments have led to economically significant innovations, such as computers, the Internet, airplanes, automobiles, nuclear energy, and radar. As the 21st-century economy becomes more dependent on information, investments in R&D are likely to continue the upward trend that began in World War II (Dickson 1988). Literally millions of scientists are employed in universities, research institutions, private laboratories, or other organizations that conduct research (National Science Foundation 1997). It is estimated that there are more scientists alive today than all of the scientists who have lived during the past 2,500 years of human history (Dickson 1988).

Science's increased economic, social, and political influence carries added ethical responsibilities. Although laws and regulations, institutional and journal policies, and professional codes of conduct can provide valuable guidance for scientists, they have significant limitations. First, laws, regulations, policies, and codes do not cover every situation that may arise in research. For example, none of these rules say anything about authorship order on a scientific paper, which is often important. Second, the rules need to be interpreted and applied to particular situations. For example, to apply a prohibition against fabricating data to a particular study, one must understand particular details concerning the study's methodology and assumptions. Second, these different rules sometimes conflict. For example, funding agency and journal requirements to share data may conflict with the duty to protect confidential information concerning human research subjects. Fourth, the rules themselves need to be evaluated and critiqued. For example, when a journal revises its policies pertaining to authorship, it must draw insights or inspiration from something beyond those policies (such as ethical considerations). Policies and other rules do not stand on their own: They must be based on more fundamental goals or concerns.

For these and other reasons, it is important for science students and working scientists to have a fuller understanding of research ethics. It is not enough to try to be familiar with a list of rules developed by governments, institutions, journals, or other organizations. To make responsible decisions involving ethical issues, one must also understand the deeper rationale for ethical rules and standards and how to deal with ethical dilemmas and problems in a rational way. To help achieve these goals, we provide an overview of ethics and ethical decision making.

WHAT IS ETHICS?

Ethics can be understood as (1) standards of conduct and as (2) an academic discipline that studies standards of conduct and ethical decision making. Ethics as an academic discipline is concerned with answering age-old questions about duty, honor, integrity, virtue, justice, and the good life (Frankena 1973). Scholars and scientists study ethics from a normative or descriptive point of view. The questions addressed by normative ethics have to do with how one *ought* to live or how society *ought* to be structured. These are the traditional questions addressed by philosophers, theologians, and political theorists. Various disciplines in the social and behavioral sciences, including psychology, neurobiology, sociology, and anthropology, take a descriptive approach to ethics and attempt to describe and explain ethical beliefs, attitudes, emotions, judgments, decisions, and behaviors (de Waal 2009; Haidt 2007; Miller 2008). Although the facts discovered by descriptive ethics have some bearing on normative questions, they cannot, by themselves, provide complete answers to normative questions because questions require normative answers.

For example, suppose that someone is trying to decide whether to cheat on her income taxes. Her question might be, "Should I cheat on my income taxes?" Suppose that a social scientist conducts a study showing that 65% of people cheat on their income taxes. This scientific study still would not answer the person's question. She wants to know not how many people cheat, but whether *she* should cheat. The fact that most people cheat does not justify cheating. The person asking the ethical questions is requesting a normative justification for a particular course of action, but scientific studies do not provide this. Science delivers facts and explanations, not values and justifications.

The study of normative ethics can be subdivided into theoretical ethics, which studies general theories, concepts, and principles of ethics; meta-ethics, which studies the meaning and justification of ethical words, concepts, and principles; and applied (or practical) ethics, which studies ethical questions that arise in specific situations or areas of conduct, such as medicine or business (Frankena 1973). Research ethics is a branch of applied ethics that studies the ethical problems, dilemmas, and issues that arise in the conduct of research.

In this book, we do not explore meta-ethical issues in great depth, but we mention one issue that has some relevance for research ethics. One of the key questions of meta-ethics is whether ethical standards are universal (Frankena 1973; Pojman 1995). According to one school of thought, the same ethical (or moral) standards apply to all people at all times in all situations. A contrasting school of thought holds that different ethical standards apply to different people in different situations: There are no universal moral rules or values. We mention this issue here because in some situations in research ethics one must take a stand on this dispute (Angell 1997a, 1997b; Emanuel et al. 2000; Resnik 1998b). For example, different countries have various views on human rights, including the right to informed consent. In some countries, a woman's husband or older male relative (such as her father) provides consent for the woman. Scientists who conduct research in these countries must face the question of whether they should follow local customs concerning informed consent or Western standards, which require the individual to consent (Hyder and Wali 2006).

Returning to our focus on ethics as a standard of conduct, it is important to compare and contrast ethics and the law. Societies have had laws since ancient times. Laws are like ethical standards in several ways. First, laws, like ethics, tell people how they ought or ought not to behave. Second, ethical and legal standards share many concepts and terms, such as duty, responsibility, negligence, rights, benefits, and harms. Third, the methods of reasoning used in law and ethics are quite similar: Both disciplines give arguments and counterarguments, analyze concepts and principles, and discuss cases and rules.

However, ethics differs from the law in several important ways as well. First, the scope of ethics is not the same as the scope of law. There are many types of conduct that might be considered unethical but are not illegal. For instance, it may be perfectly legal to not give credit to someone who makes a major contribution to a research project, but this action would still be unethical because it would violate principles of fairness and honesty. We can think of ethics and law as two different circles that overlap in some areas. Because laws are enforced by the coercive power of government, societies usually make laws pertaining to a behavior only when there is a social consensus concerning that behavior. The law usually sets a minimal standard of conduct, but ethics can go beyond that standard (Gert 2007).

Second, people can appeal to moral or ethical standards to evaluate or judge legal ones. People may decide that there needs to be a law against some type of unethical behavior, or they may decide that an existing law is unethical. If we consider a law to be unethical, then we may be morally obligated to change the law or perhaps even disobey it. For example, many people who considered South Africa's system of apartheid to be unethical fought to change the system. Some of them made a conscious decision to protest apartheid laws and engaged in a kind of law-breaking known as civil disobedience.

Third, ethical standards tend to be more informal and less technical than legal standards; ethical standards are not usually legalistic. In many cases, ethical standards are not even written down, but legal standards always are.

Because ethics and the law are not the same, scientists must consider and weigh both legal and ethical obligations when making ethical decisions.

It is also important to distinguish between ethics and politics. Politics, like ethics, deals with standards for human conduct. However, political questions tend to focus on broad issues having to do with the structure of society and group dynamics, whereas ethical questions tend to focus on narrower issues pertaining to the conduct of individuals within society (Rawls 1971). Many of the controversial areas of human conduct have both ethical and political dimensions. For instance, abortion is an ethical issue for a woman trying to decide whether to have an abortion, but it is a political issue for legislators and judges who must decide whether laws against abortion would unjustly invade a woman's sphere of private choice. Thus, the distinction between ethics and politics is not absolute (Rawls 1971). Although this book focuses on the ethics of research, many of the issues it covers, such as government funding of science and research with animal or human subjects, have political dimensions.

The distinction between ethics and religion is also important for our purposes. Ethical theories and religious traditions have much in common in that they prescribe standards of human conduct and provide some account of the meaning and value of life. Many people use religious teachings, texts, and practices (e.g., prayer) for ethical guidance. We do not intend to devalue or belittle the importance of religion in inspiring and influencing ethical conduct. However, we stress that ethics is not the same as religion. First, people from different religious backgrounds can agree on some basic ethical principles and concepts. Christians, Jews, Muslims, Hindus, and Buddhists can all agree on the importance of honesty, integrity, justice, benevolence, respect for human life, and many other ethical values despite their theological disagreements. Second, the study of ethics, or moral philosophy, is a secular discipline that relies on human reasoning to analyze and interpret ethical concepts and principles. Although some ethicists adopt a theological approach to moral questions and issues, most use secular reasoning methods, concepts, and theories. While our book focuses on research ethics, many of the issues it addresses have religious aspects as well. For instance, various churches have developed opinions on specific issues arising from science and technology, such as cloning, assisted reproduction, DNA patenting, and genetic engineering.

ETHICAL THEORIES

To understand what a normative ethical theory is, it will be useful to compare normative ethical theories to scientific ones. Scientific theories include laws or generalizations that explain and predict observable phenomena. For example, the kinetic theory of gases includes the ideal gas law ($PV = nRT$), which explains and predicts how gases respond to change in temperature, pressure, and volume under certain conditions. Ethical theories include principles or norms that justify and prescribe behavior. For example, one might appeal to a theory of human rights to justify prohibitions against torture and reprimand governments for engaging in torture.

To test a scientific theory, one must produce empirical evidence (i.e., observations and data) that could support or undermine the theory. For example, measurements of continental drift and studies of volcanic activity patterns provided evidence for the plate tectonics theory. If evidence emerges that contradicts a theory, then scientists may reject the theory or modify it to account for the new evidence. For example, scientists rejected the theory of spontaneous generation of life from inert matter (such as rotting meat) on the basis of experiments showing that living organisms did not emerge from inert matter when the matter was shielded from flies and other contaminants.

Normative ethical theories are tested by appealing not to empirical evidence but to our judgments of right/wrong or good/bad in particular cases. For example, suppose that an ethical theory includes a principle like "promote human life." The theory should be able to provide a satisfactory account of judgments concerning the ethics of killing in particular situations, such as murder, self-defense, and war, and the importance of saving human lives. To test this theory, we could consider a hypothetical case (or thought experiment) where a doctor has an opportunity to use the organs from a patient to save the lives of five people. The patient is now in a persistent vegetative state as a result of a massive stroke. Before he had the stroke, he told the doctor and his family that he did not want to donate his organs because he believes that the human body is sacred. Should the doctor use the organs from the patient, against his wishes, to save the five people, or should he allow the patient to die without damaging his body? The theory implies that the doctor should take the organs, because this would promote human life. If we judge that this would be the wrong thing to do in this situation because we think the patient's wishes should be respected, then this would constitute evidence against this simple theory. If enough evidence of this sort emerges, we may reject the theory or develop a different one that does a better job of handling this and other cases. Over time, our theories can become better at systematizing our ethical judgments. This method for testing ethical theories is known as reflective equilibrium (Harman 1977; Rawls 1971).

Moral judgments are different from perceptual judgments. To make the judgment "this stop sign is red," I apply my beliefs and concepts to my sensory experience. For example, I might apply the concepts of "red" and "stop sign" to my visual experience to judge that "this stop sign is red." Although we have five senses that we use to make perceptual judgments, we have no sensory organ that provides input for moral judgments. Instead, we make moral judgments by forming a holistic impression of the situation we are presented with, based on our beliefs, concepts, and emotional reactions (Haidt 2007). For example, suppose I observe Jane Doe cutting John Doe with a knife, and I also believe that Jane is trying to kill John. I may experience revulsion, fear, anxiety, disgust, and other negative emotions. I may conclude, from this whole impression, that what is happening is wrong. However, I might not arrive at this judgment if I observe the same act of cutting (i.e., the same perceptual experience) when I believe that Jane is a skilled surgeon performing an emergency tracheotomy in an attempt to save John's life. Under these circumstances, I may experience no negative emotions, except perhaps some disgust at seeing John being cut. The difference between judging that an action is a vicious assault and judging that an action is a commendable deed is a function of my beliefs about the act.

While the analogy between ethical and scientific theories is useful, it only goes so far. Scientific theories are different from ethical ones because they have greater objectivity. Although controversies concerning scientific theories (such as evolution and global warming) abound, scientists have made considerable progress over the years and have produced many theories that are widely accepted on the basis of substantial evidence, such as the ideal gas theory, plate tectonics, general relativity, atomic theory, chemical bonding theory, and so on. Philosophers have argued about ethical theories since the time of Plato (427–347 B.C.E.) and no consensus has emerged. One reason why consensus is so difficult to achieve in philosophy is that ethical judgments are strongly influenced by social, cultural, economic, and religious biases, which play only a minor role in perceptual judgments. Two people with very different religious beliefs and cultural backgrounds can look at a stop sign and agree that it is red if they have the concepts "red" and "stop sign" in their mental repertoire, but the same two people who witness an abortion or a public execution may not agree whether it is right or wrong. While there is some rough agreement on basic ethical principles (such as "don't lie, cheat, or steal") there is little agreement about theories. The method of reflective equilibrium may help philosophers move toward some consensus on ethical theories, but there is no guarantee that this will happen.

Given the lack of philosophical consensus about philosophical theories, we will not defend any particular theory as the "correct" or "best" one. Instead, we will describe (below) several prominent theories for students and scientists to consider when making ethical decisions and reflecting on the philosophical basis of the ethical guidelines for the conduct of research. These theories capture different insights about the nature of morality (Hinman 2002). Some focus on moral rules; others focus on moral virtues. Some emphasize the good of the individual, while others stress the good of society (Beauchamp and Childress 2001).

KANTIANISM

Kantianism is a theory, developed by the German Enlightenment philosopher Immanuel Kant (1724–1804), that has been revised and fine-tuned by modern-day Kantians (Korsgaard 1996). The basic insight of Kantianism is that ethical conduct is a matter of choosing to live one's life according to moral principles or rules. The concept of a moral agent plays a central role in Kant's theory: A moral agent is a self-governing (or autonomous) person who can distinguish between right and wrong and choose to obey moral rules. For Kant, the motives of agents (or reasons for action) matter a great deal. One should do the right action for the right reason (Pojman 1995). To decide what the right thing to do is in a particular situation, one must apply a principle known as the categorical imperative (CI) to that situation (Kant 1753 [1981]). According to one version of the CI, the right thing to do in a particular situation is to follow a rule for action that could become a universal law for all people. For example, suppose that I am considering making a promise that I do not intend to keep in order to obtain money from someone. The CI implies that making this false promise would be wrong, because if everyone made false promises, no one could trust anyone and promises wouldn't mean anything anymore. So making false promises is a self-defeating rule for action that could not become a universal law. According to the respect-for-humanity version of CI, one should treat humanity, whether in one's own person or in another person, always as an end in itself, never only as a means. Making a false promise would be wrong, according to this version of the CI, because it would treat another person as a mere means to obtain something. The basic insight in this version of the CI is that all human beings have intrinsic, equal moral dignity or worth: We should not abuse, manipulate, harm, exploit, or deceive people in order to achieve specific goals. As we discuss later in this book, this concept has important applications in the ethics of human research.

UTILITARIANISM

The English philosophers and reformists Jeremy Bentham (1748–1832) and John Stuart Mill (1806–1873) developed the theory of utilitarianism in the 1800s. Utilitarians hold that the right thing to do is to produce the best overall consequences for the most people. We should maximize good consequences and minimize bad ones (Frankena 1973; Pojman 1995). Philosophers have introduced the term "consequentialism" to describe theories, such as utilitarianism, that evaluate actions and policies in terms of their outcomes or consequences (good or bad). "Deontological" theories, on the other hand, judge actions and policies insofar as they conform to moral principles or rules, and these theories do not appeal to consequences directly. Kantianism is a deontological theory because it holds that actions are morally correct insofar as they result from moral motives and conform to moral principles. Different utilitarian theorists emphasize different types of consequences. Mill and Bentham thought that the consequences that mattered were happiness and unhappiness. According to Mill's Greatest Happiness Principle, one should produce the greatest balance of happiness/unhappiness for the most people (Mill 1861 [1979]). Due to problems with defining the term "happiness," some modern utilitarians hold that one should maximize preferences, welfare, or other values. Different utilitarian theorists stress different ways of evaluating human conduct. For instance, act utilitarians argue that we should apply the principle of utility to different actions when deciding what to do, whereas rule utilitarians argue that we should apply the principle of utility to a set of rules for society and that we should follow the rules that maximize utility. A number of different approaches to social problems are similar to utilitarianism in that they address the consequences of actions and policies. Cost-benefit analysis examines economic costs and benefits, and risk-assessment theory addresses risks and benefits. In this book, we will discuss how the utilitarian perspective applies to many important ethical questions in research and science policy.

VIRTUE ETHICS

The virtue ethics approach has a long history dating to antiquity. Virtue theorists, unlike Kantians and utilitarians, focus on developing good character traits. Their key insight is that ethical conduct has to do with living a life marked by excellence and virtue (Aristotle 330 B.C.E. [1984]; Pojman 1995). One develops morally good character traits by practicing them: A person who acts honestly repeatedly develops the virtue of honesty. Although virtue theorists do not emphasize the importance of moral duties, they recognize that one way of becoming virtuous is by honoring our moral obligations or duties. For example, a person who follows the rule "be honest" will become honest. Some of the frequently mentioned virtues include honesty, honor, loyalty, courage, benevolence, fairness, humility, kindness, fairness, and temperance. We will mention the virtue ethics approach again when we discuss scientific mentoring, because good mentors should model scientific virtues, such as honesty, courage, flexibility, and fairness (Pellegrino 1992; Resnik 2013).

INTEGRITY

Integrity has become a frequently used buzzword in research ethics (Macrina 2013). Scientists, scholars, and government or institutional officials frequently talk about "threats to scientific integrity," "promoting research integrity," and so on. People use this word often without defining it clearly. What does integrity in research mean? We will distinguish between two different senses of "integrity": a rule-following sense and virtue sense. According to the rule-following sense, to act with integrity is to act according to rules or principles. Integrity in science is a matter of understanding and obeying the different legal, ethical, professional, and institutional rules that apply to one's conduct. Actions that do not comply with the rules of science threaten the integrity of research. According to the virtue approach, integrity is a kind of meta-virtue: We have the virtue of integrity insofar as our character traits, beliefs, decisions, and actions form a coherent, consistent whole. If we have integrity, our actions reflect our beliefs and attitudes; we "talk the talk" and "walk the walk" (Whitbeck 1998). We think both senses of integrity can play an important role in discussions of research ethics, and we will use them both throughout this book.

CRITIQUES OF ETHICAL THEORIES

Each of the theories we described has strengths and weaknesses. The strengths reside in their ability to provide insight into different aspects of morality. The weaknesses relate to their inability to deal with some difficult cases or provide useful guidance for decision making.

One of the main critiques of Kantianism is that it cannot deal with situations in which most people would say that we should sacrifice the rights or welfare of an individual for the common good. For example, suppose an estranged, angry husband is looking for his wife and two children, and he comes to your door asking for her whereabouts. He is carrying a gun and says that he will kill them all. You know that they are hiding in the house next door. Most people would agree that you could tell the husband a lie—"they are out of town on vacation," for example, in order to protect the wife and two children. Kantian theory seems to imply that you should not lie to the husband to save three people because this would be treating him as a mere means to saving other people. Lying is wrong as a matter of principle, even for a noble cause. Kantians have tried to interpret the theory so that it does not have this unacceptable implication, but one can construct similar examples that challenge Kantian principles (Korsgaard 1996).

One of the main problems with utilitarianism is that it does not seem to provide adequate protection for individual rights and welfare: utilitarians are apt to sacrifice individuals for the common good. For example, suppose that a 20-year-old healthy male has been admitted to the hospital for a drug overdose. He has suffered severe brain damage and will probably never be able to walk, speak, or lead a normal life again. His vital organs are in good shape, however. There are four people waiting for organs they need to live (i.e., heart, lungs, two kidneys, and a liver). They will die soon if they do not receive these organs, and no organs appear to be forthcoming. Utilitarians would favor killing the brain-damaged patient and using his organs to save four lives because this would produce a greater balance of good/bad consequences than the other options. Most people, however, would not favor this option because it would involve taking an innocent life. Utilitarians have tried to interpret their theory so that it does not have this unacceptable implication. For example, rule utilitarians would say that accepting a rule like "kill innocent people to save the lives of other people waiting for organ transplants" would not produce an overall net utility because it would make people distrust the medical profession, would devalue human life, and so on. However, philosophers have constructed other examples that challenge utilitarian thinking about ethics (Pojman 1995).The main criticism of virtue ethics is that it does not provide adequate guidance for dealing with ethical dilemmas. For example, suppose you have promised to attend your son's baseball game. Just before you leave for the game, you notice that your neighbor has just collapsed in the yard. You could stay with your neighbor and help her receive medical attention by taking her to the hospital or possibly calling an ambulance. Either of these choices will result in your missing your son's game. Acting according to different virtues would favor different choices. The virtues of loyalty would favor going to the game, since you promised you would go, but the virtue of benevolence would favor helping the neighbor. Virtue ethics theories do not include a decision procedure for dealing with conflicts like this one, because there is no method for prioritizing virtues. Virtue ethicists have tried to interpret theory so that it can provide a way of dealing with ethical dilemmas like this one, but philosophers have constructed other examples that challenge this approach. Thus, while virtue theories can provide useful guidance most of the time, they seem to break down when you face difficult ethical choices (Pojman 1995).

Examining the strengths and weaknesses of different ethical theories in detail is beyond the scope of this book. However, we think it is important for the reader to have a basic grasp of some influential theories, since they can provide some guidance regarding ethical conduct and decision making. For further discussion of the strengths and weaknesses of different ethical theories, see Pojman (1995).

ETHICAL PRINCIPLES

In addition to these different theories, moral philosophers and theologians have developed a variety of ethical principles (or general rules), which can be useful in thinking about ethical questions, problems, and decisions. There are several advantages to using ethical principles to frame ethical questions, problems, and decisions. First, principles are usually easier to understand and apply than are theories because they are not as abstract or complex as theories (Fox and DeMarco 1990). It is much easier to understand and apply a rule like "don't kill innocent human beings" than Kant's moral theory. Second, many ethical principles have widespread theoretical and intuitive support (Beauchamp and Childress 2001). The principle "don't kill innocent human beings" is implied by many different moral theories, including Kantian ethics, rule utilitarianism, and virtue ethics. Different societies around the world accept some version of this principle. In this book, we will defend a principle-based approach to ethics in research.

PRINCIPLES FOR ETHICAL CONDUCT IN RESEARCH

We will now consider some principles pertaining to a particular area of conduct: scientific research. To understand these principles, it is important to distinguish between general ethical principles and special ethical principles. General ethical principles (or morals) apply to all people in society. For example, the rule "be honest" applies to everyone, regardless of their social role. Special ethical rules, however, apply only to people who occupy specific social roles. Such social roles include professions (e.g., doctors or lawyers), positions (e.g., mayors or legislators), and relationships (e.g., parents or siblings) (Bayles 1988). The rule "do not fabricate data" applies to scientists but not necessarily to those in other social roles. As noted earlier, people who enter a profession agree to abide by the special ethical rules of the profession. Special ethical principles systematize our ethical judgments concerning particular social roles. Special ethical principles are not simply the application of general ethical principles to particular social roles: Special principles take into account the unique features of social roles. In making judgments of right and wrong pertaining to social roles, we draw on our understanding of the general principles of ethics and our understanding of a particular social role. Special ethical principles should take into account the unique features of a social role, that is, what it is and what it does. For example, a principle of honesty in science takes into account the unique features of science that require honesty, such as recording, reporting, or analyzing data. As a result, honesty in science may be different from honesty in a different social role. For example, a scientist who exaggerates when reporting data would be acting unethically, but a salesperson who exaggerates when selling a car might be acting appropriately. Though both have a duty to be honest, honesty in science is different from honesty in selling cars.

We now briefly describe some principles for ethical conduct in research (in bold) and some subsidiary rules.

1. Honesty: Honestly report data, results, methods and procedures, publication status, research contributions, and potential conflicts of interest. Do not fabricate, falsify, or misrepresent data in scientific communications, including grant proposals, reports, publications, and curriculum vitae.

2. Objectivity: Strive for objectivity in experimental design, data analysis, data interpretation, publication, peer review, personnel decisions, grant writing, expert testimony, and other aspects of research where objectivity is expected or required.

3. Carefulness: Avoid careless errors and negligence; carefully and critically examine your own work and the work of your peers. Keep good records of research activities, such as data collection, research design, consent forms, and correspondence with agencies or journals.

4. Credit: Allocate credit fairly on publications, patents, and other materials.

5. Openness: Share data, results, ideas, tools, materials, and resources. Be open to criticism and new ideas.

6. Confidentiality: Protect confidential communications, such as papers or grants submitted for publication, personnel records, proprietary information, and records that identify individual research subjects or patients.

7. Respect for colleagues: Respect collaborators, peers, students, and research staff. Do not harm colleagues; treat them fairly. Do not discriminate against colleagues on the basis of sex, race, ethnicity, religion, or other characteristics not related to scientific qualifications. Help to educate, train, mentor, and advise the next generation of researchers.

8. Respect for intellectual property: Honor patents, copyrights, and other forms of intellectual property. Do not use unpublished data, methods, or results without permission. Give credit where credit is due. Do not plagiarize.

9. Freedom: Do not interfere with freedom of thought and inquiry.
10. Protection of animals used in research: Protect the welfare of animals used in research. Do not conduct animal experiments that are unnecessary or poorly designed.
11. Protection of human research subjects: Protect the rights, dignity, and welfare of human research subjects. Obtain informed consent from competent, adult subjects; minimize research harms and risks and maximize benefits; take special precautions with vulnerable populations; and distribute the benefits and burdens of research fairly.
12. Stewardship: Make good use of human, financial, and technological resources. Take care of materials, tools, samples, and research sites.
13. Respect for the law: Understand and comply with relevant laws and institutional policies.
14. Professional responsibility: Maintain and improve your own professional competence and expertise through lifelong education and learning; take steps to promote competence in science as a whole through mentoring, education, or leadership. Report misconduct and illegal or unethical activities that threaten the integrity of your profession.
15. Social responsibility: Promote good social consequences and avoid or prevent bad ones through research, consulting, expert testimony, public education, and advocacy.

A few words about these principles are in order. First, many of these principles may seem familiar to readers who have some experience with professional codes of ethics in research (Shamoo and Resnik 2006a), government-funding requirements, oversight agencies, sponsors, or journal policies. Our principles complement but do not undermine existing ethics codes and policies. Some readers may wonder whether these principles are redundant or unnecessary, because other rules and guidelines have already been stated publicly. However, we think the principles above have several important uses, because they may cover problems and issues not explicitly covered by existing rules or guidelines, they can be helpful in interpreting or justifying existing rules and guidelines, and they can apply to new and emerging disciplines or practices that have not yet established ethical codes.

Second, the principles we describe here, like the other ethical principles, may conflict with each other or other rules or values in some circumstances. For example, the principles of openness and confidentiality conflict when a researcher receives a request to share data pertaining to human biological samples. When conflicts like this arise, researchers must

prioritize principles in light of the relevant facts. We discuss conflict resolution in greater detail below. Researchers who work for private industry
or the military may face restrictions on information sharing that conflict
with the principle of openness. In these situations, researchers must
choose between honoring their professional responsibilities and loyalty to
the organization and its goals and rules. We will discuss conflicts in more
detail below.

Third, the principles imply many different subsidiary rules. We have
already stated some of the rules above, and we will discuss others in this
book. Subsidiary rules play an important role in connecting general principles to specific decisions or actions (Richardson 2000). For example, the
principle "protection for human research subjects" implies many different
rules pertaining to informed consent that apply to particular situations
involving consent (Richardson 2000).

ETHICAL DECISION MAKING

Having described some ethical theories and ethical principles for scientific research, we are now ready to discuss ethical decision making (also
known as moral reasoning). Ethical decisions involve choices that have
ethical implications. For example, choosing between different flavors of
ice cream is probably not an ethical decision, because the choice is a matter
of personal preference, with almost no impact on other people. However,
purchasing an automobile probably is an ethical decision, because the
choice can have a significant impact on other people and the environment.
Because many of our choices have some impact on other people, and are
not simply a matter of personal preference, many of the choices we make
in life have ethical dimensions.

Ethical decisions that are particularly challenging are known as ethical
dilemmas. An ethical dilemma is a situation where two or more options
appear to be equally supported by different ethical theories, principles,
rules, or values (Fox and DeMarco 1990). A person facing an ethical dilemma may find it difficult to decide what to do. Consider Case 1 (above)
again. The student is attempting to decide whether to do anything about
problems she has noticed with a diagram in a senior investigator's published paper. She suspects there may be an error or possibly something
worse, such as data fabrication or falsification. What should she do?

There are many different ways of making decisions at the student's dis-
posal: she could consult an astrologer, psychic, a pollster; she could read
tea leaves, flip a coin, or pray; she could look for an answer on the Internet

by using Google. A rational approach to ethical decision making is different from all of these methods. A person who is using a rational approach to make an ethical decision uses his or her judgment and intellect to carefully examine the different options in light of the relevant facts and ethical values. He or she considers the interests of all of the affected parties and then examines the choice from different points of view. A rational, ethical decision need not be perfect, but it should represent a sincere attempt to do the right thing for the right reason.

Philosophers, ethicists, and other scholars have debated about three distinct approaches to rational, ethical decision making: (a) a top-down, theory-based approach; (b) a bottom-up, case-based approach known as casuistry; and (c) a mid-range, principle-based approach known as principlism (Beauchamp and Childress 2001). According to the top-down approach, to make a decision about what to do in a particular situation, one must appeal to a moral theory and infer a course of action from the theory. If the theory says to choose a particular option instead of the alternatives, then one should choose that option and implement it. The top-down approach has been popular among moral philosophers for many years. While we agree the theories can be an important part of an ethical analysis of a decision, they have significant limitations, as we have discussed earlier. Therefore, we do not recommend this approach.

In response to problems with theory-based approaches to ethical reasoning, some philosophers have defended a case-based approach known as casuistry (Johnsen and Toulmin 1988; Strong 2000). According to this method of ethical decision making, one should make decisions about particular cases by comparing those cases to previous cases. If cases are similar in relevant ways, then the decisions that one reaches should be the same. If cases are different, then one should reach different decisions. The method is like the case-based approach used in legal reasoning, in which past cases set precedents for future ones. For example, to decide whether one should exclude five data outliers from a dataset, one should compare this situation to previous cases in which the scientific community judged it was ethical to exclude data outliers. If the current situation is similar to those other cases, then excluding the data outliers is ethical and one may exclude them. If the current situation is different from those previous cases, or is similar to cases in which excluding outliers was regarded as unethical, then excluding the five outliers may be unethical (Penslar 1995). The method of casuistry is also known as situational ethics, because matters of right and wrong depend on factors inherent in the particular situation.

The casuist approach offers many useful insights for ethical decision making. First, it emphasizes the importance of understanding and appreciating the facts and circumstances concerning cases. In ethics, the details matter. For example, the difference between appropriate exclusion of outliers and falsification of a data often depends on the details concerning methodology, analysis, and communication. The difference between plagiarism and proper citation may come down to the placement of quotation marks. Second, the casuist approach emphasizes the importance of learning from the past and other cases. If we are to make any progress in ethics, we must learn from good decisions (and bad ones) (Strong 2000).

However, the casuist approach also has some flaws that hamper its ability to guide ethical decision making. First, the casuist approach has no systematic way of comparing cases (Beauchamp and Childress 2001). We need some method or procedure for determining which features of a case are relevant for ethical analysis, because cases have many features that we do not need to consider. For example, if we compare two cases where authors have excluded data from a publication, what aspects of data exclusion should we focus on? The percentage or amount of data excluded? The type of data excluded? The effect of the data exclusion on the results? To answer questions like these, we need ethical principles, rules, or methods for comparing cases, but the casuist approach does not provide these.

Second, the casuist approach does not offer satisfactory justifications for ethical decisions. People are frequently asked to justify their ethical decisions to colleagues, supervisors, governmental officials, or the public. To justify his or her conduct, a person should be able to do more than explain how she or he examined cases—the person should also be able to explain how the decision followed from a rule or principle that transcends those cases (Gibbard 1992). For example, a researcher who wants to defend herself from the charge of plagiarism should be able to do more than say that her conduct is similar to other cases that were not regarded as plagiarism; she should also be able to explain why her conduct does not fit the definition of plagiarism and therefore does not violate any rules against plagiarism.

Some proponents of casuistry have responded to objections like those mentioned above by admitting that casuistic reasoning needs to be supplemented with rules or principles. But making this admission changes the approach from a pure case-based method to one that appears to be principle based. Indeed, there would seem to be very little difference between casuistry that includes rules or principles and principle-based approaches (Iltis 2000).

We therefore favor the principle-based approach for many of the reasons noted above. Ethical principles are less controversial than ethical theories. They are also easier to interpret and apply. Ethical principles provide a framework for comparing different cases. So, the principle-based approach does not have the same problems as the other two approaches. One of the most influential books in bioethics, Beauchamp and Childress's *Principles of Biomedical Ethics* (2001), takes a principle-based approach to ethical problems in medicine and health care. We are following their example by articulating a principle-based approach to ethical problems in scientific research (Shamoo and Resnik 2006b).

The principle-based approach is not flawless, however. Because it straddles the fence between theory-based and case-based approaches, it is susceptible to attacks from both sides. Proponents of theory-based approaches argue that principle-based approaches are nothing but an amalgam of different theories, a hodgepodge. Principle-based approaches have no way of settling conflicts among principles: They lack philosophical unity and coherence (Gert 2007). Proponents of case-based approaches argue that principle-based approaches are too abstract and general to provide sufficient guidance for ethical decision making. Principle-based approaches are not practical enough (Strong 2000). We acknowledge these problems but think the principle-based approach can overcome them (for further discussion, see Beauchamp and Childress 2001).

Having made these general comments about rational, ethical decision making, we now describe a method for making ethical decisions. We do not claim to be the originators of this method, because many other writers have described methods very similar to this one (Beauchamp and Childress 2001; Fox and DeMarco 1990; Shamoo and Resnik 2006a; Swazey and Bird 1997; Weil 1993; Whitbeck 1996). Nevertheless, it will be useful to review the method here and make some clarifying comments.

A METHOD FOR ETHICAL DECISION MAKING

Our method for ethical decision making involves six steps:

Step 1: Define the problem, question, or issue.
Step 2: Gather relevant information.
Step 3: Explore the viable options.
Step 4: Apply ethical principles, institutional policies, or other rules or guidelines to the different options.
Step 5: Resolve conflicts among principles, policies, rules, or guidelines.
Step 6: Make a decision and take action.

For an illustration, consider Case 1. The student's problem, question, or issue is to decide whether to do anything about the discrepancy she noticed between the diagram and the published data. She is not sure whether she should report this as possible misconduct or whom she should contact about this. The information she could gather would be more information about the research: how it was conducted, the methodology, how the data were gathered, reported, analyzed, and so on. She could obtain this information by talking to her supervisor or other people involved with the research project. She would have several options, including doing nothing, talking to the investigator more about it, talking to other students or researchers, talking to the department head, and possibly making an allegation of misconduct. The ethical principles that apply include professional responsibility (i.e., here, duty to report conduct that violates laws, ethical standards, or institutional policies) and self-protection (she could experience adverse career consequences, such as retaliation or loss of her position or funding, if she takes some action against the investigator). The student's professional responsibility conflicts with her interest in self-protection, because she may face adverse consequences if she takes action against her supervisor. To resolve this conflict, she will need to decide whether taking some action against the investigator is worth the price she may pay. It may turn out that she has misunderstood the problem or it is an innocent mistake, in which case she may face no adverse consequences. But it is also possible that some harm could come to her if she blows the whistle. She could also face adverse consequences if she does nothing about the situation, because she is an author on the paper and might be implicated if someone else makes a misconduct allegation.

Resolving conflicts is often the most difficult part of this method, because it involves balancing different principles, policies, rules, or guidelines and deciding which one should have greater weight. Sometimes conflicts can be resolved when a legal requirement conflicts with other principles, rules, policies, or guidelines. If a particular option would require one to violate the law, then that option should not be pursued unless one has a very strong ethical reason for breaking the law, such as protecting people from harm. Sometimes one can resolve conflicts by obtaining additional information or exploring options one has not considered. In Case 1, the conflict might be resolved if the student obtains more information and discovers that she perceived a discrepancy between the data and the diagram because she did not fully understand the method of data analysis described in the paper. The conflict might also be resolved if the student contacts someone at the institution who provides advice on ethical or legal issues in research, such as a research compliance officer or a research integrity official.

However, it is frequently the case that conflicts persist even when one has considered legal requirements and one has examined all the relevant information and viable options. One strategy for resolving a difficult conflict would be to consider how ethical theories might suggest a resolution. If the student in Case 1 takes a Kantian perspective on her dilemma, she could ask whether any of the options could become a universal rule for all researchers. The option of doing nothing would probably fail this test, because if everyone decided not do anything about problems they discover with research, the entire research enterprise would collapse. Science is a self-correcting process that depends heavily on peer review, criticism, and debate. In order for science to be self-correcting, scientists need to call attention to problems they discover with research. So a Kantian perspective would favor doing something about the problem. If the student takes a utilitarian perspective on the problem, she could consider the different consequences for all those impacted by the different options, such as herself, the investigator, the institution, the scientific community, and society. While the option of doing nothing might protect her from harm, it would probably yield more bad consequences than good ones, because the scientific community could be harmed if erroneous research is published and society could be harmed if the erroneous information leads to medical decisions that place patients at risk. If the student takes a virtue ethics approach to the issue, she could ask herself what a good (or virtuous) scientist would do in the situation. The virtue ethics approach probably also would not favor the option of doing nothing, because this option would reflect a lack of courage and integrity.

Before concluding our discussion of this ethical decision-making procedure, a few comments are in order. First, this procedure is an idealization: Real-world decisions sometimes deviate from this stepwise progression. For example, some may formulate a problem and then start gathering information, only to realize that they need to reformulate the problem; some apply ethical principles and resolve conflicts simultaneously, and so on. Second, this method has limitations. This method requires decision makers to use their reasoning skills to make decisions, but other factors often play a key role in decision making, such as emotion, intuition, and even religion. Although we believe that people should try their best to use reasoning to solve ethical dilemmas, we recognize that human reasoning has limitations. If one cannot make a decision after diligently following the method we have outlined here, then it may be appropriate to appeal to some other source of guidance. Third, using this reasoning method to analyze a choice does not preclude one from bringing other reasoning methods, such as economic or legal analysis, to bear on the choice. Ethics does not have exclusive dominion over practical choices.

This concludes our first chapter. Although we may not specifically address elsewhere in this book many of the topics included in this chapter, we expect that students and teachers will be able to use the foundational material in thinking about and analyzing the cases, rules, and applications discussed throughout.

QUESTIONS FOR DISCUSSION

1. Do you think that most scientists and science students are ethical?
2. When, how, and why are scientists tempted to violate ethical standards in research?
3. What situations in science present the most difficult ethical problems and dilemmas?
4. Do you think researchers should adhere to the same ethical standards that apply to other professions, such as medicine or law? Why or why not?
5. Do you think researchers have ethical duties and responsibilities "over and above" the ethical obligations of ordinary people?
6. Can you think of any principles to add to our list of principles for ethical research conduct? What would they be, and how would they be justified? Do you think our list contains some principles that should be omitted or reworded?
7. Is reasoning the best method for making an ethical decision? Why or why not?
8. Do you think that ethical theories and principles have some bearing on practical choices and decisions? Why or why not?
9. How should one resolve conflicts among ethical principles? Do you agree with our approach to conflict resolution?
10. What ethical principles are most important in society? In science? Why?

CASES FOR DISCUSSION

CASE 1

Suppose that there is a runaway trolley heading down the tracks. Five people are tied up on the tracks and will be killed if the trolley continues its current direction. There is a switch at the tracks that can divert the trolley onto another set of tracks.

However, one person is tied up on those tracks and will be killed if you pull the switch and divert the trolley. Thus, if you pull the switch and divert the trolley you will kill one person but save five. What should you do? What would the different ethical theories (Kantianism, utilitarianism, and virtue ethics) instruct you to do?

Suppose the trolley is heading down the tracks but there is no switch. There is a very large man on a bridge above the tracks who is leaning over the edge, about to fall on the tracks. If you push the large man off the bridge before the trolley comes, he will stop the trolley. You will kill that man but save five lives. What should you do? What would the different ethical theories instruct you to do?

Suppose that the large man is a murderer who recently escaped from prison. Would this impact how you think about the situation?

Suppose the large man is a law-abiding citizen but the five people tied to the tracks are your spouse and four children. Would this impact how you think about the situation?

CASE 2

Suppose you were the first mate on a ship that has sunk and 10 people, including yourself, were able to escape on a lifeboat. The other people are presumed dead. You are hundreds of miles away from the shore and the chances of immediate rescue are slim. You are in charge of the lifeboat. There is only enough food and water for nine people for one week. One person must exit the lifeboat (with a lifejacket) to give the others a good chance of surviving. No one wants to volunteer to leave the lifeboat. The people on the lifeboat besides you are a 12-year-old boy and his father, a 6-month-old girl and her mother, an 80-year-old man, a 45-year-old female nurse, a 22-year-old crewman from the ship, a 35-year-old unemployed actress, and a 50-year-old male lawyer. Should you order someone to leave the boat? If so, who should leave? How would the different ethical theories suggest that you approach this decision?

CHAPTER 2

Misconduct in Research

Since the 1980s, well-publicized cases of research misconduct have increased public concerns and stimulated responses from government, universities, and other research institutions. Surveys indicate that the prevalence of misconduct may be larger than many researchers would like to acknowledge. This chapter discusses the definition of scientific misconduct as well as policies and procedures for reporting, investigating, adjudicating, and preventing misconduct.

In the previous chapter we provided a general overview of the ethical conduct of research, including some basic principles and a decision-making procedure. In this chapter, we begin our discussion of specific ethical issues in research by focusing on research misconduct. We believe it is important to discuss misconduct in research before considering the other topics because misconduct has more of an adverse impact on the research enterprise than any other type of behavior. Misconduct has also received considerable scrutiny from politicians and the public. To promote the ethical conduct of research, it is important to understand what misconduct is, how it is caused, and how it can be prevented.

Although breaches of scientific integrity have been part of our culture for many years, a book by two science journalists, William Broad and Nicholas Wade, *Betrayers of the Truth: Fraud and Deceit in the Halls of Science* (1982 [1993]), played an important role in focusing public attention on research misconduct. The authors recounted both historical and current cases of scientific fraud and criticized the scientific community for its indifference to the problem. According to the authors, Galileo made the data for falling objects appear better than they really were; Isaac Newton made his experimental results fit his theories better by fudging his predictions on the velocity of sound, the procession of equinoxes, and gravitational forces; John Dalton cleaned up his data on the ratios of chemical reactions, which remain hard to duplicate; Gregor Mendel manipulated the heredity ratios on his experiment with peas; Robert Millikan selectively reported oil drop data on his calculation of electronic charges; and even Louis Pasteur was guilty of announcing his anthrax vaccine before he completed his experiments (Broad and Wade 1982 [1993]; Geison 1978, 1995; Shamoo and Annau 1989).

Among the most famous historical examples of misconduct is the story of the "Piltdown Man." In 1908, skull bones were found in Piltdown, a town not far from London. The bones were presented by a brilliant young curator as being thousands of years old and belonging to a person who had the characteristics of both a monkey and a man. In 1912, it was sensational scientific news that made it to the newspapers: Here was the "missing link" to prove that man had evolved directly from apes. Forty-five years later, however, some scholars concluded that the curator had pieced together contemporary skull bones from the two different species and had aged them chemically (Barbash 1996). At the time of the discovery, the curator's colleagues had accepted his findings without critical appraisal, largely because "the researchers [had] shaped reality to their heart's desire, protecting their theories, their careers, their reputations, all of which they lugged into the pit with them" (Blinderman 1986, p. 235).

A host of contemporary cases complement these historical examples. Some of them have been widely publicized by the media, while others have appeared only as footnotes (Broad and Wade 1982 [1993]; Shamoo and Annau 1989). Scientific misconduct concerns have entered an alarming level in the world's political and economic culture (The Economist, 2013). Below are selected cases from a much larger pool.

FAMOUS CASES OF MISCONDUCT OR ALLEGED MISCONDUCT

In 1974, William Summerlin admitted to fabricating data in skin transplant experiments he was conducting at the Sloan Kettering Institute in New York. Summerlin joined the transplantation immunology laboratory of Robert Goode at Sloan Kettering in 1973. Goode was one of the country's top immunologists. Summerlin hypothesized that growing tissues in culture for several weeks prior to transplantation could prevent tissue rejection. In an experiment designed to answer critics of his work, Summerlin "transplanted" cultured skin patches from black-haired mice onto white-haired mice. While cleaning the mice, a laboratory assistant observed that alcohol could wash away the black hair color on the white mice. The assistant reported this to Goode, who suspended Summerlin and initiated an investigation. Summerlin soon confessed that he had drawn patches of black hair on the white mice with a black felt-tip pen. The committee conducting the investigation of Summerlin also found that he had fabricated data relating to several other "transplantation" experiments. The committee required Summerlin to take a medical leave of absence (for mental health problems), publish retractions, and correct irregularities in his work. The scandal ruined Goode's career even though he was innocent of any wrongdoing (Hixson 1976).

Between 1980 and 1983, Dr. Steven Breuning of the University of Pittsburgh published 24 papers funded by a National Institute of Mental Health (NIMH) grant to study powerful neuroleptic antipsychotic drugs for the treatment of retarded patients. The overseer of the grant was Dr. Robert L. Sprague, the director of the Institute of Child Behavior and Development. Breuning's results questioned the use of neuroleptics in retarded children and led to a change in their clinical management nationally (Garfield 1990). In a renewal application for a four-year extension to the grant, Breuning submitted additional new data. Sprague questioned these data and informed NIMH of his concerns. According to Sprague, NIMH's first response was slow and accusatory. Ultimately, Sprague's frustration with NIMH spilled over to the media and led to congressional hearings. Meanwhile, Breuning remained active and funded. Finally, an NIMH panel in 1987 found that Breuning had committed scientific misconduct by reporting nonexistent patients, fabricating data, and including falsified results in a grant application. The panel recommended barring Breuning from receiving any grants from the U.S. Public Health Service (PHS), including NIMH, and referred him for criminal prosecution. Breuning was convicted in 1988—the first scientist to receive such action. He was sentenced to 60 days of imprisonment and five years of probation and was ordered to pay $11,352 in restitution to the University of Pittsburgh. During this process, Sprague lost all funding for his grants and was investigated by the NIMH. He was ultimately cleared of wrongdoing (Monson 1991; Shamoo and Annau 1989; Sprague 1991, 1993; Wilcox 1992).

In a highly publicized case in 1981, Dr. John Darsee, a postdoctoral fellow at the Harvard laboratory of Dr. Eugene Braunwald, was accused of using fraudulent data in the assessment of drug therapy to protect against ischemic myocardium (Lock 1993; Wade 1981). Stewart and Feder (1991), dubbed "fraud busters" by the media, published a paper in *Nature* showing that Darsee's publications contained excessively favorable language, fabricated experimental data, and fudged control data. A committee investigating Darsee found that he fabricated or falsified data in five papers he published while at Harvard and eight papers while a graduate student at Emory University. Even though Darsee was found to have committed misconduct in research, he went on to practice medicine.

During the early 1980s, Robert Gallo, from the National Cancer Institute of the National Institutes of Health (NIH), and Luc Montagnier, from the Pasteur Institute in France, were both working on isolating a virus thought to cause acquired immunodeficiency syndrome (AIDS). They cooperated at first and exchanged cell samples infected with different strains of the virus. They agreed to publish their articles on the human immunodeficiency virus (HIV) together in *Science* in 1984, but Gallo started to receive top billing. Later, when tests revealed that the two different strains were nearly genetically identical, Montagnier accused Gallo of stealing his strain and claiming it as his own. Gallo was investigated for misconduct but exonerated. Apparently, a third, vigorous strain from Montagnier's lab had contaminated both of their samples, which explains their genetic similarity. Failure to keep good laboratory notebooks contributed to the difficulties related to the resolution of this case. The U.S. and French governments also reached an agreement naming both scientists as codiscovers and sharing patent rights between both institutes for the HIV blood test (Cohen 1991; Culliton 1990).

In 1986, Thereza Imanishi-Kari and four coauthors at the Whitehead Institute (operated by Tufts and the Massachusetts Institute of Technology) published a now-famous paper in the journal *Cell* (Weaver et al. 1986). Among the authors was the winner of the 1975 Nobel Prize in Medicine, David Baltimore. The paper claimed to show that foreign genes had stimulated the production of large amounts of antibody by the genes in normal mice, which was considered to be a remarkable achievement. However, Margot O'Toole, a postdoctoral fellow working in Imanishi-Kari's laboratory, was not able to reproduce a key part of the experiment, and she asked to see Imanishi-Kari's laboratory notebook. When O'Toole could not reconcile data recorded in the notebook with what was reported in the paper, she accused Imanishi-Kari of fabricating data. An internal investigation found no misconduct, but a congressional committee headed by Representative John Dingell that was looking into fraud in NIH-funded research began looking into the case, as did "fraud busters" Stewart and Feder. Their analysis of the case triggered an investigation by the NIH's Office of Scientific Integrity (Stewart and Feder 1987, 1991).

The story made the front pages of the *New York Times*. The NIH found that Imanishi-Kari committed misconduct, but this finding was later overturned by a Department of Health and Human Services (DHHS) appeals panel in 1996, which said there was not enough evidence to prove misconduct. Though Baltimore was not implicated in misconduct, his reputation was damaged and he resigned as president of Rockefeller University. During the congressional hearings, he defended Imanishi-Kari and described the whole matter as a witch hunt. Imanishi-Kari has maintained she did nothing wrong, except for keeping poor records (Baltimore 1991; Eisen 1991; Friedly 1996a, 1996b; Hamilton 1991; Imanishi-Kari 1991; Kevles 1996; Kuznik 1991).

In 1993, Roger Poisson, a professor of surgery at the University of Montreal, admitted to fabricating and falsifying data for patients enrolled in the NIH-funded National Surgical Adjuvant Breast and Bowel Project (NSABP) between 1977 and 1990. Poisson had altered his patients' medical data in order to ensure that they would meet the enrollment criteria for the study. NSABP investigators reanalyzed the data after removing Poisson's patients from the dataset and found that his misconduct had no impact on the overall results. The Poisson case spurred efforts to reform Canada's research ethics policies (Angell and Kassirer 1994).

In 2002, Jan Hendrik Schön, a rising star in the fields of condensed matter physics and nanotechnology at the world-renowned Bell Laboratories, was found by a group of independent investigators to have faked data in at least 17 publications (Service 2002). His publication rate was astounding: He published a paper every eight days. His publications appeared in most prestigious journals, such as *Science, Nature,* and *Physical Review Letters.* Since 2002, 28 of his papers have been withdrawn from journals. In 2004, the University of Konstanz withdrew Schön's Ph.D., after finding that his dissertation was also fraudulent. This large-scale fabrication and falsification of data is considered the most extensive scientific misconduct in the physical sciences in recent memory (Reich 2009).

In 2002, several scholars and journalists accused a University of New Orleans history professor named Stephen Ambrose of plagiarizing different works from 12 different authors in seven of his published books and his Ph.D. dissertation. Ambrose defended his actions, claiming that he did not intend to plagiarize and had forgotten to use quotation marks. Ambrose has published 24 books, including highly acclaimed accounts of World War II and biographies of Presidents Eisenhower and Nixon. Ambrose has served as a historical advisor for several movies and television shows, including *Saving Private Ryan* (History New Network 2010).

In 2004 and 2005, Woo Suk Hwang, a professor at Seoul University in South Korea, published two papers in *Science* reporting the derivation of human embryonic stem (HES) cell lines by therapeutic cloning (Hwang et al. 2004, 2005). The papers claimed that the HES cell lines produced by this process were genetically identical to the donor somatic cells. Hwang had assistance from numerous colleagues at Seoul University and other collaborators. The two papers, especially the second one, had a tremendous impact on the stem cell research field. Hwang attained international recognition for his work and became a national hero. Hwang, a veterinarian by training, had published previous papers on cloning dogs and cows. In November 2005, one of Hwang's collaborators on the 2005 paper, the University of Pittsburgh scientist Gerald Schatten, accused Hwang of misleading him about the source of the eggs used in the experiments. Hwang admitted that some of the eggs had been provided by women working in his laboratory, a practice that was legal in South Korea but regarded by many as unethical because using research subjects who are subordinates can be coercive. Hwang later admitted that each egg donor was paid as much as $1,400 (Resnik et al. 2006).

In December 2005, the editors of *Science* received an anonymous tip that two of the photos of HES cells published in the 2005 paper were duplications. Later, one of Hwang's coauthors, Sung Roh, told the media that Hwang had fabricated 9 of the 11 cell lines presented in the paper. Hwang asked for the article to be withdrawn from *Science*, and a committee from Seoul University began investigating the 2005 paper and Hwang's other publications. The committee determined that none of the HES cell lines were genetically identical to the somatic donor cells. The committee also found that Hwang had used 273 eggs, not 185 as reported, and that the cell lines in the 2004 paper were also fabricated. The committee also found that Hwang had been involved in the egg procurement process—Hwang had helped donors fill out forms and had escorted them to clinics for egg removal—and that authorship on the 2004 and 2005 papers had been granted in return for minor contributions to the research. Hwang resigned his position at Seoul University at the end of December 2005. In May 2006, Hwang and five collaborators were convicted of charges of fraud, embezzlement ($3 million), and breach of bioethics laws but their sentence was suspended (Whon and Normile 2006).

In 2006, a committee at the University of Pittsburgh examined Schatten's collaboration with Hwang. The committee found that Schatten played no role in the data fabrication but that he had shirked his authorship responsibilities by failing to carefully review the data and the manuscript. The committee also found that Schatten had accepted unusually large consulting fees ($40,000) for his role in assisting Hwang's research group (Resnik et al. 2006).

Following the Hwang affair, the editors at *Science* decided to change their peer-review policies to try to prevent similar scandals from occurring in the future. Although peer review is not designed to catch fraud, the editors were embarrassed that an obvious problem (two duplicate images) had slipped through their peer-review process. The editors decided to start giving high-impact papers extra scrutiny and to pay greater attention to digital images (Kennedy 2006). Other journals have also revisited their peer-review and misconduct policies in response to the Hwang affair. The Committee on Publication Ethics (COPE) has also developed some guidelines and rules to help journals deal with misconduct (Committee on Publication Ethics 2013).

In 2006, a group of graduate students at University of Wisconsin, after much heart-wrenching and soul-searching, alleged that their doctoral adviser, the geneticist Elizabeth Goodwin, committed data falsification. The university's investigation did confirm the allegations and referred the matter to the Office of Research Integrity (ORI). This is the saddest case that we have encountered in terms of its negative effect on the careers of so many graduate students. Three of the students with many years in graduate school quit the university. One student moved to a different university, and two others started their graduate education anew (Couzin 2006). Moreover, many faculty members were not receptive to their action. This case illustrates that the system in place to deal with misconduct is not yet accepted or handled well.

Eric Poehlman was a tenured professor at the University of Vermont (1987–1993; 1996–2001) and a professor at University of Maryland (1993–1996) and had held an endowed chair at University of Montreal (2001–2005). He resigned his position in Canada in 2005 after a lengthy investigation by the University of Vermont and the ORI found that he had falsified or fabricated data on 15 federal grant applications (totaling $2.9 million) and 17 publications (Office of Research Integrity 2005a). On March 17, 2005, Poehlman admitted his guilt and accepted a comprehensive criminal, civil, and administrative settlement. Under the terms of the settlement, he agreed that he committed scientific misconduct, that he would pay $180,000 in restitution and $16,000 to the lawyer of the whistleblower, that he would be barred for life from receiving federal grants, and that he would correct the scientific literature. On June 29, 2006, he was sentenced to serve a year and a day in federal prison. The University of Vermont investigation was prompted by allegations made by his research assistant, Walter F. Denino, who became suspicious when Poehlman made inappropriate corrections in Excel spreadsheets. In the course of the investigation, Poehlman destroyed evidence in his electronic data that showed that he had falsified documents and presented false testimony.

In 1998, the journal *Lancet* published a paper by the British surgeon and researcher Andrew Wakefield and 12 authors claiming that 12 normal children developed gastrointestinal disease and developmental regression after receiving the measles, mumps, and rubella (MMR) vaccine. The paper speculated that exposure to the MMR vaccine is a possible cause of autism (Wakefield et al. 1998). The antivaccine community seized on the paper as proof that vaccines can cause autism and other problems, and vaccination rates in the United Kingdom and other countries declined significantly. In 2004, the journalist Brian Deer began investigating Wakefield's work. In February 2004, he published an article in the *Sunday Times* accusing Wakefield not disclosing a significant conflict of interest and not obtaining ethics board approval for the study. Deer found that Wakefield's research was supported by a law firm preparing a lawsuit against MMR manufacturers and that a lawyer from the firm helped to recruit research participants (Godlee et al. 2011). In 2010, the U.K. General Medical Council (GMC) investigated Wakefield and concluded that he had acted dishonestly by failing to disclose a significant conflict of interest and that he had ordered risky medical procedures, such as colonoscopies, colon biopsies, and lumbar punctures, without appropriate pediatric qualifications or approval from his hospital's ethics committee. The GMC revoked Wakefield's medical license. In 2010, *Lancet* retracted the paper. In 2011, the *British Medical Journal* published an article by Deer alleging that Wakefield had falsified data in the study. He reviewed the medical records and found that in nine cases, unremarkable pathology results were changed to colitis. Three of the children did not have autism at all and only one had regressive autism. Five of the children had developmental problems prior to the study (Deer 2011). Wakefield continues to maintain his innocence and has sued Deer and the *British Medical Journal* for libel. He also advises antivaccine groups.

On August 20, 2010, an investigation by Harvard University determined that the psychologist Marc Hauser fabricated and falsified data in three published papers. The investigation became public after the *Boston Globe* reported the story. Investigations are supposed to be confidential until a federal agency has made a determination, but this story was leaked to the public (Wade 2010). Hauser resigned from Harvard on August 1, 2011. The ORI concluded its investigation in 2012 and determined that Hauser had fabricated data in a published paper and falsified results in an unpublished study. The ORI said that his misconduct was reckless but not intentional. Hauser's papers have been corrected or retracted (Office of Research Integrity 2012). Hauser has only admitted that he made mistakes and regrets what happened. Hauser has conducted extensive research on the biological foundations of cognition and morality and has been a very important rising star in the field. He published an influential book, ironically titled *Moral Minds*, which examines the evolution of moral behavior (Hauser 2006). Hauser's disputed experiments involved inferring monkeys' thoughts or expectations from observations of how they reacted to sensory stimuli. Hauser developed a coding system for interpreting the behavior and entering the information into a data table. Graduate students accused him of misconduct when they noticed that information he entered into data tables on monkey behavior did not match the videotaped records (Wade 2010).

U.S. News and World Report (Wecker 2012) listed the revocation of doctoral degrees (including honorary degrees) from 10 high-profile individuals. The doctoral degrees of several European cabinet members, such as the German defense and education ministers, were revoked for plagiarism (Cottrell 2013). Also, the doctoral degree of the Romanian minister of education and research was revoked for plagiarism too (Abbott 2012).

Scientists and public officials have responded to these and other highly publicized misconduct cases in a number of ways. Congressional committees have held hearings on integrity in federally funding research; funding agencies have developed policies on misconduct, conflict of interest, and other integrity issues (discussed below), required instruction in responsible conduct of research (RCR) (discussed below), and supported research on research integrity; research institutions have adopted integrity policies (discussed below) and developed RCR programs of instruction; scientists have conducted research on research integrity and have educated and mentored students in RCR; and professional societies have developed codes of conduct. In 1992, the PHS consolidated the Office of Scientific Integrity and the Office of Scientific Integrity Review into the ORI. The ORI oversees the integrity of research in PHS-funded studies. The office reviews misconduct reports made by PHS-funded institutions, conducts its own investigations, supports research on research integrity, provides guidance for investigators and institutions, and publishes educational materials (Office of Research Integrity 2011). Although misconduct continues to occur in science, most scientists are aware of the importance of dealing with the problem and taking steps to prevent it.

The most fundamental issue related to research misconduct is how to define it. We shall distinguish between two different senses of misconduct: an *ethical* sense and a *legal* sense. According to the ethical sense, misconduct is simply unethical or wrongful behavior. This could include fabrication, falsification, and plagiarism, as well as other behaviors widely regarded by scientists as unethical, such as significant violations of human or animal research regulations, misuse of confidential information in journal peer review, undeserving authorship, abuse of subordinates, theft or destruction of property, and harassment. We can think of scientific behavior as falling on a spectrum, with clearly unethical behavior at one end, ethical behavior at the other, and ethically questionable behavior in the middle. See table 2.1.

In the legal sense, misconduct is behavior that is illegal. Normally, there will be some overlap between illegal and unethical behavior, because society usually makes laws to punish behaviors widely regarded as wrong. Fabricating or falsifying data generally fits both senses of misconduct because it is unethical and illegal in many nations. Misuse of confidential information in journal peer review only fits the ethical sense because it is widely regarded as unethical but generally not illegal.

In 2001, after nearly a decade of debate, U.S. federal agencies agreed upon a common definition of misconduct in research as "fabrication, falsification, or plagiarism in proposing, performing, or reviewing research, or in reporting research results" (Office of Science and Technology Policy 2000, p. 76,262). Fabrication is defined as "making up data or results and recording or reporting them"; falsification is "manipulating research materials, equipment, or processes, or changing or omitting data or results such that the research is not accurately represented in the research record";

Table 2.1. SPECTRUM OF SCIENTIFIC BEHAVIOR

Ethical	Ethically Questionable	Clearly Unethical
Honestly reporting data/results	Overstating the significance of one's data/results	Data fabrication/falsification
Granting authorship for significant intellectual contributions research	Mentioning someone who made a significant contribution in the acknowledgments but not naming him or her as an author on a paper	Plagiarism

and plagiarism is "the appropriation of another person's ideas, processes, results, or words without giving appropriate credit" (Office of Science and Technology Policy 2000, p. 76,262). Misconduct does not include honest error or disagreement about methods, interpretations of data, or scientific issues (Office of Science and Technology Policy 2000).

The definition also sets a standard of evidence for a finding of misconduct by a federal agency. To make a finding of research misconduct, an agency must determine that there has been "a significant departure from accepted practices of the relevant research community" and that the accused person acted "intentionally, knowingly, or recklessly" and that the allegation is proven by "a preponderance of the evidence" (Office of Science and Technology Policy 2000, p. 76,262). Preponderance of evidence is a legal concept meaning roughly the conclusion or finding is more than 50% probable, given the evidence. Preponderance of evidence is a much weaker standard of evidence than the "beyond reasonable doubt" standard used in criminal law.

The federal definition focuses on three types of misbehavior: fabrication, falsification, and plagiarism (FFP). What these behaviors all have in common is dishonesty: fabrication and falsification involve lying about data or results, and plagiarism involves lying about the authorship of a work. Plagiarism also involves theft of intellectual property. Before 2001, the PHS, which funds NIH research, the National Science Foundation (NSF), and some other federal agencies, had used a broader definition of misconduct that included FFP as well as "other serious deviations" from accepted research practices (U.S. Public Health Service 2005). The "other serious deviations" category was eliminated on the grounds that it was regarded as difficult to enforce because it is vague and open ended (Resnik 2003b). Other serious deviations might include a broad array of misbehaviors, ranging from misusing confidential information in peer review to theft or destruction of property.

Although the definition of misconduct seems clear and easy to apply, this is sometimes not the case. In some situations it may be obvious that misconduct has occurred. For example, in the Summerlin, Hwang, Poisson, and Poehlman cases (discussed above) the misconduct was blatant. Some cases are more difficult to discern, such as the Imanishi-Kari, Ambrose, Gallo, and Hauser cases. It is clear that there is a continuum of behavior in conducting research, ranging from outright misconduct to honest errors. The distinction between FFP and questionable research practices (QRP) often can turn on subtle details related to the case, such as degree of deviation from the methodology accepted within the discipline (for fabrication or falsification) or the amount or type of text copied (for plagiarism). Some examples of QRP that could be FFP, depending on the situation, include the following:

- Enhancing digital images (discussed in chapter 3). This could be fabrication or falsification, depending on whether the enhancement affects the overall results.
- Excluding data from an article or presentation without a good statistical, technical, or methodological reason (also discussed in chapter 3). This could be falsification, depending on the facts of the case.
- Using statistical methods to impute (or replace) missing data values for a study. This could be fabrication, depending on the facts.
- Performing a statistical analysis in a deliberately dishonest way. This could be fabrication or falsification, again, depending on the facts.
- Poor record keeping. When scientists keep poor records, it may look like they have fabricated or falsified data when someone has difficulty reproducing the results and they cannot understand the relationship between the published results and the original data.
- Poor citation practice. When scientists or scholars paraphrase or copy text without using quotations or citing properly, it may appear that they have committed plagiarism, even if they did not intend to do so.
- Not giving credit to someone who has assisted with a research project by providing ideas, helping to collect data, or developing processes or techniques. While this might seem to be an authorship matter, it could fit the definition of plagiarism, depending on the facts of the situation.
- Self-plagiarism. This is republishing your own work without proper citation.

It is worth noting that some institutions, organizations, and governments have adopted definitions of misconduct that are broader than FFP (Buzzelli 1993; Resnik 2003b). The Wellcome Trust Fund's definition of misconduct includes FFP as well as "deliberate, dangerous, or negligent deviations from accepted practices in carrying out research" and "failure to follow established protocols if this failure results in unreasonable risk or harm to humans, other invertebrates, or the environment" (Koenig 2001, p. 2,012). China's Ministry of Science and Technology has adopted a definition of research misconduct that includes FFP as well as submitting a false résumé or violating animal or human research regulations (Zeng and Resnik 2010). More than half (59%) of U.S. research institutions have misconduct policies that go beyond FFP. Behaviors other than FFP classified as misconduct by U.S. research institutions include other serious deviations (45.4%), significant or material violations of regulations (23.0%), misuse of confidential information (15.8%), and misconduct related to misconduct (14.8%), such as interfering with a misconduct investigation (Resnik et al. 2014).

It is also important to understand that fraud is a legal concept that is distinct from research misconduct. Although people talk loosely about fraud in research to describe dishonest actions, the term has a precise legal meaning. Fraud is a "knowing misrepresentation of the truth or concealment of a material fact to induce another to act to his or her detriment" (Garner 1999, p. 292). Someone who commits misconduct may be charged with criminal fraud, and he or she may be sued in civil court for the damages caused by his or her fraud. However, an administrative finding of misconduct by a government agency does not, by itself, imply any civil or criminal liability. As noted above, very few researchers have faced criminal charges for research misconduct, although some scientists, such as Hwang from Seoul University and Poehlman from the University of Vermont, recently have. In some cases, the federal government has sued research institutions to recover damages caused by fraud committed by researchers. Civil liability for fraud can be very costly for institutions because they can be liable for "treble damages" or triple the amount of money the damages cost (Resnik 2003b). For example, if a researcher committed fraud on a $1 million grant, the university could be liable for $3 million.

DEALING WITH MISCONDUCT

Federal agencies require institutions to adopt policies for handling misconduct allegations as a condition of receiving funding. Research institutions are responsible for investigating and adjudicating misconduct allegations within their jurisdiction. Institutional policies typically include four stages: (a) initial assessment, (b) formal inquiry, (c) investigation, and (d) adjudication (see table 2.2). The initial assessment is an informal part of the process. The person making the accusation (i.e., the complainant) may contact an institutional official (such as a department head) about suspected misconduct. Some institutions allow anonymous allegations to protect the whistleblower. However, it will not be possible to maintain anonymity once a formal inquiry is initiated if testimony from the complainant is needed. The person who receives the allegation will make an initial assessment to determine whether the allegation meets the definition of misconduct, has evidential support, and is sincere (not knowingly false or malicious). If the person who receives the allegation determines that it is

Table 2.2. HANDLING MISCONDUCT ALLEGATIONS

Stage	Questions
Informal assessment	Does the allegation meet the definition of research misconduct?
	Is there evidence to support the allegation?
	Is the allegation sincere (not knowingly false or malicious?)
Formal inquiry	Does the allegation meet the definition of research misconduct?
	Is there enough evidence to warrant an investigation?
	Do any other issues need to be addressed (e.g., animal or human subjects, harassment, discrimination, intellectual property, etc.)?
Investigation	Does the preponderance of the evidence support a misconduct finding?
Adjudication	What are the appropriate penalties to administer?
Reporting	Are there any sponsors (government or private) that need to receive reports?

serious, he or she will relay it to someone higher in the administration. All misconduct allegations eventually go to the responsible institutional official, the research integrity officer (RIO).

When the RIO receives an informal allegation, he or she will also assess it to determine whether a formal inquiry is warranted. The RIO will also determine whether other issues besides misconduct are involved, such as compliance with animal or human research rules, discrimination, harassment, intellectual property disputes, and so on. If other issues are involved, the RIO will refer those issues to the appropriate institutional office. A formal inquiry is like a grand jury hearing. The goal of the formal inquiry is to determine whether there is enough evidence to move forward with a formal investigation. The RIO will appoint an inquiry committee composed of experts in the relevant research discipline who have no direct interest in the case (e.g., collaboration with either the respondent or complainant). The committee may hear testimony and review research records. The committee will usually also sequester research records to prevent them from being tampered with. If the committee determines that no investigation is warranted, the matter will end there. If the committee determines that an investigation is warranted, the RIO may appoint a committee to conduct an investigation. The investigation committee will also review evidence and make a determination. If the committee finds that the evidence does not support a finding of misconduct, the matter will end there. If the committee finds that the evidence supports a misconduct finding, the RIO will act on the committee's recommendation and impose sanctions (i.e., adjudication).

After the institutional investigation/adjudication is complete, the institution will also need to report its findings to the sponsor (if there is one), such as a federal agency or private company. If the research has been funded by a federal agency, then the institution must send its report to that agency. For example, the ORI oversees PHS-funded research, which includes NIH-funded research. Institutions must report their investigations into misconduct allegations in NIH-funded to the ORI. The ORI reviews these reports and may accept them or require additional information. The ORI can also conduct its own investigation if it is not satisfied with the institution's investigation or if it determines that it needs to conduct its own investigation to protect public health and safety. Once all the investigations are complete, the ORI will reach a formal finding (i.e., misconduct or no misconduct). If the ORI reaches a finding of misconduct, it will enter into an agreement with the guilty party. In the agreement, the ORI may require the party to correct the research record (e.g., by submitting retractions or corrections to journals), and it may bar the party from receiving federal research funding for a particular period of time. The entire process falls within the domain of administrative law, and ORI findings can be appealed to the judicial board. For example, Imanishi-Kari appealed the ORI's finding of misconduct, and the appellate board found there was not sufficient evidence to prove that she fabricated or falsified data. If research is funded by the NSF, institutional reports go to the NSF's Office of Inspector General. Research institutions may act on their own to deal with misconduct. For example, an institution could terminate a guilty party's employment or place him or her on probation.

Handling misconduct allegations is a legal process. Once a formal inquiry is initiated, the person accused of misconduct (the respondent) has legal rights to due process. The respondent has the right to obtain legal counsel, review the evidence, and call and cross-examine witnesses. The process is supposed to be kept confidential to protect the rights of the respondent and others involved in the case. Breaches of confidentiality may damage the reputation of innocent parties. The institution has an obligation to compensate an innocent respondent for damage to his or her reputation. It can take a year or more to resolve a misconduct allegation, including appeals. For example, the Imanishi-Kari case lasted 10 years.

Everyone involved in the allegation, including the complainant, respondent, witnesses, and committee members, may have to expend considerable time and energy to deal with the process. Thousands of dollars may be spent on attorneys' fees.

One of the problems with relying on institutions to conduct their own misconduct inquiries or investigations is that institutional officials may have a conflict of interest. Institutional officials may decide not to pursue an allegation in order to avoid scandal, embarrassment, or loss of funding. If the respondent is a powerful, senior investigator who receives hundreds of thousands or millions of dollars per year in grant funding, institutional officials may face significant pressure to sweep an allegation under the rug. Although federal agencies have the right to conduct their own investigations, this will not happen if they never find out about an allegation in the first place. To deal with institutional conflicts of interest related to misconduct allegations, it is important for institutional officials to be aware of the issues they face and to maintain their integrity and commitment to ethics (Resnik 2008).

Whistleblowers are often adversely affected by the process. Though institutions have policies to protect whistleblowers from direct retaliation, they may be harmed in other ways (Malek 2010). As noted above, they may have to expend considerable time and energy to pursue an allegation. They may even need to hire their own attorneys. They may develop a reputation as a troublemaker if word gets out that they accused someone of misconduct who was found to be innocent. They may even lose their position or their funding if their supervisor is found to have committed misconduct, and they may need to transfer to another laboratory or institution. In the Goodwin case (discussed above) the student-whistleblowers suffered adverse consequences to their careers. Mary Allen was one of those students. She reports that she had to move to another university and began her research over again. It took her eight and a half years to complete her Ph.D. (Allen and Dowell 2013). Deciding whether to report misconduct can pose a difficult ethical dilemma for the would-be whistleblower, because it often involves a conflict between professional responsibility and self-interest (Malek 2010). However, not blowing the whistle can also have negative repercussions, because one may be implicated in misconduct if you are involved in the research and someone else makes an allegation. You may also have a guilty conscience if you do nothing. Allen writes:

> I would make the same choice today that I made then. Many people point to
> the negative consequences for everyone involved in the case and wonder why
> would I make the same choice again? First, I think that I would have had a

guilty conscious [*sic*] if I had chosen to hide what I had learned. Someone else, another graduate student years after I left, might have had to deal with the misconduct I could have prevented. Second, I recognize that for the scientific community, honesty is best for progress. The presence of falsified data in the scientific discourse slows everyone's progress. Finally, I had a goal when I entered graduate school: to do quality science. . . . I have learned much from my path, even if it was not an easy path to take. (Allen and Dowell 2013, p. 347)

Clearly, institutions should take appropriate steps to protect whistleblowers, including helping students find a new supervisor, position, laboratory, or even university if the situation warrants.

Correcting the research record is another important issue related to misconduct. Guilty parties and journal editors have an obligation to print retractions or corrections when a paper has been affected by misconduct, so that other scientists will not rely on fabricated, falsified, or erroneous data. As noted above, federal agencies usually require guilty parties to correct the research record.

Difficulties can arise in correcting the research record, however. First, many papers, often dozens, may need to be retracted or corrected. It can take considerable time to track down every paper. In many cases, papers affected by misconduct are never retracted or corrected, and they remain in the scientific literature for other researchers to use or cite. Second, coauthors may not want to retract or correct a paper because they are concerned about how their reputation may be affected. Many journals require that all coauthors agree to a retraction or correction, because they may be concerned that they will be sued for libel if they print a retraction or correction without the consent of all the authors. Some, however, have decided to relax this requirement in order to correct the research record. In some cases, the journal will act on its own, without obtaining consent from the authors, because the editors want to protect the integrity of the research published by the journal. Third, even when editors print a retraction or correction, they usually do not honestly say why a paper is being retracted or corrected. They may say that the reason for the retraction or correction is that "data are unreliable" when the real reason is that the data were fabricated or falsified. In some cases, journals simply print "retracted" with no explanation (Resnik and Dinse 2012a).

Researchers have recently published some interesting studies of retractions and corrections related to misconduct. Steen (2011) examined 742 English-language retractions in PubMed from 2000 to 2010. Of these, 31.5% were retracted for scientific mistakes, 15.8% for duplicate publication, 15% for fabrication, 14.4% for plagiarism, 13.2% for falsification,

10.2% for ethics violations, 8.2% for unstated reasons, and 3.6% for journal error. Steen also found that the number of retractions, as well as the number due to misconduct, has been increasing. Steen conducted another, larger study of retractions to determine the real reason for retractions, because he suspected that many papers listed scientific mistake as the reason for retraction, when the real reason may have been misconduct. Steen and two colleagues examined all 2,047 articles in PubMed that were indexed as retracted. To verify the real reason for retraction, they consulted reports from ORI, Retraction Watch, news media, and other public sources for evidence of misconduct or suspected misconduct. Their research resulted in reclassification of 118 articles (15.9%) from Steen's earlier study. The reason for these retractions was changed from error to fraud. They found that 67.4% of retractions were attributable to misconduct, including fraud or suspected fraud (43.4%), duplicate publication (14.2%), and plagiarism (9.8%). They concluded that incomplete, uninformative, or misleading retraction announcements led to the previous underestimation of the role of fraud in retractions (Fang et al. 2012).

Resnik and Dinse conducted a study that confirms some of these findings. They reviewed all 208 closed cases involving official findings of misconduct handled by the ORI from 1992 to 2011, of which 75 cited at least one published article affected by the misconduct. These 75 cases cited a total of 174 articles. Of these 174 cited articles, they found both the article and a retraction/correction for only 127. Twenty of the cited articles they found (11%) were never corrected or retracted at all. Because 8 of the 127 retractions consisted of simply the word "retracted," their analysis focused on the remaining 119 articles for which a more substantial retraction or correction statement was published. The 119 statements they examined were published between 1989 and 2011 in journals with impact factors that ranged from 1 to 39. Of these 119 retraction or correction statements, only 41.2% mentioned ethics at all and only 32.8% named a specific ethical problem such as fabrication, falsification, or plagiarism. The other 58.8% described the reason for retraction or correction as error, loss of data, or replication failure when misconduct was actually at issue. Among the published statements in response to an official finding of misconduct (within the time frame studied), the proportion that mentioned ethics was significantly higher in recent years than in earlier years, as was the proportion that named a specific problem. The authors concluded that honesty and transparency require scientists to tell the whole truth when retracting or correcting an article, so that others can evaluate their work and decide whether parts of the research unaffected by misconduct can be trusted and whether any of the coauthors are at fault (Resnik and Dinse 2012a).

Journal editors should consider adopting policies pertaining to corrections and retractions. Unfortunately, the vast majority have not (Resnik and Dinse 2012a). The Committee on Publication Ethics (2014) has developed extensive guidelines for retractions and corrections, which can serve as a model for journal policies. The guidelines recommend that editors should consider retracting articles when there is clear evidence that the findings are unreliable due to misconduct or honest error. Editors may also retract articles that have been published previously. Corrections are appropriate when only a small portion of an otherwise reliable publication is misleading. Retraction notices should be freely available, published promptly in electronic and print versions, and electronically linked to the retracted article. Retraction notices should state who is retracting the article and why (e.g., for misconduct or error). Journal editors may retract articles even if some or all of the authors do not agree to the retraction.

INCIDENCE AND CAUSES OF MISCONDUCT

In their influential book, Broad and Wade (1982 [1993]) claimed that there was more misconduct in the research community than scientists want to admit. Furthermore, they said misconduct is probably greatly underreported. By the time misconduct is reported, it is probably the culmination of a spectrum of unethical activity, of which misconduct is only the end point (LaFollette 1994a, 2000). Therefore, one may surmise that the reported cases of misconduct are but the "tip of the iceberg" (American Association for the Advancement of Science–American Bar Association 1988). Richard Smith, the editor of the *British Medical Journal* from 1997 to 2004, claims that scientific misconduct is much more prevalent than the scientific community acknowledges or knows: "Most cases are probably not publicized. They are simply not recognized, covered up altogether; or the guilty researcher is urged to retrain, move to another institution, or retire from research" (Smith 2006a, p. 234).

Although scientists, politicians, and the public regard the problem of scientific misconduct as extremely important, the scientific community still lacks solid evidence concerning the incidence of misconduct. Estimates of the misconduct rate, based on surveys that asked researchers whether they know about misconduct that has occurred, range from 3% to 32% (Steneck 2000). One survey of scientists found that 32% suspected a colleague of plagiarism (Tagney 1987). Another study showed that the reported incidence of fraud affected 0.01–0.1% of all published research (Glick 1992). A 1993 survey of science students and faculty estimated that the percentage of questionable research studies, including fraud, may range from 6% to 12%. The results further showed that 44% of the responding students and 50% of the faculty reported being exposed to two or more types of misconduct or questionable research practices, and 6–9% reported having direct knowledge of plagiarism or data falsification (Swazey et al. 1993).

A survey of 3,247 scientists by Martinson et al. (2005) found that 0.3% (3 out of 1,000) admitted to falsifying or cooking research data during the previous three years. The survey also found that scientists admitted to engaging in other unethical activities in the last three years, including ignoring major aspects of human subjects requirements (0.3%), using someone else's ideas without obtaining permission or granting proper credit (1.4%), and unauthorized use of confidential information in connection with one's own research (1.7%). Steneck (2000) estimated the rate of misconduct by extrapolating from confirmed cases: With 200 confirmed cases of misconduct involving NIH funds in 20 years, this works out to a misconduct rate of 1 out of 100,000 researchers per year. However, because this estimate relies on confirmed cases of misconduct, it is susceptible to a large underreporting bias.

Fanelli (2009) conducted a systematic review of and meta-analysis of survey research pertaining to the incidence of misconduct. He included 21 surveys in the systematic review and 18 in the meta-analysis. He found that 1.7% of scientists have admitted to fabricating or falsifying data at least once and that 33.7% admitted to questionable research practices. Also, 14.12% of scientists said that they had observed colleagues falsifying data, and 72% said they had witnessed colleagues engaging in questionable research practices.

Most methods of measuring the misconduct rate from surveys or other reports of misconduct probably underestimate or overestimate the rate of misconduct. To see why this is so, consider how one might attempt to measure the rate of tax fraud. One could mail out surveys and ask people if they have ever committed fraud, but who would want to admit to this, even on an anonymous survey? One could ask people if they know of someone who has committed tax fraud, but why would they have access to this information? Most people probably will not learn about tax fraud because someone who commits fraud will try to keep it secret. Or they could claim to know about something that never happened, because they have based their opinion on rumor or hearsay. One could also estimate the rate of tax fraud based on the rate of convictions for tax fraud, but many people get away with tax fraud without ever being indicted, and many people who are indicted are never convicted. Given difficulties like these, we believe that the only way to get a good estimate of the rate of misconduct is to randomly audit research procedures and research data (Loeb and Shamoo 1989; Shamoo and Annau 1987) to be discussed later—other methods would introduce underreporting or overreporting biases.

Regardless of what the exact rate of misconduct turns out to be, misconduct is still a very important concern for researchers, because it undermines trust, trustworthiness, integrity, and accountability in research (National Academy of Sciences 1992). For example, murder is still regarded as a serious crime worthy of public attention even when the murder rate is low. Thus, those who maintain that misconduct is not an issue in science because it is so "rare" do not understand the seriousness of the crime. Moreover, given the growing influence of money in research, misconduct may be more common than people think.

The etiology of scientific misconduct is probably as complex as any other form of deviant human behavior. The theories of the 19th-century French philosopher Emile Durkheim and the 20th-century American sociologist Robert K. Merton (1973) provide a theoretical framework for its genesis (Garfield 1987; Zuckerman 1977a, 1977b). According to these theories, the values and norms pertaining to the conduct of science ordinarily become internalized during the period of education and are reinforced later with a system of social control that includes both rewards and sanctions. Deviant behavior is likely to occur when values break down and an individual's aspirations and goals come into conflict with society's structure and controls.

Although it is tempting to blame misconduct on the occasional "bad apple," it probably results from a variety of factors, such as the following:

- The pressure to produce results in order to publish or obtain and maintain funding;
- Career ambitions, interests, and biases of individual scientists;
- Stress, mental illness, and other psychological factors;
- Financial, political, and institutional influences;
- Cultural differences concerning the understanding of ethics;
- Inadequate education, training, supervision, and oversight at all levels of research;
- Increased complexity of the research environment;
- Poor communication among members of the research team; and
- Difficulties related to managing large research groups. (American Association for the Advancement of Science–American Bar Association 1988; Institute of Medicine 2002; Krimsky 2007; Loeb and Shamoo 1989; National Academy of Sciences 1992; Shamoo 1989; Shamoo and Annau 1987)

Education and mentoring in the responsible conduct of research (RCR) are the two main strategies that institutions have pursued to prevent misconduct and promote integrity. Education can take many different forms, including formal courses, seminars, workshops, lectures, brown-bag lunches, online learning modules, and mentoring. Mentoring takes place when supervisors have informal discussions with students about RCR and serve as role models for ethical behavior. This book is designed to be used in research ethics courses.

The NIH began requiring graduate students receiving PHS funding to receive RCR instruction in 1989. Since then it has extended mandatory training to include postdoctoral fellows and other trainees and intramural researchers. The NIH requires that RCR instructional programs provide eight hours of education in key topic areas, including misconduct, data management, authorship, collaboration, mentoring, publication, peer review, animal research, human research, and social responsibility (National Institutes of Health 2009a). In 2009, the NSF began requiring RCR instruction for all undergraduate students, graduate students, and postdoctoral researchers supported by NSF funds. Though the NSF does not mandate content or hours of instruction, institutions must submit a training plan to the NSF for approval (National Science Foundation 2009). We also refer the reader to an article written by David Wright and his colleagues from the ORI on the history of development of RCR educational initiatives (Tamot et al. 2014).

U.S. research institutions have complied with and in many cases gone beyond these requirements. Of U.S. research institutions, 52.1% require individuals not mandated by NIH or NSF to receive RCR instruction, including students in selected programs (23.6%), all students participating in externally funded research (12.5%), and all graduate students. Also the same study shows that only 8.2% of faculty involved in research with human subjects had any training (Resnik and Dinse 2012b). In addition, Titus, in an extensive survey on 5,100 medical school researchers, found that only 5.6% of researchers are able to correctly distinguish seven or more of nine scenarios depicted as likely misconduct (Titus 2014). Although the United States has taken the lead in RCR instruction, other countries have begun to implement educational requirements for research ethics (Resnik and Master 2013a; Zeng and Resnik 2010).

The primary reason for requiring and promoting RCR education and mentoring is to foster ethical behavior in research (Hollander et al. 1996; Steneck and Bulger 2007; Vasgird 2007). An ORI survey of 2,910 researchers regarding research integrity measures used in biomedical research laboratories indicates that there is a need for more educational material, written laboratory research guidelines, assessment of outcome measures, and electronic data recording with an audit trail (Office of Research Integrity 2003). A pilot study based on interviews of 23 senior researchers and research administrators found that they favor education and training being imparted by researchers to students, with an emphasis on professional development and practical wisdom (Deming et al. 2007). Koppelman-White (2006) argues that mentoring is more effective than classroom education when it is discipline specific and evolving.

Evidence concerning the effectiveness of RCR education and mentoring is inconclusive, however. Some studies have shown that RCR education can improve knowledge of ethical norms, raise awareness of ethical issues and concerns, enhance ethical reasoning skills, and influence ethical attitudes. However, no studies have demonstrated that RCR education has a positive impact on ethical behavior (Antes et al. 2009, 2010; May and Luth 2013; Plemmons et al. 2006; Powell et al. 2007). Two different surveys cast some doubts on the effectiveness of the current process of RCR education. Anderson et al. (2007) found that formal courses in RCR were ineffective in reducing unethical behavior among research scientists funded by NIH but that mentoring did have a positive effect on behavior. Another, more limited survey (Funk et al. 2007) of those who received an NIH training grant fellowship found that ethics training had no effect on their ethical behavior and knowledge concerning authorship and publication. It is clear from these studies that further research is needed to understand the impact of education and mentoring on ethical behavior in research.

In addition to education and mentoring, policy development is another key strategy for preventing misconduct and promoting integrity (Institute of Medicine 2002). Policy development is important for setting a standard of behavior within the institution. Students, professors, or research staff who have questions about how to deal with ethical issues can often find guidance in institutional policies. Federal agencies require institutions to develop policies pertaining to many different areas of RCR, including misconduct, conflict of interest, laboratory guidelines and biosafety, animal research, human subjects research, and equal employment opportunity. Many institutions have developed policies that address other RCR areas, such as record keeping, data ownership, publication, authorship, mentoring, and intellectual property (see, for example, Duke University 2013; National Institutes of Health 2009b).

Compliance and oversight are other important strategies for preventing misconduct and promoting ethical behavior. Compliance and oversight activities include various measures to ensure that researchers are complying with institutional policies and government laws and regulations. Many institutions have offices of research compliance or research ethics/integrity to ensure that rules are followed. These offices are in charge of developing and publicizing policies; supporting educational activities; overseeing various committees that deal with ethical issues and compliance issues, such as committees that review animal or human research; making reports to university leaders, federal agencies, and sponsors; and receiving reports of noncompliance, including misconduct.

Journals have begun using computer programs to check articles for plagiarism and self-plagiarism. The programs compare submitted articles to published articles in a database to detect similarity. Because a certain amount of similarity may not constitute plagiarism, articles flagged for potential plagiarism by the programs must still be examined by human beings to determine whether the similarity is appropriate, given the context of the research. Hundreds of cases of plagiarism have been discovered in this fashion (Butler 2010).

Finally, data auditing is another important strategy for preventing misconduct and promoting ethical behavior. At research institutions that do not have any kind of data audit system in place, the main way that unethical or illegal conduct is discovered is through whistleblowing. This is a very poor way of detecting illicit activity. Suppose that the Internal Revenue Service (IRS) never audited tax records. If this were the case, then cheating would be much more prevalent than it already is because taxpayers would have little reason to think they would be caught (Shamoo 2013). One need not audit every taxpayer to deter cheating. The IRS audits only about 1% of individual tax returns and focuses its efforts on returns it judges to be suspicious (Taylor 2013).

Data auditing is a common practice in private industry, because companies often have hundreds of millions of dollars at stake in research (Glick 1993). Problems with data quality and integrity, such as fabrication/ falsification, errors, or irreproducibility, can jeopardize applications for drug approval or intellectual property claims. Although academic institutions audit animal and human research studies to ensure compliance with rules and regulations, no institutions that we are aware of audit data. Data audits are looked upon with suspicion in academic research, because scientists do not want to allow outside parties to examine their research records, perhaps because they are afraid of what auditors might find. Others may object that auditing interferes with their academic freedom. However, we do not find these objections to be compelling. If scientists are conducting research at the public's expense, then the public should be able to examine their records to ensure that their work is trustworthy. Also, academic freedom does not imply a right to conduct research that is fabricated, falsified, or otherwise untrustworthy.

The idea of data auditing was first introduced in the late 1980s as an approach to the prevention of misconduct (Glick 1992; Glick and Shamoo 1991; Loeb and Shamoo 1989; Rennie 1989a, 1989b; Shamoo 1988; Shamoo and Annau 1987). It was patterned after experience in the financial field, where cooperative experience between auditor and corporate executives is the norm. Auditors have total access to records, and personnel answer questions forthrightly.

In 1991, J. Leslie Glick and Adil E. Shamoo (one of the authors of this textbook) published a prototypical example of how data audits can work in the scientific world. Shamoo, an experienced biophysicist, agreed to have his work audited by Glick, a much-audited biotechnology corporate executive as well as an experienced scientist with a scholarly interest in data auditing. The audit was a retrospective evaluation of a research project that culminated in the publication of a paper in 1983. The ground rules were that Glick had total access to any records, could ask any question, and could arrive at any conclusion. The audit process involved tracking the data from the published paper back to the original raw data in the laboratory notebooks. At the conclusion of the audit, a report was written providing the details of the audit process and its results (Glick and Shamoo 1991).

Some have objected that academic institutions do not have the money or resources to support data auditing. However, one only needs to audit a small percentage of studies in order to deter misconduct and encourage integrity. Moreover, data audits could be supported through the regular funding process. Grant proposals could include funds for a data audit (Shamoo 1988; Shamoo and Dunigan 2000). Glick (1992, 1993) has argued that a scientifically conducted data audit can become an effective management tool in saving the public not only from poor data but also from unnecessary expenses. He estimated that 10–20% of all research and development data funds result in questionable data because of inappropriate research activities ranging from sloppy work to outright misconduct. If a data audit were to result in a 50% reduction of questionable data production, there would be a savings of $5–10 per audit dollar spent. Twenty years into the data audit program, the public would save $40–90 of research expenditure per audit dollar (Glick 1992).

Subsequent to the introduction of the proposal for data audits, Grimlund and Doucet (1992) developed detailed scientific statistical auditing techniques for research data based in part on financial auditing methods.

The key new element in this technique is the development of stratified sampling for rare events. Two years later, Doucet and Grimlund collaborated with others, including one of the authors of this textbook (Doucet et al. 1994; Shamoo 1988), to apply their statistical technique to existing data in toxicology that had been audited using a 100% random auditing method. They found the stratified method to be faster, more reliable, and more economical than 100% random auditing, because fewer actual data were audited.

Additional activity pertaining to data audits includes a 1992 report by the ORI (Price and Hallum 1992) on their use of several data analysis methods to detect scientific misconduct, including statistical auditing and sampling techniques. Similarly, a statistical approach that identified lack of randomness in detecting fabricated data was published by Mosimann et al. (1995). Data can be audited on a random basis or for cause. A for cause audit would be appropriate when research has come under suspicion.

QUESTIONS FOR DISCUSSION

1. Based on the current information available about the incidence and significance of misconduct, do you think the press has exaggerated its implications? Does the process currently mandated by the federal government adequately manage the issue? How could it be improved? Do you think more or fewer regulations are needed to manage scientific misconduct?

2. What comments do you have on the causes of scientific misconduct? Which factors do you think are the most important? Do you think that the etiology of scientific misconduct resides primarily within the individual or within the system?

3. Can you give an example of possible scientific misconduct from your own experience or ones that you have heard about? How was it dealt with? How should it have been dealt with?

4. How would you evaluate the process (inquiry, investigation, etc.) for the management of misconduct described in the text? Is it fair to the accused? To the accuser? To the university? To the public? Can you think of any changes that would improve the procedures?

5. If you were charged with scientific misconduct, would you hire legal counsel? If so, at what stage in the process?

6. Do you think that it could be possible to fully protect a whistleblower? What would be the essential safeguards of an effective policy for protecting whistleblowers?

7. Is a data audit contrary to the personal liberty of scientists? Is it destructive to the principles of the scientific method? Could a data audit stifle creativity and engender distrust? What system would you design to ensure scientific integrity?

CASES FOR DISCUSSION

CASE 1

Ms. Watson is a graduate student in Dr. Parker's molecular entomology lab. They are working on understanding proteins in spider silk. Dr. Parker has prepared a paper claiming that Protein SM plays a key role in strengthening spider silk. Because the paper includes some of Ms. Watson's data, he asks her to read it and sign the authorship form prior to submission. When Ms. Watson reads the paper she discovers that Dr. Parker did not report 6 out of 12 experiments she had done that undermine support for the hypothesis, and she can find no clear explanation for this omission in the methods section. The paper also includes data from 24 other experiments done by other students for a total of 30. She asks Dr. Parker why he did not report these six experiments, and he says they were poorly executed. Somewhat dismayed, she presses him further on this point, but he puts her off and says that they can talk about it later. He wants her to go ahead and sign the journal's author agreement form so they can submit the paper to meet a deadline for a special issue of the journal on spider silk.

- Did Dr. Parker falsify data? What additional information do you need to know to make this determination?
- What should Ms. Watson do?
- Should she sign the authorship agreement form?
- Who can she talk to at her institution about this issue?

Suppose that Ms. Watson tells Dr. Parker she cannot sign the author agreement form until she has a better explanation of why 6 of her 12 experiments were dropped. Dr. Parker tells her that he does not have time to go into more detail and he says he will publish without her experiments. She will be removed from the paper.

- What should Ms. Watson do now?

CASE 2

A graduate student interviewed homeless people as part of a larger NSF grant that had been obtained by his mentor. The study was to be the core of his Ph.D. thesis.

However, the intended sample size of 50 was proving even more difficult to obtain than he had expected. Despite his most diligent efforts and the help of a social worker who had recently joined the grant team, he was able to recruit only 44 subjects. The prospect for getting more seemed dim. He was more successful, however, in his rapport with the social worker, and they began living together. Still, he was faced with the practical academic problem of completing his thesis. The conclusions that he could make from the statistical data from his 44 subjects supported his hypotheses. Nevertheless, he was still short on subjects. His solution to the problem was to use statistical techniques to impute data for the four remaining, nonexisting subjects, based on the average data from the 44. His conclusions were basically the same whether he used 50 or 44 subjects, but he presented all 50 for his thesis and did not disclose his imputation method. Within a year he had defended his thesis successfully and received his Ph.D. He submitted two papers based on his thesis to a refereed journal and they were accepted for publication. He took a job at another college in the area so that his living arrangements could remain the same. A year later, after a nasty fight, he broke off his relationship with the social worker. Unbeknownst to him, she had been aware of the data imputation. In anger, she wrote a letter to the NSF. The NSF informed the university and requested a report.

- Did the student fabricate data? What additional information do you need to make this determination?
- What responsibility does the social worker have for the actions of the graduate student?
- Should the graduate student's mentor have known what was going on in the activities of her grant?
- Does the mentor bear any responsibility for her student's actions?
- Can the university and the NSF take action even though the Ph.D. degree has already been given?
- Assuming a guilty verdict, what do you consider appropriate sanctions in this case?

CASE 3

A biostatistician is reviewing the data for a clinical trial conducted at a university medical center on methods for using genomic analysis in order to select the best form of chemotherapy for treating cancer. The research is supported in part by the NIH and a biotechnology company. The methods were patented by the lead investigator, a well-established, highly funded oncologist. The investigator transferred patent rights to the university and the biotechnology company. The NIH, the university, and the biotechnology company have a Cooperative Research and Development Agreement (CRADA) to develop and test the methods. The investigator receives royalties from the patent and owns stock in the company. The company sponsors $5 million dollars of research at the university each year. The biostatistician becomes suspicious of the data after the lead investigator makes some changes to a data sheet. All of the changes tend to support his hypothesis (i.e., the methods work). The biostatistician suspects that the lead investigator has been fabricating or falsifying data. She asks the investigator if she can see the case reports from the patients treated as part of the study so she can verify the quality of the data. The investigator does not allow her to see the case reports, but she is able to obtain them (without his permission) from a research nurse. After reviewing the case reports, she notices that the data sheets do not match the case reports, and she decides to report the issue to the department chair. When the department chair brushes off her concerns, the biostatistician brings the matter to the attention of the university's RIO, the vice president for research. After the RIO also dismisses the biostatistician's concerns, she reports the issue to the institutional review board (IRB), which oversees human subjects research at the university. The IRB decides to review the case and temporarily suspends the study and makes a report to the RIO. After the RIO learns about the suspension of the study, he is very upset and places the biostatistician on administrative leave for insubordination. He orders the IRB to restart the study.

- Did the lead investigator fabricate or falsify data? What additional information would you need to make this determination?
- Did the biostatistician act appropriately in pursuing this allegation?
- Should the biostatistician have access to the case reports?
- Should the research nurse have given her access?
- What can the biostatistician do at this point if she wants to pursue the allegation?
- Does the university have a conflict of interest in this case?
- Would it be best for an outside party to review this case?
- Did the RIO perform any actions that were unethical or illegal?
- Should the IRB inform any federal agencies about the RIO's actions?

CASE 4

An assistant professor of philosophy submits an article to a top-tier journal criticizing the use of Bayesian statistics to determine stopping points for clinical trials. The review takes a long time (nearly a year). The professor receives a rejection letter from the journal with little comment. About a month after receiving the rejection letter, the professor notices that a paper published in another journal is remarkably similar to the one he wrote that had been rejected. The paper uses many of the same phrases he used in the rejected paper, develops similar arguments, and draws the same conclusions. He needed to publish this paper to support his tenure case, but now he doubts that he can. He suspects that his work was plagiarized but he does not know what to do.

- Was this a case of plagiarism? What more information or evidence would you need to prove plagiarism?
- What can the professor do? Should he contact the journal editors? The author of the other paper?

CASE 5

A new assistant professor was accused of misconduct by a technician at the university where she had trained. The accusation was that she published a questionable abstract for a national meeting based on research that was supported by an NIH grant. The problem was that the abstract contained data that the technician could not find in any of the laboratory notebooks. The technician also determined that these data had never been used in any other full-length published paper but had been part of the professor's Ph.D. dissertation. The technician discussed his concerns with the professor's former mentor, who in turn called the professor. Subsequently, the professor said that she was not able to find the data and claimed that it must have been misplaced. The technician made an official complaint to both the ORI and the university.

- Did the professor fabricate data? What additional information do you need to make this determination?
- If the grant had been from a non-NIH source, would the university still have jurisdiction over this issue?
- What, if any, is the mentor's responsibility for the action of his former graduate student, either while she was a student or during the preparation of this abstract? Does the mentor have any obligations beyond his call to his former student?
- How do you assess the technician's response, including both the scope of his fact-finding activities and his decision making regarding his complaint?
- Now that the complaint has been made, what do you think should be the response of the assistant professor? The mentor? The ORI? The university?
- How could the situation in this case have been prevented?

CASE 6

An associate professor at a large university submitted a major grant proposal to the NIH. During the grant review at the study section, a reviewer noticed that the p-value calculated for the table was based on eight experiments. However, the methods section had stated that the experiments had been conducted four times in duplicate. A preliminary inquiry by the study section staff raised further questions about the authenticity of the data. The executive secretary of the study section felt compelled to write to the university's grant office for clarification, with a copy to the ORI. The university responded by conducting an inquiry. The faculty member admitted that she always uses the number of experiments times the number of replicates to obtain the total number of experiments. The university chose not to proceed with the investigation. Instead, it warned her to stop using such methods. The university informed the ORI of its decision.

- What went wrong here, and what preventive remedies would you recommend?
- Did the professor fabricate or falsify data? What additional information would you need to make this determination?
- Do you think the university's action was appropriate? Why or why not?
- Now that the case is in the ORI's hands, should it accept the university's decision?

CASE 7

A newly appointed assistant professor applied for his first NIH grant. A member of the study section noticed that parts of the proposal looked unusually familiar. The reason was that entire paragraphs in the methods and the perspective/significance sections had been lifted from her own grant proposal that she had submitted last year. Although it was obvious that the new assistant professor had not been a member of last year's review process, the current reviewer knew that the submitter's department chair and former mentor had been a member of that study section. The reviewer called the department chair to find out what had happened. The chair reluctantly told her that he had showed the grant proposal to his then postdoctoral fellow for an opinion because he was too busy to read it thoroughly.

- Did the assistant professor do anything wrong when he agreed to read the grant proposal?
- Besides the assistant professor, does anyone else share responsibility for what happened?
- Was it appropriate for the member of the study section to first call the chair? Did the study section member have other alternatives?
- If the university hears about these events, what should it do?
- Was this a personal or a systemic failure? Why?

CASE 8

An administrative assistant, after leaving her current job to take other employment in the same institution, accused her former boss of falsifying a letter of support from a collaborator. The letter was appended to an NIH grant proposal. The assistant wrote directly to the ORI, which requested that the university initiate the misconduct process. An inquiry found that the professor had actually falsified the letter. However, the collaborator had verbally agreed to write such a letter of support but was unable to do so because of travel commitments. If the researcher had waited until the collaborator had come back, he would have missed the grant submission deadline. Based on the collaborator's confirmation that the agreement of collaboration had already been made, the university found that there was no scientific misconduct.

- Although the professor falsified the letter, the university found that scientific misconduct had not occurred. Do you agree with this action? What are the implications of this action? In what way does the professor's falsification of the letter meet or not meet the definition of misconduct?
- Could the professor have handled his dilemma differently?
- What other options did the assistant have when she discovered the falsification of the letter? Did she make a good choice?

CASE 9

Three economics professors published an influential book on consumer choice behavior. One of the professors copied several paragraphs from the book almost word for word and published them in a review article, without using quotation marks or citing the book.

- Did the professor commit plagiarism?
- Would it be plagiarism if he cited the book but didn't use quotation marks?

CASE 10

A physics professor decided to repeat a controversial experiment pertaining to the electrical properties of a material composed of ceramics and glass, with the assistance of two graduate students and a technician. The professor published a paper showing that he was unable to reproduce the experimental results, and he proposed some possible explanations for replication failure. In the paper, she copied most of the materials and methods section from the previous paper nearly word for word, without using quotation marks. She cited the original paper but did not quote it.

- Is this plagiarism?

CHAPTER 3

Data Acquisition and Management

Data play a key role in testing scientific theories or hypotheses and form the backbone of scientific inference. The different steps of research should be monitored carefully, and research design should include built-in safeguards to ensure the quality, objectivity, and integrity of research data. This chapter addresses ethical issues pertaining to data acquisition and management, including hypothesis formation, research design, data collection, data analysis, data interpretation, data storage, and data sharing.

Scientific research is the systematic attempt to describe, explain, and understand the world. Though different disciplines study different aspects of the natural world, they share some common methods that are designed to produce objective knowledge by subjecting hypotheses or theories to rigorous tests (see table 3.1). Ideas that cannot be tested, such as metaphysical theories, ideological claims, and private intuitions, are not scientific. Some (but not all) tests involve experiments. In an experiment, a researcher attempts to reduce the number of variables and control the conditions in order to understand statistical or causal relationships between variables or parameters. For an experiment to be rigorous, a researcher must describe it in enough detail that other researchers can obtain similar results by repeating the experimental conditions (Cheny 1993; Kirk 1995; Kitcher 1993; Popper 1959; Resnik 2007; Shamoo and Annau, 1987).

All test results in science, whether from controlled experiments, field observations, surveys, epidemiological studies, computer models, or meta-analyses, should be open to public scrutiny and debate. Peer review, with some limitations, is one of science's most important methods because it promotes the public scrutiny of hypotheses, theories, and test results (see chapter 7 for further discussion). Once a hypothesis or theory becomes well established, it may be said to be a "fact." For example, the idea that the sun is the center of the solar system is now accepted as a fact, but it was a hypothesis during the time of Copernicus (1542 [1995]). Well-established generalizations, such as Newton's laws of motion and the ideal gas laws, are known as laws of nature (Giere 1991; Hempel 1965; Popper 1959; Resnik 1998a).

Data (or recorded observations) play a key role in testing scientific theories or hypotheses and form the backbone of scientific inference. Data can take many forms, including observations recorded by scientists in laboratory notebooks, field notes, entries into electronic notebooks or spreadsheets, outputs from machines (such as optical scanners, gas chromatographs, or automated DNA sequencers), photographs, x-rays, video or audio recordings, transcribed interviews, digital images, computer printouts and databases, historical documents, and case reports in clinical trials. Data include the primary (or original or source) data, which are drawn directly from the experiment or test. These include entries in a laboratory notebook, field notes, computer printouts, photographs, machine outputs, and so on. Secondary (or derived) data are data based on primary data, such as spreadsheets derived from entries into laboratory notebooks, or figures or diagrams based on machine outputs. Data are different from research materials, such as chemical reagents, biological samples (blood, tissue, urine, etc.), cell lines, slides, gels, rocks, laboratory animals, and others. To illustrate the difference between data and materials, consider a project to sequence an organism's genome. The materials would include biological samples from the organism (blood, tissue, cells, etc.). The data would include the genomic information derived from these materials (i.e., deoxyribonucleic acid [DNA] sequences, such as GTTAGATTCCA, etc.). In this chapter we will examine various ethical issues pertaining to the acquisition and management of data that arise at different stages of research.

PROBLEM SELECTTION

Ethical issues arise at the very first stage of research, because problem selection is often affected by funding and politics (Resnik 2007, 2009a). Though most scientists choose problems based on their curiosity and professional interests, research costs a great deal of money, and scientists usually end up working on problems that sponsors are willing to pay for. In the private sector, profit plays a major factor in funding decisions.

Table 3.1. STAGES OF SCIENTIFIC RESEARCH

1.	Select a problem or question to investigate.
2.	Review the relevant literature.
3.	Propose a hypothesis to solve the problem or answer the question.
4.	Design and plan experiments or other procedures to test the hypothesis.
5.	Collect and record data.
6.	Analyze data.
7.	Interpret data.
8.	Disseminate results.

A drug company will consider how a research project is likely to affect its bottom line in making funding decisions. For example, a company may prefer to fund research on a drug for a common illness, such as hypertension, than to fund research on a treatment for a rare disease, because it will make more money from treating a common illness. Though some private companies, such as Bell Laboratories, have sponsored basic research, most focus on applied research pertaining to their products or services. Scientists who conduct research for private companies will need to come to terms with their research agendas.

Politics can affect funding in many different ways. First, politics usually impacts a funding agency's research priorities. The National Institutes of Health (NIH), for example, establishes different priorities for research on different diseases, such as cancer, HIV/AIDS, and so forth, and for research pertaining to different areas of study, such as aging, mental health, and allergies. Second, politics sometimes impacts specific research projects. For example, since the 1980s the U.S. government has banned the use of federal funds for research on human embryos. In 2001, the G. W. Bush administration imposed significant restrictions on research involving human embryonic stem cells, though the Obama administration lifted some of these restrictions in 2009 (Obama 2009; Resnik 2009a). In 2003, a congressional committee held a hearing on 198 NIH-funded research projects on human sexuality, HIV/AIDS, and drug abuse that the Traditional Values Coalition said was a waste of the taxpayers' money (Resnik 2009a). Third, disease-specific advocacy bolstered by lobbying from the pharmaceutical industry influences the area of research as well as the amount of funding to a specific area. Though we believe that public funding of research should be as free as possible from politics, we call attention to this issue so that scientists can be mindful of how the choice of a research topic may impact one's ability to receive funding. We will discuss funding issues again in chapters 5, 7, and 12.

LITERATURE SEARCH

The literature search can be an important early step in the overall project. This is an important step for the investigator because it can save a great deal of time and money by eliminating a flawed objective or a hypothesis. It can also help researchers to learn whether their projects may make an original or worthwhile contribution or whether they merely repeat previous work or would result in knowledge that has little value. A literature search can also help researchers learn about previously used methods, procedures, and experimental designs and can place the project's experimental design and protocol within the known realities of the subject matter. A thorough literature search can allow researchers to give proper credit to others who have already worked in the area. Failing to acknowledge other relevant work is arrogant and self-serving and is a type of plagiarism or serious bias if one knowingly or unknowingly claims to be the originator of someone else's idea (Resnik 1998b; Shamoo 1992).

An inadequate literature search in clinical research can lead to tragic results. Ellen Roche died while participating in an experiment designed to produce a mild asthma attack in healthy (nonasthmatic) volunteers at Johns Hopkins University. Roche inhaled hexamethonium, a blood pressure medication used in the 1950s and 1960s. Roche developed a cough and breathing difficulties and was put on a ventilator. She died because of extensive lung damage produced by the hexamethonium. An Office of Human Research Protections investigation of Roche's death determined that this tragedy probably could have been avoided if the principal investigator, Alkis Togias, had consulted articles published in the 1950s (and cited in subsequent publications) warning of lung damage due to inhaling the hexamethonium. Togias did a standard PubMed search on hexamethonium and consulted current textbooks, but this literature search did not include references from the 1950s (Savulescu and Spriggs 2002).

HYPOTHESIS FORMATION

After selecting a problem and reviewing the literature, researchers should formulate a hypothesis (or hypotheses or theories) to test. They may also need to formulate aims or objectives for the research project. It is important for hypotheses, aims, and objectives to be testable, because an important part of the scientific method is subjecting hypotheses to rigorous tests. If a hypothesis is not testable, researchers may waste time and money collecting data that have no clear value. To ensure that a hypothesis is testable, researchers need to state it clearly, avoiding ambiguous terms. They also need to derive predictions from the hypothesis for different tests (e.g., "hypothesis H predicts chemical X will increase the rate of tumor formation in laboratory mice"). If the predictions occur, they may confirm the hypothesis; if they do not, they may disconfirm it. In the past, most research projects were hypothesis-driven, that is, researchers formulated hypotheses prior to gathering data. Today, research is often data-driven, that is, researchers formulate hypotheses after gathering data. For example, researchers in the fields of genomics and proteomics may analyze large datasets in order to discover statistical associations among different variables. In psychology, sociology and epidemiology researchers often conduct cross-sectional studies to obtain some baseline data pertaining to a population.

One of the problems with data-driven research is that it may lead researchers to make up post-hoc hypotheses to explain patterns in the data. To avoid this problem, researchers must ensure that hypotheses in data-driven research are testable. They may also want to conduct more tests to provide additional, independent evidence for or against their hypotheses.

RESEARCH DESIGN

The design of experiments is one of these crucial steps in preserving the integrity, quality, and objectivity of the research project. In this stage of research, scientists should clearly describe experiments or other tests (e.g., surveys, focus groups, etc.) they will perform, the materials they will use, and the procedures, methods, and protocols they will follow. They should also describe their plan for collecting, recording, and analyzing the data, including the use of any statistical methods. The research should be described in sufficient detail so that someone not involved in the project can evaluate it and repeat the work. The research design should be based on one's previous research, existing literature, laboratory manuals, and other appropriate sources. Researchers should follow appropriate standards in applying methods and should keep records of what methods they use and how they use them. During initial tests, researchers should use and identify standard (or well-established) methods, but they can modify these methods to suit new experimental applications or testing procedures. It is important for researchers to note changes they make and to state the reasons for them. Furthermore, researchers should not make changes in the middle of a test or experiment, because this will bias or corrupt the data. All accidental changes, such as dropping a test tube, should be noted in the laboratory notebook. Researchers should not pick and choose among experiments or tests to achieve a desired result. However, they may do so if they recognize a variable inherent in the protocol that was not first recognized in earlier stages of the project. For example, in testing a new drug in humans, researchers may realize that an unanticipated side effect should be recorded and could therefore change the protocol and then design a new experiment that measures this side effect. However, researchers should record these decisions and discuss them in detail at the same time and place where the experiments are recorded, derived, or manipulated.

Because it is easy to employ research designs that tend to bias the data and results, scientists should be mindful of how biases may affect their work and they should take steps to minimize the potential for bias. Since biases may operate at a subconscious level, researchers may not even be aware that their studies may be flawed. Scientists, like all human beings, are susceptible to self-deception (Broad and Wade 1982 [1993]). Because it is not always possible to see the biases in one's own work, it is important to solicit critical feedback from colleagues prior to the initiation of a study and also after its completion. Biased research wastes time, money, and effort, and it can also involve the unnecessary use of human or animal subjects. Sound experimental design is also one of the key ethical principles of research with animals and human subjects (Irving and Shamoo 1993; Levine 1988). Because no amount of statistical analysis or interpretation can overcome a design flaw, data that result from a flawed design are virtually useless, and using them can be unethical (Irving and Shamoo 1993; Resnik 2000).

Since there are many different ways that biases can affect research, we cannot discuss them all here. We will, however, call attention to some common biases. First, sometimes the experimental conditions may affect the data. For example, an in vitro experiment to determine how a chemical affects cell signaling may be affected by many different factors that scientists may not be aware of, such as subtle changes in temperature, humidity, PH, electrolytes, impurities in the chemical, or the growth medium. Montagnier's misconduct allegation against Gallo (discussed in chapter 2) probably resulted from a vigorous HIV strain that contaminated different cell lines used by two researchers. Temperature, feeding, and other living conditions (such as overcrowding) may affect how labora-tory animals respond to stimuli. Environmental factors (such as privacy, time of day) may affect the answers that human subjects provide during interviews. Second, a poor statistical design may impact research out-comes. A common statistical problem is inadequate sample size. For exam-ple, if scientists find that there is no difference between how a potential neurotoxin affects 20 laboratory mice, as compared to 20 controls, the sample size may not be large enough to demonstrate that the chemical has no neurological effects. One may need a larger sample to reach conclusions that have statistical significance. Third, exclusion/inclusion criteria may bias outcomes in clinical research involving human subjects. For example, testing an erectile dysfunction drug on healthy male subjects aged 18–50 may overestimate the efficacy of the drug in the general population, be-cause many of the men who take the drug will be over 50 and will have health problems (such as a decline in stimulus response due to obesity or hypertension or other unknown factors). Fourth, survey questions may introduce subtle biases. For example, a question like "Do you think that President Obama is not doing enough to deal with the country's crippling federal deficit problem?" may generate a different response from this question worded slightly differently, "Do you agree or disagree with the way President Obama is dealing with the federal deficit?" Fifth, private companies may intentionally introduce biases into their experimental de-signs in order to promote their economic interests (Crossen 1994; Porter 1993; Resnik 2007). We will discuss biases related to privately funded re-search in greater depth in chapters 5 and 9.

COLLECTING, RECORDING, AND STORING DATA

After one has designed a research project, the next step is to collect, record, and store the data. Scientists should keep accurate records of all aspects of the research project, including data, protocols, and methods (including any changes); drafts of manuscripts; and correspondence with institutional officials, funding agencies, and journal editors. Good scientific record keeping is important for ensuring the quality and in-tegrity of research for numerous reasons. First, good record keeping is essential for conducting your own research. Members of the research team need access to records to conduct experiments or tests, analyze data, make reports, draft manuscripts, and so on. Second, good record keeping is important for authentication of your work by outside parties, such as peer reviewers, or scientists who want to reanalyze your data or replicate or build on your work. Third, good record keeping is crucial for investigating allegations of research misconduct and other problems. Indeed, good scientific records can be your best defense against a misconduct allegation. If other scientists have trouble replicating your results, they may suspect that you have committed misconduct if you keep poor records (see the Imanishi-Kari case, discussed in chapter 2). Fourth, detailed and accurate record keeping is essential for proving ownership of legal claims related to patents and copyrights (we discuss intellectual property in greater depth in chapter 8). Fifth, good record keeping is legally required for research that is submitted to the Food and Drug Administration (FDA) and other regulatory agencies. Sixth, good record keeping is needed for accurate auditing and quality assurance. Although this may sound strict to some, we believe that research records can be viewed as quasi-legal documents analogous to medical records, business inventories, or investment accounts (Shamoo 1989, 1991a, 1991b).

Although different disciplines, laboratories, and research groups have different record-keeping styles and formats, the following guidelines apply generally. First, records should be accurate and thorough. Records should include what was done (i.e., data and results), how it was done (i.e., methods and materials), when it was done, why it was done, who did it, and the next steps. Records should be signed and dated. If laboratory notebooks are used, all additive information directly relevant to the raw data, such as derived data, tables, calculations, or graphs, should be either done directly in the notebook or taped thoroughly on an adjacent page in the notebook. If this is not feasible, files can be used; providing clear identification of the data and the page where the data were derived from is essential. Ideally, entries should also be signed (or initialed) and dated. If electronic notebooks are (or other types of electronic records) are used, these should include an electronic date trail to allow for accurate information concerning the identity of individuals who enter data and entry time (Schreier et al. 2006).

Second, records should be well organized. Researchers should be able to keep track of their records and know where and how they are kept. A laboratory data notebook should be bound and the pages numbered consecutively. Loose-leaf notebooks are hazardous and may tempt a beginning researcher or technician to tear off pages with mistakes. If electronic notebooks are used, these should be properly filed and linked to other records. Large collaborative projects involving different laboratories, research groups, or institutions sometimes hire a data manager to help organize and keep track of all the data (Schreier et al. 2006).

Third, records should be clear, legible, and recorded in the language collectively used by the research group (e.g., English). All entries in a laboratory notebook should be made legibly with permanent, nonerasable ink. Researchers should draw a line through a mistaken entry, without making it completely illegible, and should not use correction fluid (Schreier et al. 2006).

Fourth, records should be secure. Paper records should be stored in a secure place. Electronic records should be protected against unauthorized use or hacking. Access to research records should be restricted to members of the research team or to institutional officials who have the right to review them. Although many researchers take data with them when they change jobs, we strongly recommend that research institutions keep copies of all raw data while allowing individuals to have copies. Some universities follow the example of private industry and treat research data as the property of the institution. Keeping the data within the institution is important so that future interested parties can check the original data against derived data, graphs, or published results (Schreier et al. 2006).

Fifth, records should be backed up as a safeguard against destruction or theft. Data recorded on older formats (such as computer diskettes) should be transferred to newer formats (such as CDs or computer servers) so that they will be readable (Schreier et al. 2006).

Sixth, records should be kept for the appropriate length of time. Keeping records for seven years from the time of a last expenditure report or publication is a good general rule, although some records (such as FDA-regulated research records) may need to be kept longer (National Academy of Sciences 1994; National Institutes of Health 2008b; Shamoo and Teaf 1990). In the event that a federal agency or sponsor audits and inquires about the data, data storage should be automatically extended for the needed length of time.

Although it is important to store research records and materials, storage introduces problems of space allocation. Some of these problems can be handled by transferring records to digital formats, but computer storage space may also be limited. Few universities have provisions for storing records or materials in centralized facilities. We recommend that research institutions develop archives for records and materials and require researchers to make deposits on a regular basis. The federal government can and should provide funding to develop resources for data storage, such as GenBank, which stores genomic data. Researchers who create banks for storing biological samples may have to deal with space allocation issues.

Seventh, supervisors, mentors, laboratory directors, and other scientists who are responsible for mentoring students or leading research groups have responsibilities related to good record keeping. Supervisors and mentors should instruct students on how to keep good records for their research projects. They should have regular meetings with members of the research team to review data and address concerns. Laboratory directors should provide some record-keeping rules within their laboratory (Schreier et al. 2006).

Eighth, quality assurance procedures should be used to correct errors related to data entry or processing. Primary data are usually processed through many stages, depending on the type of research, before they are presented as graphs, charts, or tables or in a publishable form. As data are processed, the risk of introducing (intentional or unintentional) biases, adjustments, or errors increases (Grinnell 1992; Shamoo 1989, 1991a, 1991b).

Some recent studies indicate that academic researchers are not doing a good job of record keeping. In a survey of 1,479 researchers funded by the NIH (2007a), Martinson et al. (2005) found that the most prevalent (27.5%) self-reported inappropriate behavior was "inadequate record-keeping." Moreover, one in ten had withheld details in publications, used an inadequate experimental design, or dropped data. At 90 major research institutions, 38% of research integrity officers reported encountering problems with research records during misconduct inquiries and investigations, which often delayed investigations or made them impossible to complete (Wilson et al. 2007). In a survey conducted at the National Institute of Environmental Health Sciences (NIEHS), 31% of 243 researchers said that they had encountered poor record keeping at the NIEHS (Resnik 2006).

DATA ANALYSIS

The analysis of data in modern science involves the application of various statistical techniques, such as correlation, regression, analysis of variance (ANOVA), t-tests, and chi-square tests. These techniques provide a way of drawing inductive inferences from data and distinguishing any real phenomena or effects from random fluctuations. A responsible researcher will make every attempt to draw unbiased inferences from data. Statistical practices vary a great deal across different disciplines. Most fields have accepted practices for data analysis, and it is prudent for researchers to follow these norms (Resnik 2000). There is nothing inherently unethical in the use of unconventional statistical methods. It is important, however, to be forthright in clearly stating the method of analysis, why it is being used, and how it differs from others. It is unethical to fail to disclose important information relevant to the data analysis, such as assumptions made concerning populations or parameters or computer programs used (Resnik 2000).

Given the complexities of data analysis, it is easy to introduce biases or other errors in the analysis and to misrepresent the data (Bailar 1986). The failure to provide an honest and accurate analysis of the data can have as significant an impact on research results as recording data improperly. Moreover, research indicates that statistical errors are fairly common in science (DeMets 1999). Thus, this step is crucial for ensuring the objectivity, integrity, and quality of research. Some aspects of data analysis that raise ethical concerns include excluding outliers, imputing data (i.e., using a statistical method to fill in missing data), editing data, analyzing databases for trends and patterns (or data mining), developing graphical representations of the data, and establishing the statistical and practical significance of the data. While none of these areas of data analysis are inherently deceptive, biased, or unethical, researchers must be sure to follow good statistical practices and honestly describe their statistical methods and assumptions to avoid errors in data analysis (American Statistical Association 1999). Intentionally misrepresenting the data can be regarded as a type of misconduct (Resnik 2000).

A problem common in many research disciplines is deciding whether to report and analyze all of the data collected as part of a research project. It may be the case that not all of the data collected as part of a study are relevant to the overall results. For example, some data may be corrupted due to human or experimental error. Some data may be statistical outliers (generally two standard deviations from the mean) that may skew the analysis. Sometimes researchers may decide to take a project in a different direction so that not all of the data collected will be relevant to the results. Researchers may also conduct small pilot studies to establish the feasibility of a larger study. Honesty is an important ethical concern when one is deciding whether to report or analyze all of the data. As noted in chapter 2, exclusion of data that impact one's overall results is a type of misconduct known as falsification. However, reporting and analyzing all of the data collected as part of a study may also be problematic if the data are not relevant. Researchers must use good judgment when dealing with these issues.

Consider the case of the physicist Robert Millikan (1868–1953), who won the Nobel Prize in Physics in 1923 for measuring the smallest electrical charge (i.e., the charge on an electron). Millikan's famous oil-drop experiment involved spraying oil drops through electrically charged plates. When a drop was suspended in the air, the electrical force pulling up on the drop was equal to the force of gravity pulling it down. Millikan was able to determine the charge on an electron by calculating these forces. In his paper describing this experiment, Millikan said that he had reported all the data. However, the science historian Gerald Holton (1978) examined Millikan's laboratory notebooks and found that Millikan did not report 49 out of 189 observations (26%) that were marked as "poor" in the notebook. Though some commentators, such as Broad and Wade (1982), have argued that Millikan's work was fraudulent, a plausible explanation for his conduct is that he had a good understanding of his experimental apparatus and was therefore able to determine when it was not working properly. The "poor" results he excluded may have involved oil drops that were too big or too small for accurate measurements. However, one could argue that Millikan should have discussed this issue in the paper and that it was dishonest to claim that he had reported all the data.

Another area of concern is the treatment of digital images, such as pictures of proteins from gel electrophoresis or cell structures. Computer programs, such as Photoshop, can enhance the quality or clarity of digital images. In some cases, researchers have manipulated images in order to deceptively change the image to produce a desired result. To deal with this potential problem, many journals have adopted requirements for the submission of images for publication (Couzin 2006). Journals usually require researchers to submit the original images so they can be compared to the enhanced images. The Office of Research Integrity has special instructions on its website for forensic tools to detect fraud in images (Office of Research Integrity 2007b). Researchers should be aware of and use these tools when necessary. While it is acceptable to use image-manipulation technologies to make it easier for researchers to perceive patterns in an image, it is not acceptable to manipulate an image in order to mislead or deceive other researchers. The *Journal of Cell Biology* has adopted the following guidelines, which we endorse:

> No specific feature within an image may be enhanced, obscured, moved, removed, or introduced. The grouping of images from different parts of the same gel, or from different gels, fields, or exposures must be made explicit by the arrangement of the figure (i.e., using dividing lines) and in the text of the figure legend. If dividing lines are not included, they will be added by our production department, and this may result in production delays. Adjustments of brightness, contrast, or color balance are acceptable if they are applied to the whole image and as long as they do not obscure, eliminate, or misrepresent any information present in the original, including backgrounds. Without any background information, it is not possible to see exactly how much of the

original gel is actually shown. Non-linear adjustments (e.g., changes to gamma settings) must be disclosed in the figure legend. All digital images in manuscripts accepted for publication will be scrutinized by our production department for any indication of improper manipulation. Questions raised by the production department will be referred to the Editors, who will request the original data from the authors for comparison to the prepared figures. If the original data cannot be produced, the acceptance of the manuscript may be revoked. Cases of deliberate misrepresentation of data will result in revocation of acceptance, and will be reported to the corresponding author's home institution or funding agency. (*Journal of Cell Biology* 2007)

DATA INTERPRETATION

If all researchers interpreted the data in the same way, science would be a dry and dull profession. But this is not the case. Many important and heated debates in science, such as research on firearm violence, studies of intelligence tests, and studies of global warming, involve disputes about the interpretation of data. Sometimes an important discovery or advance in science occurs as the result of a new interpretation of existing data. Of course, challenging a standard interpretation of the data is risky: Those who challenge the existing paradigm either go down in flames or win the Nobel Prize. Most challenges to the existing paradigm turn out to be wrong. But those few times that the new interpretation is correct can change and advance our knowledge in a revolutionary fashion. For example, Peter Mitchell won the Nobel Prize for his chemiosmotic theory. He advanced the notion that a proton gradient across the mitochondrial membrane is the driving force to synthesize adenosine triphosphate (ATP) from adenosine diphosphate (ADP) and inorganic phosphate. The chemiosmotic theory was originally considered heresy because it contradicted the long-held theory of a phosphorylated intermediate for the synthesis of ATP.

The path of a trailblazer is full of hazards. Most researchers, despite their image as being open-minded and liberal, resist new ideas and stick to generally accepted standards. Although revolutions do occur in science, most research conforms to the model of "normal" science—science that falls within accepted standards, traditions, and procedures (Kuhn 1970). It is often the case that researchers who have new interpretations are scoffed at before their ideas are accepted. For example, the idea of continental drift was viewed as ludicrous, as was the idea that a bacterium could cause ulcers. However, if researchers can find new ways of interpreting data, they should be encouraged to do so. Their new interpretations will be more readily accepted (or at least considered) if they properly acknowledge the existing paradigm (Resnik 1994).

Even within the existing paradigm, the interpretation of the same data can take very different pathways, none of which are likely to be unethical. As we discussed in chapter 2, there is an important distinction between misconduct and disagreement. Just because one researcher disagrees with another's interpretation does not mean that one of them is being dishonest (Resnik and Stewart 2012). It is especially important for researchers with new interpretations to be even more careful about documenting and leaving a thorough paper trail of their data, so that other researchers will be able to understand their interpretations and not dismiss them as resulting from fraud or error. Ensuring the integrity of research data does not mean straitjacketing the investigator's creativity and latitude in introducing new ideas and interpretation. However, prudence suggests that all interpretations of data should be consistent with the existing knowledge. If the interpretation of new data is inconsistent with existing knowledge, an honest discussion of the differences is in order.

One common ethical problem with data interpretation is what we will call "overreaching." Researchers overreach when they claim that their data are more significant or important than they really are. This problem often occurs with industry-funded pharmaceutical research (Resnik 2007). For example, suppose that a study shows that a new analgesic medication is 2% more effective at reducing arthritis pain compared to acetaminophen and 4% more effective than aspirin. However, the new medication also increases systolic and diastolic blood pressure by 10% in about 30% of the people who take it. Because its patent has not expired, the new medication will be much more expensive than acetaminophen or aspirin. The researchers would be overreaching if they claimed that the new medication is superior to acetaminophen and aspirin, because the medication brings a marginal improvement in pain relief but has some dangerous side effects. Overreaching can be an ethical problem in clinical research if it causes physicians to prescribe new medications to their patients without considering costs or side effects (Angel 2004). Overreaching can be a significant issue in research with public policy implications if it supports unwise decisions.

PUBLISHING DATA

We discuss publication issues in more detail in chapters 5, 7, and 9. For now, we simply note that researchers have an obligation to disseminate work for the obvious reason that science cannot advance unless researchers report and share results. Dissemination can include publication in peer-reviewed journals, monographs or other books, and web pages, as well as presentations at professional meetings. The important ethical consideration is that research should be disseminated to colleagues and the public for scrutiny and review. Indeed, researchers who receive grants from the government or private funding agencies are usually required to specify a plan for disseminating their research in the grant proposal and to report to the agency about publications that result from the grant (Grinnell 1992). However, researchers who work for business and industry or the military often sign agreements to not publish results or to withhold publication until they obtain approval from management (Blumenthal 1997; Gibbs 1996). For instance, researchers working for the tobacco industry did not publish their work on nicotine's addictive properties for many years (Resnik 1998b). Pharmaceutical companies have also suppressed data pertaining to their products (Resnik 2007).

SHARING DATA AND MATERIALS

As noted in chapter 1, openness is a key principle in research ethics. Scientists should share data, results, methods, and materials to (a) promote the advancement of knowledge by making information publicly known; (b) allow criticism and feedback as well as replication; (c) build and maintain a culture of trust, cooperation, and collaboration among researchers; and (d) build support from the public by demonstrating openness and trustworthiness. While openness is considered by many people to be a fundamental part of academic research and scholarship, the real world of research does not always conform to this ideal. Although researchers share data within the same team of collaborators working on a common project, they rarely share data with noncollaborators and often do not welcome requests to share data with other researchers in the field, much less with people from outside the research community. The resistance to data sharing is especially high among researchers who have concerns about intellectual property, such as potential patents or trade secrets, but resistance is also high among researchers who want to protect their own interests in claiming priority (to be first) for discoveries or publishing original research.

Several recent studies have documented problems with data sharing in biomedical science. In a survey by Campbell et al. (2002) of academic geneticists concerning their experiences with data withholding, 47% stated that at least one of their requests to share data or research materials related to published research had been denied in the last three years; 28% reported that they had been unable to confirm published research due to refusals to share data or materials; and 12% said that they had denied a request to share data or materials. Of those who refused to share data or materials, 80% said they refused because sharing required too much effort; 64% said they refused to share to protect someone else's ability to publish; and 53% wanted to protect their own ability to publish (Campbell et al. 2002). Another survey (Blumenthal et al. 2006) found that 32% of biomedical researchers had engaged in some type of data withholding during the last three years and that data withholding is common in the biomedical sciences.

Although refusals to share data and materials appear to be common, especially in biomedical sciences, some organizations have adopted policies that require researchers to share data and materials following publication. Many government granting agencies, such as the NIH and National Science Foundation (NSF), encourage or require researchers to share data and materials. The NIH expects intramural and extramural researchers to share data as widely and freely as possible (National Institutes of Health 2003). The NIH also has policies that encourage or require funded researchers to share reagents and model organisms (e.g., transgenic animals). The NIH also requires researchers to state their plans to share data, reagents, or organisms in their grant applications or to explain any proposed restrictions on sharing (National Institutes of Health 1998a, 2003). The NIH has a genome-wide association studies (GWAS) policy that establishes a repository for all GWAS data obtained with NIH funding (National Institutes of Health 2009c).

Many scientific journals have also created policies that require researchers to share supporting data or materials as a condition of publication. Many journals have websites where researchers can deposit data and other supporting materials that do not appear in a published article. For example, *Science* requires researchers to share data and materials. The journal asks researchers to deposit large databases on a publicly available website prior to publication and to share data and materials after publication (*Science* 2007).

While the progress of science thrives on sharing data and materials as soon as possible, there are some legitimate reasons to refuse to share data or materials, at least temporarily, such as the following:

1. To protect a researcher's interests in publishing articles from the data or materials. If a researcher collects data or develops materials for a project, she should not have to share the data or materials until she is ready to publish, since sharing prior to publication may impact her ability to publish. But once a researcher has published, she has an obligation to share. A difficult question arises when a researcher has acquired

a large database and hopes to publish a series of papers from the database. Should the researcher be required to share the whole database as soon as she publishes the first paper from it? If she must share the whole database with other investigators, this could jeopardize her ability to publish other papers from it, because the other investigators might beat her to it. One way of handling this dilemma is to allow a researcher to publish a specific number of papers from her database before releasing the entire database to the public. Another solution is for researchers with databases to collaborate with other researchers when they share data, so that they both can receive publication credit. Difficult questions also can arise with sharing research materials, since sharing materials with others can jeopardize one's prospects of publishing articles based on those materials. Also, if the materials are in limited supply and cannot be re-created, then researchers must decide how to allocate the materials. For example, a blood sample is a limited quantity—once it has been used up, it is gone. To protect their own ability to use the sample in research, investigators need to decide carefully whom to share it with.

2. To protect intellectual property claims. Sometimes investigators are conducting research that may be patentable. Sharing data or other information related to the research prior to submitting a patent application can jeopardize the patent. Thus, researchers may refuse to share data in order to protect potential patents. It is important for society to protect patent rights to stimulate invention and private investment in R&D (Resnik 1998b). We discuss intellectual property issues in more depth in chapter 8.

3. To protect a researcher's reputation. Researchers may not want to share data because they are not ready to present it to the public. They may need to do quality-control checks on the data or analyze it. A researcher may fear that his reputation could be damaged if he publishes data prematurely and there are problems with it. Charles Darwin [1809–1882] waited more than 20 years to publish his theory of evolution by natural selection so that he could solidify the arguments and evidence in favor of the theory and anticipate objections.

4. To protect confidential information pertaining to human subjects (discussed in more depth in chapter 11), trade secrets (discussed in more depth in chapter 5), or national security (discussed in more depth in chapter 12).

5. To avoid wasting time, effort, and money. Sometimes it takes a great deal of time, effort, or money to share data or materials with other researchers. There are significant costs with answering requests, shipping

materials, taking care of animals, and synthesizing chemicals. One way of dealing with this problem is to deposit data on a public website or to license a private company to make data or materials available to other researchers. Whenever data or materials are shared, a reasonable fee can be charged to cover the costs of sharing.

6. To avoid being hassled by industry or political interest groups. Sometimes industry representatives will request data in order to reanalyze the data or reinterpret the results. For example, if a study finds that exposure to a pesticide increases the risk of Parkinson's disease, the manufacturer of the pesticide might want to acquire the data to reanalyze it or challenge the study. Political interest groups, such as animal rights activists, may also request data or other information to harass or intimidate researchers. While these requests can sometimes be legitimate attempts to advance scientific knowledge, they often are not.

Researchers who are considering refusing a request to share data or materials should use their good judgments to make an ethical choice. While the default ethical standard should be to share data and materials as soon as possible once research is completed, researchers may decide not to share data and materials in cases where other concerns (such as protecting confidentiality or career interests) outweigh the ethics of openness.

In the United States, if federally funded researchers refuse to share data (or other information), outside parties may still be able to obtain the data under the Freedom of Information Act (FOIA). Other countries, such as the United Kingdom, have similar laws. FOIA allows the public to gain access to recorded information gathered or generated using federal funds, including scientific research records. To gain access to information under FOIA, one must send a request in writing to the head of the appropriate federal agency asking for the records that are sought. One must also specify the records being sought and explain why they are being sought. The agency should respond to this request within 20 days by sending the documents, promising to send the documents within a reasonable time, or explaining why they cannot be sent. The agency may charge a reasonable fee for sending the records. There are some exceptions to FOIA: Agencies can refuse to share records pertaining to national security or foreign relations, agency rules or practices, confidential business information, information related to personal privacy, some types of law enforcement records, and information pertaining to the supervision of financial institutions. Federal authorities have determined that some of these exceptions apply to federally funded scientific research. For example, researchers do not have to disclose confidential information pertaining to human subjects. They also do not have to disclose information protected by trade secrecy law, including information pertaining to potential patents (U.S. Department of Justice 2007).

Some scientists have objected to FOIA on the grounds that it could subject them to harassment from people who want to interfere with their work (Macilwain 1999). Although it is important for researchers to be free from harassment from industry representatives, political activists, or other parties, we do not think that researchers who receive public funds can be completely shielded from this threat. It is difficult to know in advance whether any particular request for information would be harassment of researchers. Without having this knowledge in advance, any policy short of answering all requests for data would be arbitrary and possibly biased.

Public access to federally supported research has reached the public domain in the past few years. In an editorial, the *New York Times* (2013) opined that if we (i.e., the public) paid for it we should have access to it. The U.S. government has instructed all federal agencies with more than $100 million in expenditures on research to have a plan submitted to the government on how it will provide public access to the data. Berman and Cerf (2013) have proposed that public access to the data should be the result of private-sector partnerships.

QUESTIONS FOR DISCUSSION

1. How would you characterize scientific research? In your opinion, what is the most crucial part of research?
2. How would you list the steps in carrying out research? Are there some steps you could skip? Why? Is there a particular order to doing the steps?
3. Can scientific research incorporate quality control and quality assurance methods? Would this stifle creativity or increase workload?
4. Can you give an example of how one might modify data to suit inappropriate goals in the steps of research?
5. Can you give an example of an experimental design that would bias the data?
6. What principles or rules do you follow related to research record keeping?
7. Do you keep good records? Could someone reproduce your work from your research records (laboratory notebook, etc.)?

8. How is a lab notebook like (or not like) a business or medical record?
9. Can you give an example of an ethical or scientific issue you have faced concerning data analysis or interpretation?
10. When would you be justified in refusing to share data?

CASES FOR DISCUSSION

CASE 1

A medical student has a summer job with a faculty mentor at a research university. The student is bright, hardworking, and industrious and hopes to publish a paper at the end of the summer. He is the son of a colleague of the mentor at a distant university. The student is working on a cancer cell line that requires three weeks to grow in order to test for the development of a specific antibody. His project plan is to identify the antibody by the end of the summer. The student has written a short paper describing his work. The mentor went over the primary data and found that some of the data were written on pieces of yellow pads without clearly identifying from which experiment the data came or the data. She also noticed that some of the experiments shown in the paper's table were repeated several times without an explanation as to why. The mentor was not happy about the data or the paper, but she likes the student and does not want to discourage him from a potential career in research.

- What is the primary responsibility of the mentor?
- Should the mentor write a short paper and send it for publication?
- Should the student write a short paper and send it for publication?
- If you were the mentor, what would you do?
- Should the mentor or her representative have paid more attention to the student's work during the course of the summer?

CASE 2

A graduate student at a research university finished her dissertation and graduated with honors. Her mentor gave the continuation of the project to a new graduate student. As usual, the mentor gave the entire laboratory notebook (or computer disk) to the new graduate student, who had to repeat the isolation of the newly discovered chemical entity with high-pressure liquid chromatography (HPLC) in order to follow up the chemical and physical characterization of the new compound. The new graduate student found that if he followed the exact method described in the laboratory notebooks and published by the previous student, he could obtain the new chemical entity but not at the same HPLC location as published, but slightly shifted to the left, and there was a different peak at the location stated. However, the new student discovered that if the ionic strength is doubled, he could find the same chemical at the same location in accordance with the previous student's dissertation. The new student discussed with the mentor how he should proceed. The mentor replied, "Why make a fuss about it? Just proceed with your slightly different method and we can move on."

- What are the responsibilities of the new student? Should the new student refuse to accommodate the mentor's request?
- Should the new student have read more thoroughly the relevant laboratory notebooks prior to starting the experiment? Should there have been a paper trail of the error in the laboratory notebook? Do you think the error was intentional, and does it matter?
- If the laboratory notebook does not reveal the error, is it then misconduct? Does it indicate that a better recording of the data would have been helpful?
- Can you propose a reasonable resolution to the problem?

CASE 3

A new postdoctoral fellow in a genetic research laboratory must sequence a 4-kDa fragment. After the sequence, he is to prepare a 200-base unit to use as a potential regulator of a DNA-related enzyme. The 4-kDa fragment is suspected to contain the 200-base unit. The sequence of the 200-base unit is already known in the literature, but not as part of the 4-kDa fragment and not as a potential regulator. The fact that the 200-base unit is known is what gave the mentor the idea that it may have a functional role. The new postdoctoral fellow tried for three months to sequence the 4-kDa fragment, without success, and so simply proceeded to synthesize the 200-base unit without locating it within the fragment. After two years of research, the 4-kDa fragment appeared to play a key regulatory role in an important discovery, but at this time the mentor learned that the postdoc never sequenced the original 4-kDa fragment. The mentor could never find a "good" record of the attempts to sequence the 4-kDa fragment.

- What impression do you gather about how this mentor runs the laboratory?
- Should there be records of sequence attempts of the 4-kDa fragment?
- Are there reasons to suspect that data may have been fabricated?
- How should the mentor proceed?
- If you were the new postdoc, what steps you would take to ensure proper records of your work?

CASE 4

A graduate student prepared for her thesis a table showing that a toxic substance inhibits an enzyme's activity by about 20%. She has done 12 experiments. The mentor looked at the data and found that one of the data points showed an inhibition of 0% and that this point is the one that skewed the results to a low level of inhibition with a large standard of deviation. The mentor further determined with the student that the outlier is outside the mean by 2.1 times the standard derivation and that it is reasonable not to include it with the rest of the data. This would make the inhibition about 30% and thus make the potential paper more in line with other research results and hence more "respectable." The mentor instructed the student to remove the statistical outlier from the data.

- Should the student simply proceed with the mentor's instructions?
- Should the mentor have been more specific regarding what to do with the outlier? In what way?
- Can you propose a resolution? Should the outlier be mentioned in the paper?
- How should this laboratory handle similar issues in the future? Should each laboratory have an agreed-upon standard operating procedure, or SOP, for such a statistical issue?

CASE 5

A social scientist is conducting an anonymous survey of college students on their opinions on various academic integrity issues. The survey is administered in four different sections of an Introduction to Sociology class. The survey includes 20 questions in which respondents can use a Likert scale to answer various questions: 1 = strongly agree, 2 = agree, 3 = neither agree nor disagree, 4 = disagree, and 5 = strongly disagree. The survey also includes 10 open-ended questions that ask for respondents to state their opinions or attitudes. The social scientist distributes 480 surveys and 320 students respond. A graduate student helps the social scientist compile the survey data. When examining the surveys, the student encounters some problems. First, it appears that eight surveys are practical jokes. The persons filling out these surveys wrote obscene comments and for many questions added extra numbers to the Likert scale. Although some of the 20 Likert-scale questions in these surveys appear to be usable, others are not. Second, in 35 surveys, the respondents appeared to have misunderstood the instructions on how to use the Likert scale. They answered "5" on questions where it would seem that "1" would be the most logical answer, given their written comments. Third, on 29 surveys, the respondents wrote their names on the survey, when they were instructed not to do so.

- How should the researchers deal with these issues with their data?
- Should they try to edit/fix surveys that have problems?
- Should they throw away any surveys? Which ones?
- How might their decisions concerning the disposition of these surveys affect their overall results?

CASE 6

A pharmaceutical company conducts five small (20 subjects) phase I studies on a new drug to establish its safety in healthy individuals. Three of these studies had a p-value < 0.05, indicating significant results; two had a p-value > 0.05, indicating nonsignificant results. As it so happens, undesirable side effects were observed in both studies with the nonsignificant results but not in the other studies. The researchers report all their results to the FDA but they do not report all of these results in a publication. The publication only reports significant results.

- Are there any design problems with these studies?
- Is there an ethical responsibility to report all of the data? Would it make a difference if the subjects were not human (i.e., animals)?
- Is not reporting nonsignificant results falsification?
- What are the responsibilities of the researchers to this company, to themselves, and to society?
- Should there be a federal mandate to report all side effects to the public?

CASE 7

Dr. Heathcliff is a toxicologist testing the effects of an industrial compound that is used in manufacturing plastic food containers and that functions like testosterone in the body. The study involves two groups of laboratory mice: one is fed the compound each day, and a control group is not fed the compound. The main outcome measure is aggressive behavior, which is known to be linked to testosterone activity. He completes that study and finds that the animals fed the compound displayed significantly more aggressive behavior than the control group. He submits the paper for publication the following week. A technician assisting with the experiment discovers that the heating system in the area where animals are kept was malfunctioning one of the nights prior to their main set of observations, which took place that following morning. The temperature in the cages where the animals were kept was as much as 5°C higher than normal, according to the maintenance crew. The technician informs Dr. Heathcliff about this problem, who replies that "the temperature probably didn't make any difference since the animals were at normal temperature in the morning. And besides, the control group was not unusually aggressive; only the experimental group displayed above normal aggression."

- Should Dr. Heathcliff inform the journal about this issue?
- Should he include information about the temperature issue in the methods or discussion section of the paper?
- Should he withdraw the paper?
- Should he repeat the experiments?
- Would it be unethical to publish the paper in its present form?
- Would this be misconduct (i.e., data fabrication or falsification)?
- What should the technician do?

CASE 8

A graduate student in physics is writing a thesis that develops a mathematical model of gamma ray bursts. The student conducts a literature review on the subject as a background to her research. In conducting this review, she searches various computer databases for articles and abstracts relevant to her work, for the past five years. She gathers many abstracts and papers. For much of the research, she reads only abstracts and not the full papers. Also, she does not include some of the important work on gamma ray bursts that took place more than five years ago.

- Should the graduate student read the full articles, not just abstracts?
- If she cites an article in a publication or in her thesis, should she read the full article?
- If she cites a book, should she read the full book or only the part that she cites?
- Should the graduate student include articles published more than five years ago?

CASE 9

Dr. Reno is a junior investigator who has just received her first major NIH grant. She has used NIH funds to create a transgenic mouse model to study depression. The mouse has a genetic defect that leads to an underproduction of serotonin. She has used the model to show how a compound found in an herbal medicine increases serotonin levels in mice and also produces effects associated with normal (i.e., nondepressed) behavior, such as normal levels of exercise and normal sleep patterns. Dr. Reno applies for a patent on this compound with the intent of eventually testing it on human subjects. She also publishes a paper in a high-impact journal describing her work with the mouse model. Almost immediately after the paper appears in print, she receives dozens of requests from researchers who would like to use her transgenic mice in their own research. Dr. Reno is flattered but also overwhelmed. She has barely enough mice for her own work, and she doesn't want to turn her laboratory into a factory for producing mice for someone else's research.

- How should Dr. Reno deal with these requests to share transgenic mice?
- Does she have an obligation to share the mice?

CASE 10

Drs. Kessenbaum and Wilcox are conducting a long-term, observational study of the health of pesticide applicators. The protocol calls for an initial health assessment, including a health history, physical exam, and blood and urine tests. The researchers will collect a DNA sample from cheek scrapings and collect dust samples from the applicators' clothing and hair and underneath their fingernails. After the initial health assessment, the applicators will complete yearly health surveys and undergo a full health assessment every four years. The researchers will follow the subjects for at least 25 years. Their work is funded by the NIH. Drs. Kessenbaum and Wilcox have been conducting their study for 15 years, and they have compiled an impressive database. They have already published more than a dozen papers from the database. Whenever they share data, they require researchers who request it to sign elaborate data-sharing agreements, which spell out clearly how the data will be used. The agreements also specify the kinds of studies that can be published using the data, which allows Drs. Kessenbaum and Wilcox to protect their interests in publishing on certain topics. In the past month, they have received some requests to access their database. One request has come from a pesticide company, another has come from a competing research team also studying the health of pesticide applicators, and another has come from a radical environmental group with an antipesticide agenda.

- How should Drs. Kessenbaum and Wilcox handle these requests to access their database?
- Should they refuse to share data with the pesticide company or the environmental group?
- Is it ethical to require people who request data to sign elaborate data-sharing agreements?

CHAPTER 4
Mentoring

Effective mentoring can play a key role in preventing misconduct and promoting research integrity. This chapter explores various issues related to mentoring, including such moral dimensions as proper training, setting an example, trust, accountability, and collegiality. The chapter also addresses policies designed to promote effective mentoring.

As we noted in chapter 2, effective mentoring can play a key role in preventing misconduct and promoting research integrity. Mentoring is important in helping students learn how to deal with most of the ethical issues and concerns discussed in the book, ranging from data management and authorship to publication and social responsibility. Mentors can teach students about research norms and practices and can provide students with examples of how to behave ethically in research. Mentors can model different scientific virtues, such as honesty, openness, objectivity, fairness, integrity, flexibility, conscientiousness, resourcefulness, and social responsibility (Macrina 2013; National Academy of Sciences 1992; Resnik 2012a; Swazey and Bird 1997; Weil and Arzbaecher 1997).

Mentoring traces its history back to ancient Greece. The word "mentor" comes from the name of a man who was the adviser to King Odysseus and the teacher to Telemachus in Homer's *Odyssey*. Mentor provided education and moral guidance to his students. Following this model, a mentor was an older male teacher who had a close relationship with an adolescent young man. Socrates, the father of philosophy, mentored Plato and many other students in Athens. Plato created his own school and mentored many students, including Aristotle, who made important contributions to physics, biology, philosophy, logic, politics, and literary theory. Today, mentoring is a very important component of the research enterprise. In academic institutions, mentors not only transmit knowledge and skills to students but also teach attitudes, traditions, values, and other things that cannot be learned in formal courses. Mentors serve as role models and teach their students by example.

Most people have different mentors at different times for different reasons. A mentor could be a family member, a pastor, a coach, a friend, a teacher, a business leader, a policeman, or anyone a student knows and admires. In science, a mentor is usually a senior researcher who supervises a number of different graduate students. Usually students' graduate advisers or thesis advisers are also their mentors, but many research students obtain mentoring from senior researchers who have no formal advising responsibilities (Weil and Arzbaecher 1997). Many students consider more than one person to be their mentor, but, unfortunately, some students have no one whom they would consider a mentor. Researchers who can benefit from mentoring include undergraduate, graduate, and postdoctoral students; technicians; and junior-level professors (National Academy of Sciences 1992, 1997; National Institutes of Health 2002).

Mentors in science interact with their students in many ways. Some of the most important activities include the following:

1. Teaching students how to do research: Mentors help students learn the techniques, methods, and traditions of research. They show students how to design and conduct experiments; formulate research questions and hypotheses; collect, record, analyze, and interpret data; and write up results. They help students understand important work in their discipline, ongoing controversies, and areas of research that need further study (Macrina 2013).

2. Critiquing and supporting students' research and teaching: Mentors read students' lab notebooks, research protocols, and manuscripts, and they scrutinize students' research designs and data analyses. They may attend classes that the students teach, read students' evaluations of teaching, and provide feedback on teaching style and technique. Although it is very important for mentors to criticize students, they also need to offer support and encouragement, and they need to carefully tread the line between constructive and destructive criticism. Mentors need to guard against discrimination, favoritism, and excessively high (or low) expectations when critiquing students (Macrina 2013).

3. Promoting their students' careers: Mentors help students form professional contacts, look for jobs, and submit job applications; they write

letters of recommendation; help students prepare for job interviews; and provide career advice (Macrina 2013).

4. Helping students understand the ethical, legal, social, and financial aspects of research: Mentors teach their students about research rules and regulations, such as animal care and use regulations, human experimentation regulations, and laboratory, biological, and radiation safety rules and regulations. They also help students understand the social structure of the research environment, including relationships with colleagues, students, administrators, funding agencies, and the public. They help students understand the funding of research, including how to write grant applications and obtain scholarships and fellowships.

5. Involvement in students' personal lives: Although mentors should maintain professional distance from their students, they should not ignore their students' personal lives. For example, if mentors are aware of psychological, personal, medical, or legal problems that are affecting their students' work, they should help their students find the proper resources or help. Mentors can listen to their students' problems and support them in difficult circumstances. Even though it is important for mentors to be aware of their students' personal lives, judgment and discretion should be used so that the relationships remain professional and do not become too personal. Mentors should avoid becoming too involved in their students' personal lives so that they can maintain a measure of objectivity and fairness.

This list shows that mentors perform many important duties for their students. Mentors are more than mere teachers: They are also advisers, counselors, and often friends. Because students usually also work for mentors as teaching or research assistants, mentors also serve as employers and supervisors. These different roles may sometimes conflict. For instance, mentors may give students so much work to do that they do not have adequate time for their own research. In these cases, a mentor's role of employer/supervisor conflicts with the role of teacher. Or a mentor may believe that it is in the student's best interests to transfer to a different university to work with someone who has more expertise in that student's chosen area of research but yet may hesitate to convey this advice to the student if the mentor needs him as a research or teaching assistant.

Steiner et al. (2004) surveyed 139 primary care fellows of the National Research Service Award from 1988 through 1997 regarding their subsequent career development and research productivity. The fellows indicated whether during the fellowship they had no sustained and influential mentorship, influential but not sustained mentorship, or influential and sustained mentorship. Steiner et al. found that those with sustained and influential mentorship were more engaged in research, were publishing more often, were more likely to be the principal investigator on a grant, and were more likely to provide good mentorship to others.

Because the mentoring relationship depends on mutual respect and trust, students and mentors have ethical duties toward one another. Students should listen to and appreciate the guidance and advice from the mentors, ask for help when they need it, and work diligently on their research projects. Mentors should provide guidance, advice, and other forms of help to their students; protect their students from harm and exploitation; and treat their students fairly. Both parties should communicate honestly, maintain confidentiality concerning private matters, and respect each other's choices and values.

To better understand the ethical dimensions of the mentor–student relationship, it is important to realize that mentors have more power, experience, knowledge, and expertise than their students and that students depend on their mentors for education, training, advice, and often employment (Macrina 2013; Weil and Arzbaecher 1997). Given their minimal power, experience, knowledge, and expertise and the high degree of dependency, students are highly vulnerable. It is very easy for mentors to manipulate, control, or exploit their students, because students often may be unable to prevent or avoid such abuses of power. Thus, the mentor–student relationship resembles other professional relationships where one party is highly vulnerable, such as the doctor–patient relationship and the lawyer–client relationship. These relationships are sometimes called fiduciary relationships because the powerful party is entrusted with protecting the interests of the vulnerable party. This is different from a contractual relationship in which both parties need only look out for their own interests (Bayles 1988).

Unfortunately, various forms of exploitation are fairly common in mentoring. Mentors sometimes do not protect their students from harm or treat them fairly. For instance, mentors often do not give students proper credit for their work. They may fail to give students acknowledgments in papers or include them as coauthors (Banoub-Baddour and Gien 1991). They may fail to list students as first authors when students make the most important contribution to the research. In some of the more egregious cases, mentors have stolen ideas from their students without giving them any credit at all (Dreyfuss 2000; Marshall 1999a, 2000). One well-known case of this type of exploitation involved the famous scientist Robert Millikan (discussed in chapter 3) and his student Harvey Fletcher.

Millikan began his experiment by trying to measure the electric charge on water droplets. When the experiment was not working well, Fletcher suggested that Millikan use oil droplets instead. Millikan took this advice but did not acknowledge Fletcher's contribution in his paper describing these experiments (Holton 1978). A more recent case involved Carolyn Phinney and her former mentor, Marion Perlmutter, a University of Michigan professor. Phinney had developed an instrument to measure psychological effects when she worked as a research assistant for Perlmutter. Perlmutter incorporated Phinney's work into a grant application and began claiming the instrument as her own. She also refused to return Phinney's laboratory notebooks. In 1997, Phinney won a $1.67 million lawsuit against Perlmutter and the University of Michigan (Grossman 1997).

Mentors may also overwork their students by assigning them too many experiments to run, too many papers to grade, too many undergraduate students to tutor, and so on. If students are assigned too much work, they will not have enough time for their own education and research. In recent years, graduate students have formed unions to deal with poor working conditions. Postdoctoral students often face especially demanding and exploitative working conditions. They are usually nontenured researchers who are paid through "soft money," that is, money from research grants. Postdoctoral students are paid much less than regular faculty members even though they have doctoral degrees and often do just as much research or teaching. They also do not receive the usual benefits package (e.g., health insurance), and they have little job security (Barinaga 2000). Although some postdoctoral students enjoy their work, others feel mistreated or exploited. Given their vulnerability, it is very hard for these students to complain about working conditions or about their mentors, because they face the real threat of retaliation. For example, a mentor could refuse to work with the student any longer, recommend that the student be expelled from the program, or encourage his colleagues not to work with the student.

Other examples of ways in which mentors may mistreat their students include the following:

- Giving students misinformation or poor advice
- Intimidating or harassing students
- Discriminating against students
- Showing favoritism to one or more students
- Failing to help students advance their careers
- Not recognizing when students are having psychological troubles that require counseling

Given the importance of the mentor–student relationship for scientific research, and the kinds of problems that routinely arise, many universities and professional organizations have developed programs and policies aimed at improving mentoring (National Academy of Sciences 1997; National Institutes of Health 2002). Some of these policies include the following:

1. Train researchers how to be good mentors (Pfund et al 2006).
2. Reward researchers for effective mentoring: Most universities do not emphasize or even consider mentoring skills when they review faculty for hiring and promotion, but this needs to change if we want to improve mentoring (Djerassi 1999).
3. Provide mentors with enough time for mentoring: Professors who do not have adequate time for mentoring will do a poor job of mentoring. Professors who have heavy mentoring responsibilities should be released from other administrative or teaching obligations.
4. Develop clear rules concerning workloads, teaching duties, research opportunities, authorship, time commitments, and intellectual property: Many of the problems that occur in mentoring are due to poor communication. Communication can be improved by clearly defining expectations and obligations (Macrina 2013).
5. Establish procedures and channels for evaluating mentoring and for allowing students and mentors to voice their grievances.
6. Ensure that students who "blow the whistle" on mentors are protected: A whistleblower is someone who reports unethical or illegal conduct. Whistleblowers often face retaliation. To avoid this, whistleblowers must be protected. (See the discussion of whistleblowing in chapter 2.)
7. Promote a psychologically safe work environment: Students and mentors both need to have an environment that is free from sexual, religious, ethnic, and other forms of harassment (National Academy of Sciences 1992). Sexual harassment is unethical and can also be illegal. Although most researchers agree on the need to protect students and others from sexual harassment, there are disputes about the definition of sexual harassment as well as the proper response to sexual harassment (Swisher 1995). For further discussion, see Resnik (1998b).
8. Promote a nondiscriminatory work environment: Racial, ethnic, sexual, religious, and other types of discrimination are also unethical and often illegal. Women have for many years labored under the yoke of sex discrimination in science. Although women have made significant gains in some sciences, such as anthropology, biology, and medicine, women are still vastly underrepresented in engineering and physical science. Racial and ethnic discrimination continue to be a problem

in science as more minorities enter the workplace (Johnson 1993; Manning 1998). Although African Americans have historically been the most frequent victims of discrimination, Asian Americans also experience discrimination (Lawler 2000). Scientists should be judged by the quality of their research, education, and character, not by the color of their skin, their national origin, their religious views, or their gender. Effective mentoring cannot take place when discrimination affects the laboratory (for further discussion, see Resnik 1998b).

9. Promote a diverse workforce: Because mentors serve as role models as well as advisers and friends, one could argue that it is important to promote diversity in science in order to enhance mentoring and education. Science students have different gender, racial, ethnic, and religious characteristics. The scientific workforce should reflect this diversity so that students can benefit from having role models with whom they can identify (Holden 2000; Mervis 1999). An excellent way to promote the effective mentoring of women in science is to hire and promote more women scientists (Etkowitz et al. 1994), which will also encourage more women to study science. This same "diversity" argument also applies to racial and ethnic diversity, which raises the question of affirmative action in science: Should hiring and promotion of scientists be decided based on a person's racial or ethnic features? This is a complex legal, moral, and political question that we do not explore in depth here. We favor a weak form of affirmative action that increases the diversity of the workforce without compromising quality. Racial, ethnic, and gender considerations should be treated as one factor among many that can enhance diversity. Other factors might include geography, socioeconomic status, and life experiences. Affirmative action should not be used to promote incompetence or tokenism (Resnik 2005).

QUESTIONS FOR DISCUSSION

1. What do mentors do for students?
2. What are the qualities of a good mentor? A good student?
3. Can you describe how you are being mentored? Do you think you are being treated well? Would you like your mentor to treat you differently?
4. What types of problems can arise when the same person is a supervisor and a mentor?
5. Is the mentor–student relationship like a physician–patient relationship?
6. How can universities encourage good mentoring?

CASES FOR DISCUSSION

CASE 1

A postdoctoral fellow got into a severe conflict with her mentor. Her mentor provided her salary from his grant resources, and she was working on one of his primary projects. She found another job and took all three laboratory notebooks with her when she left. The mentor was very angry when he found out. He asked her to return the lab notebooks immediately or she would be accused of theft. He claimed the lab notebooks belonged to him and to the university, but he invited her to copy the books for her use. She returned the notebooks after making copies. Two years later, the mentor learned that she had published a paper without mentioning his name anywhere, but his grant was acknowledged.

• What should the mentor do?

CASE 2

A graduate student worked for a year with an adviser on replicating a new small protein. He spent part of the year developing the methodology before conducting the replications. However, the graduate student did not like his adviser and moved to a different adviser within the same department, who happened to be the director of the graduate program in that department. The student's new research program was in a different area from the previous work. A year later, the student learned that a subsequent student of his former mentor had used his method for replicating the protein in subsequent research and that they were writing a paper without listing him as a coauthor. He protested but was told that the new graduate student had to do the whole thing all over again and that they were not using his data. The student argued that the new technique used to collect the data was a novel technique developed by him and not available in the open literature. The student's former adviser, after meeting with everyone including the director, reluctantly agreed to publish at a later date a small technical paper on the technique, naming the student as a coauthor. The first paper will still appear, much sooner, and without his name. The student agreed, under protest, but he knew his life would be difficult if he insisted on a different outcome.

• Should the student have been listed as an author on the paper?
• What would you have done under these circumstances?
• Should the first adviser have done what he did?
• What should the new student have done, and what should he do now?

CASE 3

Dr. Trotter is a molecular geneticist who applies Darwin's principle "survival of the fittest" to his laboratory environment. Each year, he hires two new postdoctoral students for one year. He assigns them both to work on the same experiment. Whoever finishes the work first, with reproducible results, will get to be an author on a paper; the loser will not. He runs several such contests during the year. At the end of the year, the postdoctoral student who has the best results will be hired for a three-year position, and the loser will be terminated.

- What do you think about Dr. Trotter's policy?
- Is it ethical?

CASE 4

Sarah Parker is a doctoral student in entomology. Her mentor, Dr. Russell, is one of the world's experts on fire ants. He is very busy, as he supervises five students and often gives invited lectures. He also provides advice for agricultural groups on controlling fire ants. He rarely meets with Ms. Parker in person and provides most of his comments on her thesis by email. He encourages students to work independently so they will learn how to deal with problems on their own. Ms. Parker's thesis defense is next week. One of the members of the committee says that he cannot approve her thesis because she does not have enough data pertaining to one of her studies of fire-ant mating. Ms. Parker is very upset when she learns about this, because Dr. Russell had assured her that she was ready to defend. It will take her several months to collect the additional data, which will put her career plans on hold.

- Do you see any problems with Dr. Russell's mentoring approach?
- How could this problem have been prevented?
- Should Ms. Parker have requested that Dr. Russell provide her with more help? How should she have gone about this?

CASE 5

Dr. Feldman is a professor of history at Page University. He specializes in the U.S. Civil War. Brad Cooper was a graduate student who had been working with Dr. Feldman for three years. He completed his master's degree with Dr. Cooper. He was planning to write a doctoral thesis, under Dr. Parker's direction, on surgical techniques developed in the Civil War, but then he decided he would like to go to medical school.

Dr. Feldman was disappointed that Mr. Cooper made this decision, because he felt that Mr. Cooper had some promise as a historian. Mr. Cooper had extensive discussions with Dr. Feldman about a potential doctoral thesis on surgical antiseptic techniques. Unbeknownst to Mr. Cooper, Dr. Feldman began working on the ideas that they had discussed, and she did extensive historical research on surgical antiseptic techniques used in the Civil War. Mr. Cooper received a magazine in the mail from Page University that featured Dr. Feldman's research and mentioned an article she had recently published on surgical antiseptic techniques used in the Civil War. He looks up the article and finds that he is not mentioned in the acknowledgments. Mr. Cooper is very upset about this because he thinks he should have received some credit for his ideas.

- Did Dr. Feldman do anything wrong?
- Did she commit plagiarism? What additional information would you need to make this determination?
- What can Mr. Cooper do at this point?
- Would it be difficult to prove a plagiarism case against Dr. Feldman?
- How could this unfortunate turn of events have been avoided?

CASE 6

Ms. Holloway was a psychology graduate student working under the direction of Dr. Truman at a large research university. During her second year in the program, Ms. Holloway suffered from a bout of severe depression and withdrew from the university for a semester. After resuming her studies, Ms. Holloway was doing well and seemed to be making good progress on her thesis. However, Ms. Holloway's work degraded during her second semester back at the university. She missed several meetings of the research group and was late for some of her teaching sessions with the Introduction to Psychology students. Other students noticed that she kept to herself and seemed distant and emotionally detached. Dr. Truman sent Ms. Holloway an email warning her that her performance was not acceptable and that she needed to make a better effort on her research and teaching or she could lose her position. The next day, Ms. Holloway committed suicide.

- Did Dr. Truman act unethically?
- Was he a bad mentor?
- What could he have done to help prevent Ms. Holloway's suicide?
- Did he have a responsibility to be aware of her personal problems?

CASE 7

Dr. Fitzgerald is a professor of geology at a large public university. He supervises three graduate students: Tom Turpin, Wendy Price, and Melissa Macintyre. Dr. Fitzgerald has known Mr. Turpin since he was a young boy because Mr. Turpin's father is a friend and colleague at the university. Dr. Fitzgerald took an instant liking to Mr. Turpin and they have gone on several fishing trips with Mr. Turpin's father in the last year. Ms. Price and Ms. Macintyre have begun to resent this relationship and they feel that Dr. Fitzgerald is showing favoritism to Mr. Turpin. They have noticed that Dr. Fitzgerald is eager to introduce Mr. Turpin to colleagues at professional meetings. They also believe that Dr. Fitzgerald has assigned Mr. Turpin research projects that are more exciting and fulfilling than the projects they have been asked to work on. Dr. Fitzgerald also recommended Mr. Turpin for a graduate student award but did not recommend them.

- Is Dr. Fitzgerald showing favoritism to Mr. Turpin?
- Is Dr. Fitzgerald acting unethically?
- What can Ms. Price and Ms. Macintyre do about this situation?
- How could these problems have been avoided?

CASE 8

Mr. Goldman is a toxicology graduate student in Dr. Miller's laboratory. He is conducting experiments that involve exposing cells to a nanomaterial thought to be toxic because it has chemical and physical properties similar to asbestos. Mr. Goldman weighs the material in powder form and mixes it with a solution. When the material is in a powder form, it may become airborne and could be breathed in. For his protection, Mr. Goldman wears a mask and gloves and uses a negative pressure hood to prepare the solution. However, Mr. Goldman has done some reading about safety procedures related to the preparation of this material, and most laboratories use a glove box for preparation, as this greatly reduces the risk of inhalation. Mr. Goldman asks Dr. Miller if he can obtain a glove box to use in preparing the material. Dr. Miller responds that this is unnecessary and that he will be adequately protected if he follows the procedures they are using. He also says that he does not have enough money in his grant to pay for a glove box.

- Is Dr. Miller acting unethically?
- What should Mr. Goldman do about this situation?

CHAPTER 5

Collaboration within Academia and with Industry

Collaboration is essential to scientific research. Collaboration may occur among researchers working in different institutions, scientific disciplines, or countries. Collaboration raises many different ethical, legal, and practical issues that researchers should address, including authorship, publication, conflict of interest, data management, roles and responsibilities, regulation, oversight, and deadlines. International collaborations can lead to a variety of ethical problems and concerns because different members of the research team may have different understandings of research norms, procedures, and traditions, and they may have different cultural, educational, legal, and political backgrounds. Collaborations between academia and industry can create various ethical problems and concerns because academic values may conflict with corporate values and interests.

Collaboration is a defining feature of modern science. Although many great historical figures in science, such as Archimedes, Galileo, Newton, William Harvey, and Gregor Mendel, managed to do a great deal of work without collaborating significantly, today's scientists must interact with many different colleagues. Researchers work together on projects and share data, ideas, equipment, computers, methods, reagents, cell lines, research sites, personnel, and many other technical and human resources. Researchers collaborate with people from different departments, institutions, disciplines, and nations. Collaborations may involve graduate students, postdoctoral students, technicians, and junior and senior researchers. As noted in chapter 3, the National Institutes of Health (NIH) and National Science Foundation (NSF) have adopted policies about sharing data and materials in order to promote collaborative work. The agencies have also funded research centers across the United States to encourage scientists from different institutions to work together. Collaborations can range in size from small studies involving only a few researchers from two different institutions, to multicenter clinical trials involving dozens of researchers from about twenty institutions, to large-scale endeavors involving hundreds of scientists from around the globe, such as the Human Genome Project (Grinnell 1992; Macrina 2013; Mervis 2002). Collaborations can take place within academia or between academia and industry.

Successful collaborations in science require a high degree of trust, collegiality, fairness, and accountability. Trust is important because researchers need to trust that their collaborators will keep the agreements, perform according to expectations, behave ethically, and so on (Whitbeck 1998). Many different factors can undermine trust, including selfishness, incompetence, negligence, unfairness, careerism, and conflicts of interest. As noted in chapter 2, the collaboration between Gallo and Montagnier related to the discovery of HIV broke down because they had problems trusting each other.

Collegiality, one of the sociologist Robert Merton's (1973) norms of science, which also include universalism, disinterestedness, originality, and skepticism, is important in maintaining a social environment that promotes trust. The norm of collegiality requires researchers to treat each other with the respect accorded to a friend or ally in pursuit of a common goal. Colleagues help one another and provide constructive criticism. Behaviors that can undermine collegiality include harassment (sexual or otherwise); racial, ethnic, or sexual discrimination; verbal abuse; personal grudges; theft; and jealousy.

Fairness is important because collaborators want to ensure that they receive a fair share of the rewards of research, such as authorship or intellectual property rights, and they do want to be unfairly burdened with some of the more tedious or unpleasant aspects of research (Resnik 1998a, 1998b). Although research is a cooperative activity, researchers still retain their individual interests, and they expect that those interests will be treated fairly. Plagiarism and undeserved authorship are extreme violations of fairness. Fairness is also very important in other issues relating to collaboration, such as peer review and personnel decisions.

Last but not least, accountability is important because when many people work together, it is especially important to know who can be held accountable for the successes or the failures of a project (Rennie et al. 1997). Modern research involves a division of intellectual labor:

Different people do different jobs in research, such as designing experiments, gathering data, analyzing data, and writing papers (Kitcher 1993). Many research projects encompass research techniques, methods, and disciplines so different from each other that no one person can be responsible for or even knowledgeable about all the different aspects of the project. For example, the study of a new DNA vaccine may involve enzyme kinetics, X-ray crystallography, reverse transcriptase, electron micrographs, recombinant DNA, polymerase chain reactions, clinical trials, pharmacology, microbiology, immunology, and statistical analysis. Because so many people are doing different jobs, it is often hard to keep track of all of these different laborers, the standards governing their work, and the products of their labor. Leading a research team can be in some ways be like managing a small organization. Like any organization, problems relating to communication and supervision can occur in scientific research. Indeed, many of the problems related to misconduct in science often boil down to poor communication and supervision (Broad and Wade 1982 [1993]; LaFollette 1992; National Academy of Sciences 1992).

In any research project, different people need to be held accountable for different parts of the project as well as the whole project itself. Accountability is often confused with responsibility, but we distinguish between these two concepts (Davis 1995a). A person is responsible for an action if he or she deserved to be praised or blamed for the action. A person is accountable for an action if he or she is obligated to give an account (or justification) of the action and bear the consequences of the action. For example, if a 10-year-old boy breaks a neighbor's window with a rock, he would be responsible, but his parents would be held accountable, because they would be obligated to apologize to the neighbor for his actions and to pay for repairing the window.

In a large research project with many collaborators, different people may be held accountable for the project as a whole or for its various parts. A person who was not responsible for some aspect of the project, such as recording data, may still be held accountable for the project as a whole. For example, in the stem cell fabrication case discussed in chapter 2, the U.S. collaborator on the South Korean team, Schatten, was not responsible for fabricating data but he was responsible for his role in the research and could be held accountable for failing to pay closer attention to what his colleagues were doing. Clearly, accountability and responsibility are both essential in research, but it is also important to keep these notions distinct. We will return to the topic of accountability again in chapter 6 when we discuss authorship.

International collaborations can lead to various ethical problems and concerns because different members of the research team may have different understandings of research norms, procedures, and traditions, and they may have different cultural, educational, legal, and political backgrounds (Anderson and Steneck 2012; National Academy of Sciences 2011). For example, collaborators from different countries may have different ideas concerning authorship that could lead to disputes about whether certain individuals should or should not be named as authors on a paper. Some collaborators on a project may come from a country that practices censorship, which may limit their ability to freely express their political, social, or economic opinions. As a result of differing legal standards, a new invention or discovery may be patentable in one country but not another. A method of consenting human research subjects, such as allowing a husband to consent for his competent, adult wife, may be culturally appropriate in one country but not another. The Singapore Statement on research integrity, mentioned in chapter 1, can help provide some guidance for international collaborations (Resnik and Shamoo 2011). Wahlberg et al. (2013) studied the China and South Korea collaboration. The authors suggest that any future collaboration should pay close attention to accountability, clarity, and ethical capacity.

RECOMMENDATIONS FOR RESEARCH COLLABORATION

To help deal with ethical problems and issues arising during collaboration, we recommend that collaborators discuss important research issues before and during their collaborative work:

1. Extent of the collaboration: How much of a commitment of time, effort, and money is involved in the collaboration?
2. Roles and responsibilities: What is the role of each collaborator? Who is responsible for different parts of the collaboration?
3. Data management: Who will have access to data? How will records be kept, stored, secured, analyzed? How will data be shared? Will any data be confidential? Will any data be placed on public websites?
4. Materials: Who will have access to research materials? How will these be stored and shared?
5. Intellectual property: Will a patent application be submitted? Who will have patent rights? Copyrights?
6. Funding: How will the project be funded? Who will apply for funding?

7. Conflicts of interest: Are there any financial or other interests affecting the research that collaborators should know about?
8. Deadlines: Are there any institutional, funding, or other deadlines relevant to the project?
9. Authorship: On what basis will authorship be decided? Who will be an author? Who will receive acknowledgment?
10. Publication: Will the research be published? When will publication take place? Where will results be published? Who will write the first draft of the paper? Who will be the corresponding author? Will presentations be made at any scientific meetings?
11. Media relations: Is the research likely to generate media interest? Is there a plan for discussing research results with the media or the public?
12. Regulations: Which regulations, laws, or institutional policies pertain to the project? How will conflicts of rules be settled?
13. Oversight: Are there any committees, such as institutional review boards, animal care and use committees, or biosafety committees, in charge of overseeing the research? Do any submissions need to be made to these committees? Who will make these submissions?
14. Closure: What will bring the collaboration to a formal end?

Some researchers deal with these issues by signing agreements that formalize the terms and conditions of the collaboration. Collaboration agreements can play an important role in helping researchers avoid misunderstandings and disputes. Formal agreements can be very useful in large, complex collaborations, but they are often not necessary in smaller ones. Many researchers prefer a verbal understanding or an email exchange to a contract. Moreover, even when researchers have signed a formal agreement they will need to continue discussing issues related to the collaboration, because the direction of the project may shift over time, responsibilities may change, and so on. Collaborative research raises a number of different ethical issues that we cover in other chapters in this book, such as authorship, intellectual property, and conflict of interest. Below we will focus on ethical issues pertaining to collaborations with industry.

ACADEMIC–INDUSTRY COLLABORATIONS

To better understand academic–industry collaborations, it will be useful to briefly review the history of industry involvement in scientific research.

The development of the steam engine is an early example of a highly successful collaboration between science and industry. During the 17th and 18th centuries, thermodynamics emerged as an important science, as scientists sought to understand how heat can be generated, stored, transferred, and used. Thomas Newcomen, Thomas Savery, and other scientists had worked on different versions of a steam engine. James Watt (1736–1819), a mechanical engineer at the University of Glasgow, improved the efficiency of the engine and obtained a patent on his invention in 1769 from the British government. Watt collaborated with the entrepreneurs John Roebuck and Matthew Boulton. Roebuck made two-thirds of the initial investment required to develop the steam engine but went bankrupt. Boulton bought Roebuck's share of the patent and helped to market this new product. Watt's steam engine was initially most useful in draining mines but was later used for machinery in factories. Watt and Boulton made a considerable sum from the steam engine, which was the product of scientific ingenuity and private investment and marketing (Burke 1995).

The modern industrial laboratory was developed in mid-19th-century Germany, when the dye industry hired chemists to produce synthetic dyes, such as aniline red, blue, purple, and black. Synthetic dyes invented by August Hofmann (1818–1982), William Perkin (1838–1907), and other chemists helped to fuel the industry. The development of the petroleum industry in the 19th century, as exemplified by the contributions of George Bissell (1821–1884) and Benjamin Silliman (1779–1864), followed a similar pattern. Business leaders began to realize the economic value of using scientific methods and concepts to solve technical and practical problems (Dickson 1988).

An important marriage between science and private industry began in the 1920s at the University of Wisconsin, when Professor Henry Steenbock (1886–1967) discovered that he could activate vitamin D by irradiating food. He patented his discovery, hoping to benefit his own university and ensure quality of the manufacturing process (Bowie 1994). The Board of Regents of the University of Wisconsin rejected Dr. Steenbock's offer to share in the profits of the invention, because they believed that the results of academic research should be made freely available to other scientists and the public. A group headed by some of the school's alumni started a nonprofit foundation, the Wisconsin Alumni Research Foundation (WARF), to provide additional funding for research and development (R&D). WARF was responsible for thousands of patent disclosures and hundreds of license agreements, and it had an income of millions of dollars (Bowie 1994). The foundation gave 15% of invention royalties to the inventor and 85% to the foundation in order to disburse research grants to university faculties. Although WARF was formally not part of the University of Wisconsin, it was for all practical purposes a part of the university, because university officials controlled the foundation, and its functions commingled with university functions. To make money, WARF attempted to obtain monopolistic control over vitamin D synthesis and negotiated and enforced narrow license agreements that prevented poor people from having access to vitamin D. For example, WARF claimed that its patent applied to vitamin D produced by sunlight, and WARF refused to license other companies to use its vitamin D irradiation process to develop other food products, such as oleomargarine. In the early 1940s, the courts ruled that the vitamin D made by the sun is not patentable. WARF later surrendered the vitamin D patent as well as the oleomargarine production patent (Bowie 1994).

Before World War II, the U.S. government did not invest heavily in research. Indeed, in the 1930s Bell Laboratories conducted more basic research than any university (Dickson 1988). During the war, the government began funding large-scale research programs, such as the Manhattan Project and the development of radar, jet airplanes, and computers. After World War II, it became clear to many people involved in government and in science policy that science and technology helped the Allies win the war and that continued investment in R&D would be a key pillar in national security and defense (Dickson 1988; Guston 2000). Federal investments in R&D grew from less than $1 billion in 1947 (or less than 0.3% of the gross national product) to $3.45 billion in 1957 (or 0.8% of the gross national product). A crucial turning point occurred in 1957, when the Soviet Union launched Sputnik, convincing many politicians that America was in grave danger of losing its scientific and technological edge over the Russians. From that period onward, federal funding of R&D grew steadily at 5–10% a year, and the government made more extensive use of scientific advisers. Federal support of R&D climbed to $26 billion in 1965, then leveled off from 1966 through 1976, and then climbed again to $40 billion in 1985 (Dickson 1988). During this period, the federal government became the leading sponsor of R&D in the United States, but this pattern changed in the 1980s, as private industry increased its investments in R&D. In 1980, private industry and the federal government each sponsored about 48% of research, but the percentage has shifted, and private industry is now once again the leading sponsor of R&D (American Association for the Advancement of Science 2013; Jaffe 1996; Resnik 2007). In 2012, industry sponsored 61.8% of all U.S. R&D, followed by the federal government (31%), universities (2.9%), and other governmental agencies and nonprofits (4.3%) (American Association for the Advancement of Science 2013; see table 5.1). The biggest supporter of federal research

Table 5.1. U.S. R&D FUNDING, 1954–2009 IN BILLIONS OF FY 2012 DOLLARS
(DATA FROM AMERICAN ASSOCIATION FOR THE ADVANCEMENT
OF SCIENCE 2013)

Year	Total	Federal	Industry	University	Nonprofits	Other Govt.
1954	39.7	21.9	16.8	0.3	0.4	0.3
1959	78.6	51.4	25.6	0.4	0.7	0.5
1964	113.0	75.5	34.8	0.7	1.2	0.8
1969	132.5	77.6	51.0	1.2	1.6	1.1
1974	131.1	67.9	58.5	1.5	1.9	1.3
1979	148.1	72.8	69.8	2.1	2.1	1.3
1984	197.8	89.9	101.0	2.9	2.6	1.4
1989	236,0	100.6	124.7	4.7	3.9	2.1
1994	244.4	87.8	143.3	5.7	5.3	2.3
1999	325.3	89.0	218.5	7.5	7.5	2.8
2004	361.7	109.6	228.7	9.5	10.5	3.4
2009	419.8	130.4	259.3	12.0	14.2	3.9

in 2012 was the Department of Defense ($68 billion), followed by the NIH ($28.4 billion), the National Aeronautics and Space Administration ($10.6 billion), and the NSF ($5.5 billion) (American Association for the Advancement of Science 2013; see table 5.2).

After World War II, universities and colleges began to proliferate and expand around the United States, fueled by an increasing number of students seeking higher education. The GI bill allowed soldiers returning from the war to obtain an education during the 1940s and 1950s, and the baby boom generation increased enrollments during the 1960s and 1970s. Throughout the United States, state governments helped fund expansion of the higher education system, and the federal government contributed by funding R&D. However, many state colleges and universities began facing financial difficulties in the 1970s due to increasing enrollments but insufficient or shrinking state funds (Bowie 1994). In response, these institutions sought to increase revenues from traditional sources, such as tuition, fees, and donations from alumni. Universities (and to a lesser extent colleges) also began to try to obtain additional revenues from sources related to R&D, such as grants, contracts, entrepreneurial activities, and intellectual property rights. These very same economic pressures exist today and help explain why universities have become increasingly involved in commercial activities (Bok 2003; Bowie 1994). At the same time, many academic leaders have sought to expand their institutions and enhance their economic strength and overall status by building ties to the

Table 5.2. U.S. GOVERNMENT FUNDING BY AGENCY IN 2012 IN BILLIONS OF FY 2012 DOLLARS (DATA FROM AMERICAN ASSOCIATION FOR THE ADVANCEMENT OF SCIENCE 2013)

Department of Defense	68,036
National Institutes of Health	28,458
National Aeronautics and Space Administration	10,566
Department of Energy	10,332
National Science Foundation	5,478
U.S. Department of Agriculture	2,177
Department of Commerce	1,359
Health and Human Services (non-NIH)	1,307
Veterans' Administration	1,131
Department of Transportation	857
Department of Interior	765
Department of Homeland Security	773
Environmental Protection Agency	532
Other	1,442
Total	133,213

private sector. Public and private institutions have both taken a strong interest since the 1970s in increasing revenues related to research activities.

The first major corporate investment in a university came in 1974, when Monsanto and Harvard Medical School entered into a 12-year joint venture, whereby Harvard received $23 million for research and Monsanto received all of the patent rights from the venture. Also, Monsanto received a first look at research results prior to publication. The university formed a committee to "protect academic freedom" and the "public good" (Culliton 1977) to review publication delays. The Harvard/Monsanto agreement was kept confidential until 1985, reflecting the university's discomfort at that time with its collaboration with industry.

In 1981, Edwin Whitehead, president of Technicon, a medical diagnostics company, contributed $120 million to establish the Whitehead Institute at MIT. The mission of the institute was to conduct biomedical research with potential applications in medicine and biotechnology. Whitehead himself retained control of faculty appointments at the institute. Faculty also held appointments at MIT. When the institute was formed, faculty at MIT objected to the commercial ties between the university and private corporations and the potential conflicts of interest (COIs). Despite these concerns, researchers at the institute have made important contributions to basic and applied biomedical science (Teitelman 1994).

In 1982, Monsanto negotiated an agreement with Washington University in St. Louis, Missouri. Monsanto gave $23.5 million to Washington University Medical School for research in the area of biotechnology. The agreement stipulated that royalties from patents and licenses would be split three ways among the university, the medical school, and the principal investigator's laboratory, but none would be paid directly to the investigator (Bowie 1994). It was claimed that excluding investigators from receiving royalties would avoid COIs among the faculty members, but this arrangement intensified the university's COI, because this would increase the university's financial interests. Monsanto received first rights of refusal to patents and the right to review publications. In 1994, the Scripps Research Institute entered a $20 million-per-year agreement with the Swiss pharmaceutical company Sandoz. Under this arrangement, Sandoz funded research conducted at Scripps in exchange for first-refusal rights to almost half of Scripp's research results (Beardsley 1994).

Another example of corporate investment into a university illustrates how the instability of the corporate model can affect academic life. In the mid-1980s, the Italian drug company FIDIA planned to give Georgetown University $3 million a year for 20 years (a total of $60 million) for research on neuroscience, to be housed in an institute within the university (Bowie 1994). The institute would primarily be devoted to basic research. FIDIA presumably would have received in return a strong connection to the best and brightest in this field, credibility, and the first rights of refusal on patents. Unfortunately in 1993, FIDIA filed for bankruptcy in Italy, and its contributions to Georgetown were reduced to a few million dollars. The university had to downscale its efforts to build its program and hire investigators.

During the 1980s, the United States passed two laws that greatly increased academic–industry collaborations and promoted the transfer of technology from the public to the private sector (Dickson 1988). The Bayh-Dole Act allowed researchers to assign inventions developed with federal funds to a university or business. Prior to the enactment of this law, inventions developed with the help of government funds had to be assigned to the federal government. Because the government grants only inclusive licenses on its inventions, private companies were not very interested in developing products covered by government patents, because private companies want exclusive licenses, which give them more control over the market. The Technology Transfer Act of 1986 allowed private companies and universities that plan to develop products with the support of government funds to sign Cooperative Research and Development Agreements (CRADAs) with the government. CRADAs specify how data and materials will be used and delineate intellectual property rights. As a result of this legislation, universities began more actively pursuing patents and formed technology transfer offices. They also began investing in professor-initiated startup companies to develop and license new technologies (Dreyfuss 2000). (We will discuss intellectual property in greater depth in chapter 8.)

The Bayh-Dole Act helped to promote the rapid growth of the pharmaceutical and biotechnology industries during the 1980s. In response to the rapid growth of the biotechnology and university–industry partnerships in the field, *Scientific American*, not known as a radical journal, published an article titled "Big-Time Biology" (Beardsley 1994). The article raised serious concerns regarding the rapid growth of biological sciences into an industry and how it is affecting university culture. An example to illustrate the modern complex relationship between private gains, universities, and researchers (Ready 1999) involves Dennis Selkoe, a researcher at Harvard Medical School who founded California-based Athena Neurosciences. The company is based on Selkoe's own research and has already earned him millions of dollars. Athena Neurosciences manufactures a controversial blood test for Alzheimer's disease. Without disclosing his relationship to the company, he was one of the endorsers of an NIH report for the new Alzheimer's disease test (National Institutes of Health 2008b). A Harvard panel concluded that he did not violate the university's COI policy, but he did agree to publish a disclosure statement in the same journal that published his original work. Apparently, Selkoe routinely wrote about Alzheimer's disease without reporting his affiliation with Athena. He also had a $50,000-per-year consulting contract and served on the board of directors. As another example, in 1997 the University of California at Irvine found out that their cancer researchers had failed to inform the U.S. Food and Drug Administration (FDA) about a side effect of a drug they had developed. These researchers had investments in the company that hoped to sell the drug (Ready 1999). The university shut down the laboratory.

The amount of university research funding from industry continues to rise, and universities themselves are engaged in building their own corporations by joint ventures and equity arrangements. In 1997, U.S. corporations spent $1.7 billion on university research (Shenk 1999). The survey data available from 1994 indicate that 90% of companies involved in life sciences had relationships with university research; 59% of those corporations supported university research directly, at about $1.5 billion, accounting for 11.7% of all R&D funding at universities (Blumenthal et al. 1996a). The survey further indicates that more than 60% of companies involved in university research received patents and products from the data generated. According to Dustira (1992), industry support to R&D in the biomedical field rose from 31% in 1980 to 46% in 1990, while at the same time the contributions of the NIH dropped from 40% to 32%.

The Association of University Technology Managers (AUTM), representing more than 300 university and research institutions, claimed that, in 1998 alone, 364 startup companies resulted from technology transfer activities within these institutions. The total number of startup companies since 1980 now exceeds 2,500 (Press and Washburn 2000). AUTM also claims that these technology transfer activities generated $34 billion in 1998, supporting 280,000 American jobs. If one looks only at the global impact of the biotechnology industry, it is clear that this industry is becoming a new force in the world's economy, supporting millions of high-paying jobs and promoting economic activity, investment, and development (Enriquez 1998). The political economy of the 21st century will undoubtedly be shaped by biotechnology (Carey et al. 1997).

Many academic researchers now have financial ties to private companies other than research funding. Krimsky et al. (1996) examined the financial disclosure statements from 1,105 authors whose publications appeared in 14 scientific and medical journals. They found that 34% of lead authors had financial interests related to their research, such as stock ownership, service on company advisory boards, consulting arrangements, or intellectual property. Because some researchers may not disclose their financial interests to journals, Krimsky's study may underreport the extent of financial interests in research. Also, many universities or university foundations own intellectual property rights and stock in companies that sponsor research on campus (Resnik and Shamoo 2002).

ETHICAL ISSUES PERTAINING TO ACADEMIC–INDUSTRY COLLABORATIONS

Collaborations between academia and industry can lead to many different ethical problems and concerns because academic values may conflict with corporate values and interests (Bowie 1994; Davis 1995b; Dickson 1988; Krimsky 2003; Resnik 2007; Rule and Shamoo 1997; Washburn 2006). Here are some examples:

- The main goals of academic institutions are to educate students; to advance human knowledge through research, scholarship, and creative activities; and to conduct public service. Private, for-profit corporations, on the other hand, aim to maximize profits and to produce goods and services. Nonprofit corporations also seek to produce goods and services, and they seek financial growth and stability.

- Academic institutions emphasize openness and the free exchange of data and ideas. Private corporations, on the other hand, often use secrecy to protect confidential business information and proprietary interests.
- Academic institutions emphasize academic freedom, free speech, and free thought. Private corporations, on the other hand, conduct research for specific purposes and may impose restrictions on public communications in order to protect the interests of the corporation.
- Academic institutions emphasize honesty and objectivity in research. Private corporations may endorse and promote these values in principle, but also as a means of complying with the law, for enhancing market share, or for ensuring the quality of goods and services.
- Academic institutions emphasize knowledge for its own sake; corporations emphasize the utilization of knowledge for the sake of profit or other practical goals.
- In capitalistic countries, private corporations compete with different companies on the free market. To compete on the market, corporations must produce high-quality goods and services; invest wisely in technology, equity, infrastructure, and R&D; and make effective use of human, financial, and technical resources. Academic institutions, on the other hand, have not traditionally competed with each other in the free market in the same way that corporations have. Many of these institutions are subsidized by government funds and have monopolistic control over local markets.
- Private corporations have obligations to stockholders, customers, employees, the government, and the community. Academic institutions have obligations to students, faculty, staff, alumni, the government, and the community.

SECRECY

One of the most important ethical concerns pertaining to academic–industry collaborations is industry's desire for secrecy. Academic scientists generally follow the principle of openness and are interested in publishing and sharing data and results. Companies treat data, methods, and results as proprietary information. They often refuse to share this information in order to gain or maintain a competitive advantage, protect intellectual property, avoid negative publicity that could affect their products, or cover up violations of laws or ethical guidelines (Rosenberg 1996). For example, for many years the tobacco industry claimed that smoking is not addictive, while secretly conducting research on the addictive properties of nicotine. In 1994, a congressional committee on commerce and industry held hearings on the tobacco industry. The committee heard testimony from two scientists who worked for Philip Morris: Victor DeNobel and Paul Mele. Although DeNobel and Mele had signed confidentiality agreements with Philip Morris that prohibited them from talking about their research or publishing data or results without prior approval, the committee released them from this agreement so they could testify. The scientists told the committee about their research on nicotine addiction and how the company was manipulating nicotine levels in order to make cigarettes more addictive (Hilts 1994; Resnik 2007).

There have been some well-known cases of companies taking action against scientists who have violated confidentiality agreements by publishing or disclosing data without their permission. In 1995, Boots Pharmaceuticals made Dr. Betty Dong, a pharmacologist at the University of California, San Francisco, withdraw a paper on drugs used to treat hypothyroidism that had been accepted for publication in the *Journal of the American Medical Association* (JAMA). Boots had funded her research in the hopes that she could show that its product, Synthroid, was superior to three generic alternatives. Synthroid is a brand name for levothyroxine, which was manufactured in 1987 by Flint Laboratories and later bought by Boots. The sale of Synthroid generated nearly $500 million dollars annually (Weiss 1997). To Boots's dismay, Dong's study showed that several generic drugs were just as safe and effective as Synthroid and also less expensive. In response, Boots tried to reinterpret her data and spent several years trying to discredit her research. Because Dong had signed an agreement with Boots not to publish the results without written consent from the company, Boots invoked this clause in the contract to prevent Dong from publishing the paper in the JAMA. The company threatened to sue Dong if she violated the agreement, so she withdrew her submission. In the meantime, the company published a more favorable article in another journal. Boots eventually relented, and two years later, the *New England Journal of Medicine* published Dong's findings (Altman 1997; Shenk 1999; Wadman 1996; Weiss 1997).

In the 1990s, Nancy Olivieri, a physician at the University of Toronto (UT) and Toronto General Hospital (TGH), conducted research on deferiprone, a drug used to treat thalassemia, a disease in which the body makes an abnormal form of hemoglobin. The manufacturer of the drug, Apotex, sponsored her research. Shortly after publishing an article in the *New England Journal of Medicine* showing that the drug is effective at treating thalassemia, Olivieri noticed that some of her patients had dangerous levels of iron in their livers, which could lead to a heart attack or death. Olivieri informed the TGH's research ethics board about the problem, so that research subjects could be warned about this risk. Apotex terminated the study and withdrew all the supplies of deferiprone from the hospital's pharmacy. The company also threatened to sue Olivieri if she discussed this problem with the drug with anyone. UT and TGH, which were negotiating a donation agreement with Apotex, denied there was a problem with the drug, tried to discredit her work, and attempted to have Olivieri dismissed from her position. Fortunately, some of Olivieri's colleagues intervened on her behalf, and she was cleared of all charges of wrongdoing (Resnik 2007). Universities have learned some important lessons from these episodes and most now carefully examine contracts with corporate research sponsors to ensure that scientists are allowed to publish data and results even if the company objects.

There is evidence that academic researchers also practice secrecy for various reasons, other than pressure from industry. Blumenthal et al. (1997) surveyed 2,167 life science faculty and found that 19.8% had delayed publication of an article for at least six months to protect a scientific lead, slow dissemination of undesired results, or deal with intellectual property disputes. Also, 8.9% said they refused to share research results in the last three years. Campbell et al. (2002) surveyed 1,849 geneticists and other life scientists and found that 47% had been denied a request to share data, information, or materials from published research in the last three years. Twenty-eight percent said they had been unable to confirm published research as a result of their inability to obtain data, and 12% said they had refused requests to share data from published research within the last three years.

As mentioned several times above, openness is vital to scientific progress and is one of the most important academic norms. Some fear secrecy will have broad effects on research and academic life (Bok 2003; Washburn 2006). A climate of secrecy can interfere with collegiality and have a detrimental impact on students, who may become involved in secret research that they cannot discuss with other students or professors. Some argue, however, that academic researchers may influence industry to promote greater openness in industry-sponsored research (Davis 1991). So far, it does not appear that the academic researchers are winning the battle for openness. Moreover, many researchers may not feel that they can criticize the industry's secrecy policies because they do not want to jeopardize their own funding or risk the wrath of university administrators. As noted in chapter 3, researchers have reasons to keep data and results confidential even if they are not receiving funds from industry. For example, they may want to protect their own intellectual property or their own interests in publication and priority. In any case, the conflict between secrecy and openness in research bears watching. We need to find ways to promote openness while protecting private interests. In discussing cases of how secrecy has prevailed to the detriment of research progress, Steven Rosenberg, at the time the chief of surgery at the National Cancer Institute, remarked, "This is the real dark side of science" (quoted in Press and Washburn 2000, p. 42).

SUPPRESSION OF DATA/RESULTS

Another issue is the suppression of data/results by industry. Private corporations are interested in publishing data and results that are likely to promote their economic interests. If publishing all of the data tends to erode support for its products, a company may decide to selectively publish data. For example, in 1999, the FDA approved Rofecoxib (Vioxx), a drug manufactured by Merck, as a treatment for arthritis and acute or chronic pain. One of the benefits of the drug is that caused fewer gastrointestinal problems than other nonsteroidal, anti-inflammatory pain medications. As early as 2001, scientists at Merck suspected that Vioxx might have adverse cardiovascular effects, such as heart attacks or strokes. The company sponsored a clinical trial named VIGOR to compare Vioxx to other pain medicines. The trial showed that Vioxx patients had five times the risk of a heart attack or stroke compared to patients taking Naproxen. Merck scientists said this was due to protective effects of the other drugs, but this interpretation is implausible. The VIGOR study was published in the *New England Journal of Medicine* in 2001, but it did not include all the cardiovascular risk data. Merck did not publish this data, although it submitted it to the FDA. The FDA does not disclose research submitted by companies because it treats it as confidential proprietary information. Eleven out of 12 VIGOR investigators had financial ties to Merck. In 2001, the FDA warned Merck that it had misrepresented Vioxx's safety profile, and in 2002 it issued a black box warning on the drug. Another study published in 2005 showed that Vioxx had twice the cardiovascular risk compared to placebo. The study was stopped in 2002 to protect patients taking

Vioxx from cardiovascular risks. Merck withdrew the drug in 2004 due to safety and legal liability concerns. Before it was withdrawn, Vioxx had $2.5 billion in annual sales. As many as 50,000 people had a heart attack or stroke while taking Vioxx, and thousands have sued Merck (Resnik 2007). The fact that tens of thousands of people had a heart attack or stroke while taking Vioxx does not prove that the drug caused all of these adverse events, however, because other causal factors, such as the patient's underlying illness, may have played an important role.

In 2004, a systematic review of antidepressant medications, serotonin reuptake inhibitors (SSRIs), found that some of these drugs increase the risk of suicide when prescribed to teens and children. The review included data that had not been previously published but was available through the Committee on Safety in Medicines, a U.K. government agency similar to the FDA. Parents, patients, researchers, and others accused the manufacturers of intentionally hiding these data from the public. Lawsuits followed against GlaxoSmithKline (Paxil), Pfizer (Zoloft), Eli Lilly (Prozac), and Wyeth (Effexor). New York Attorney General Eliot Spitzer sued Glaxo for fraud. In response to problems with data suppression, journals and the FDA now require registration of clinical trials on a public database, which allows investigators and physicians to obtain basic information about trials that are being conducted, including research design, methodology, endpoints, inclusion and exclusion criteria, and results. Clinical trial databases make data available, however (Laine et al 2007; Resnik 2007).

RESEARCH BIAS

Bias is a third key concern in academic collaborations with industry. For an example of research bias related to industry, consider the controversy over calcium-channel blockers. In 1995, Psaty et al. published results of a population-based case–control study of hypertensive patients and the risk of myocardial infarction associated with calcium-channel blockers versus beta-blockers versus diuretics. With 335 cases and 1,395 controls, they found that the risk of myocardial infarction was increased by 60% among users of calcium-channel blockers with or without diuretics. With 384 cases and 1,108 controls, they found that the use of calcium-channel blockers was associated with about a 60% increase in the risk for myocardial infarction compared with beta-blockers. Because the study was supported by federal funds, several pharmaceutical companies who manufacture beta-blockers requested all of the documents, including original data, under the Freedom of Information Act (Deyo et al. 1997). The companies hired several academic consultants to analyze the research, and the consultants wrote scathing critiques of the study. The companies even attempted to interfere with the publication of the article (Deyo et al. 1997).

Following the controversy of calcium-channel blockers, Stelfox et al. (1998) conducted a survey of literature published from March 1995 through September 1996 on the subject. They demonstrated a strong association between authors supporting the safety of calcium-channel blockers and their financial ties with pharmaceutical companies. Stelfox et al. classified the authors into three categories: critical, neutral, and supportive of the safety of calcium-channel blockers. They found that 96% of supportive authors had ties to the manufacturers, compared with 60% and 37% of neutral and critical authors, respectively. Earlier, Davidson (1986) obtained similar results that demonstrated a link between industry funding sources and favorable outcomes for new therapies.

Subsequent research has demonstrated a strong connection between sources of funding and research results (Angel 2004; Krimsky 2003; Resnik 2007). Cho and Bero (1996) and Cho (1998) found that the overwhelming percentage of articles with drug-company support (90%) favor the company's drug, compared with those without drug-company support (79%). Friedberg et al. (1999) reported that only 95% of new cancer drug studies sponsored by the company developing the new drug reached favorable conclusions, compared with 62% of studies on the same drugs sponsored by other organizations. In the dispute over second-hand smoke, articles sponsored by the tobacco industry indicated that second-hand smoke has no ill health effects, whereas studies sponsored by other organizations supported the opposite conclusion (Bero et al. 1994). Ridker and Torres (2006) studied 349 randomized clinical trials related to cardiovascular disease and found that 67% of trials funded by for-profit organizations, compared with 49% of trials funded by not-for-profit organizations, favored a new treatment over the standard of care. The authors also found that in medical device studies, 50% of trials with not-for-profit sponsors favored the new treatment compared with 82% of trials with for-profit sponsors. Bekelman et al. (2003) reviewed 37 papers on financial relationships and their influence on research and found that there is a statistically significant relationship between industry sponsorship and pro-industry results. A similar review by Sismondo (2008) of 19 articles also found a strong correlation between the source of funding and research outcomes.

A plausible explanation for these associations between sources of funding and research outcomes is that financial interests have affected the judgments and decisions made by companies and investigators (Agnew 2000; Resnik 2007). Companies may manipulate research outcomes through funding decisions. For example, a company could sponsor a number of studies on its product with the expectation that some of these studies will yield favorable results. If preliminary results indicate that a study is not likely to produce favorable results, the company could defund the study and not publish the data (Resnik and Elliott 2013). As noted above, a company may also decide to suppress data or results when a study is completed. Companies and investigators may also attempt to manipulate research designs or skew data analysis to obtain favorable outcomes (see our discussion of research design in chapter 3), or even fabricate or falsify data (see our discussion of misconduct in chapter 2) (Resnik and Elliott 2013). While research bias also occurs in the public sector, the economic incentives to conduct biased research are stronger in the private sector and therefore pose a hazard for university–industry relationships. Moreover, the penalties for bias, such as loss of funding or tenure or a damaged reputation, are potentially more damaging to academic researchers than to private researchers or corporations.

Although research bias is often deliberate, it may also operate at a subconscious level. People may not be aware of how financial or other interests are impacting their judgments and decisions. Studies have shown that financial or other interests can exert subconscious influences on thought processes (Katz et al. 2003). Additionally, even small interests can have an effect. People can be influenced by small gifts and small sums of money. Pharmaceutical companies give small gifts, such as pens, notepads, and free lunches, because they are trying to influence physicians' behaviors. Physicians often deny that they could be influenced by something as small as a pen, but studies indicate otherwise (Katz et al. 2003). We discuss financial interests in research in more detail in chapter 9.

ADVERSE IMPACTS ON BASIC RESEARCH

A fourth concern is that relationships with industry may steer academic institutions away from basic research toward applied research. Although many universities emphasize applied research as a part of their mission, basic research is an essential activity that should not be neglected in order to achieve short-term economic or practical goals (Bowie 1994; Brown 2000; Zolla-Parker 1994). Basic research helps scientists develop theories, concepts, laws, and models that have wide-ranging impacts even when they do not have immediate practical value. For example, engineers use basic principles of chemistry and physics every day in their work, and physicians depend on a basic knowledge of anatomy and physiology. Corporations can influence academic institutions by sponsoring research on campus; donating money for equipment, buildings, centers, and laboratories dedicated to a type of applied research (such as drug development or information technology); and giving money for special academic appointments (such as endowed chairs) with the understanding that they will have some input into these appointments. All of these activities can influence faculty interests in research and education at the university, which can have a trickle-down effect on graduate and postdoctoral students. As corporate funds continue to flow into a university, it may lose its commitment to basic research and knowledge for its own sake and may become more interested in applications and profits. The curriculum can also become transformed from one that emphasizes education in critical thinking and the liberal arts to one that emphasizes the training of students for careers in business, industry, or the professions. Talented faculty who might normally be involved in teaching may be encouraged to conduct research so the university can increase its revenues from contracts and grants (Brown 2000). Corporate dollars can transform an academic institution into a private laboratory and technical training school.

BENEFITS OF ACADEMIC–INDUSTRY COLLABORATIONS

Although academic–industry collaborations can lead to ethical issues and concerns, we do not think these problems can or should be solved by prohibiting these relationships, because academic–industry collaborations provide important benefits. Academic institutions benefit in several ways. First, private corporations provide universities with billions of dollars each year to support research and education. It is not likely that other sources of funding, such as the government, could compensate for the loss of private money. Second, the knowledge and expertise obtained from the private sector can be useful in generating ideas for research or education. For example, a professor teaching a course in bioengineering may consult with leaders in the private sector to help prepare her students for real-world problems. Knowledge about private industry's plans for new products can be especially useful in clinical research. For example, academic researchers can investigate the molecular mechanisms of a new drug being tested by a pharmaceutical company. Collaborations with industry play an important role in the NIH's Roadmap for Medical Research, which emphasizes the importance of translating basic discoveries made in the laboratory into medical applications (National Institutes of Health 2008b). Third, many institutions also appoint people from the private sector to boards and committees in order to obtain advice in preparing students for careers in business, industry, or the various professions. Industry leaders often provide key advice on research and education as consultants to colleges and universities.

Industry benefits from having access to top-notch university facilities, equipment, and researchers. Although many companies already hire their own excellent researchers and have state-of-the-art facilities and equipment, universities also still have economically valuable resources. While research has become increasingly privatized in the last two decades, many of the world's top researchers are still employed by universities, not by private companies. Corporations may also benefit from good publicity and visibility in their association with universities or colleges.

Society benefits from this private investment in academic institutions, which have helped to expand and support universities, have created higher-paying jobs, and have contributed to economic development. About eight million people in the United States are employed in R&D, and approximately 6% of the U.S. economy is directly related to R&D (Resnik 2007). Society also benefits from the goods and services produced by academic–industry collaborations, such as new drugs, medical devices, and information technologies. And society benefits from the increases in productivity resulting from academic–business collaborations. The increased productivity is evident from a survey indicating that industry-supported university research produced four times more patents per dollar than did industry research and increased the rate of the technology transfer from laboratory to useful products (Blumenthal et al. 1986, 1996a, 1996b). Francisco J. Ayala, a prominent biologist and once a member of a presidential committee on science and technology, stated that biotechnology is "contributing to the economic welfare of the nation, and it has by and large benefited academic progress. The benefits have far outstripped harms that may have occurred" (quoted in Beardsley 1994, p. 93).

MANAGING THE UNIVERSITY–INDUSTRY RELATIONSHIP

Although this chapter has discussed many negative aspects of the academic–industry relationship, we would like to temper this impression. As noted above, there are many benefits of the university–industry interface. Moreover, it is hard to imagine how the modern research enterprise could proceed without some type of collaboration between academia and industry. For the last few hundred years, ties between universities and private corporations have grown stronger as research has increased in its practical relevance, economic and commercial value, complexity, and cost. Changes in the financial and economic aspects of research have transformed universities from institutions that focus on education and basic research to institutions that also have commercial ties and interests and conduct applied research. Although it is important to preserve and promote values traditionally associated with academic institutions, it is not realistic to expect that we can return to an earlier era. Instead of romanticizing about the "good old days" or complaining about corruption within the current system, we should develop practical policies for ensuring that university–industry relationships benefit both parties as well as society (Resnik 2007).

Based on the discussion in this chapter as well as preceding and subsequent ones, we recommend the following guidelines for university–industry relationships (for further discussion, see Resnik 2007; Resnik and Shamoo 2002; Rule and Shamoo 1997):

1. Develop and implement policies for managing individual and institutional COIs (we discuss this at greater length in chapter 9).
2. Develop and implement policies pertaining to other areas of concern, such as misconduct (discussed in chapter 2), data management (chapter 3), and intellectual property (chapter 8).
3. Pay careful attention to contracts signed with private industry to ensure that companies are not allowed to suppress the publication of data or results and that academic investigators have access to all of the data, materials, and protocols they need to conduct research. Contracts should allow companies to review data and results prior to publication but not to prevent publication.
4. Be especially wary of involving students in secret research conducted for industry: Students enroll in universities for education and career advancement and should not be exploited as a cheap source of labor for commercial research. Because students should be allowed to discuss their work with their colleagues and teachers, no student master's or doctoral thesis should involve secret research. Some involvement in private research can help students learn and advance their careers, but great care should be taken in involving them in this work.
5. Use contracts and agreements to set the terms for university–industry collaborations, such as intellectual property rights, publication, sharing of data and resources, research oversight, auditing, and use of funds.
6. Maintain a strong commitment to basic research on campus through faculty appointments, curriculum development, and funding strategies.

QUESTIONS FOR DISCUSSION

1. What is scientific collaboration? Why is it important in science?
2. Have you been involved in collaborative work with researchers in other departments or institutions? Was this a positive experience?
3. What are some of the challenges of international research collaborations?
4. Would you add anything else to our list of recommendations for collaboration?
5. What are some of the ethical challenges involved in academic–industry collaborations?
6. Have you taken part in research that involved collaborations with industry? Were these experiences acceptable to you?
7. Can you give some examples of the benefits of academic–industry collaborations that are not listed in this chapter?
8. What proposals do you have for managing university–industry relationships?

CASES FOR DISCUSSION

CASE 1

Two research teams, one led by Dr. Weaver and the other led by Dr. Klein, have been attempting to identify a pathogen they believe is responsible for a disease with symptoms that include chronic fatigue, joint pain, dizziness, muscle weakness, and periodic fevers. They have presented papers at scientific meetings on their preliminary research but neither team has made a breakthrough yet. Both teams are aware of each other's work and have been competing for priority. Dr. Weaver emails Dr. Klein and asks him if the two teams could collaborate in order to advance this research. The teams would both share biological samples and data as well as credit for the discovery of the pathogen if they are able to isolate and identify it. Dr. Klein is intrigued by this offer but he doesn't want to share credit with Dr. Weaver.

- Should the two teams collaborate on this research project? What factors should be considered in making this decision?
- What sorts of issues should the teams discuss prior to collaborating?
- Should they draft a collaboration agreement?

CASE 2

Dr. Chen has been studying diabetes in laboratory mice. She recently attended a scientific meeting and learned about a new genetically engineered diabetic mouse developed by Dr. Wu using NIH funds. The mice are more prone to developing type II diabetes than normal mice. After the meeting, Dr. Chen emails Dr. Wu and asks him if he could provide her with some of his transgenic mice for a study on the impact of an endocrine-disrupting compound on diabetes progression. Dr. Wu says that he is interested in sharing the mice but wants to learn more about the proposed study. He also asks Dr. Chen for a copy of her curriculum vitae. Dr. Wu notices that Dr. Chen has a good publication record, although most of her publications have appeared in lower and middle-tier journals. Dr. Wu agrees to send the mice on the condition that he will be named in the acknowledgments section of any papers using the mice in research. Dr. Chen agrees to this condition and Dr. Wu sends the mice. After six months of work, Dr. Chen has some interesting results. She makes a presentation at a scientific meeting and meets a section editor for the *New England Journal of Medicine*, who encourages her to submit her work for a special issue on diabetes. She is very excited about the prospect of publishing her work in a top-tier journal and she emails Dr. Wu again to thank him for his help. Dr. Wu asks her to send a copy of the paper she is planning to submit, and Dr. Chen sends him a draft to read. Dr. Wu is impressed with the work and asks to be named as a coauthor on the paper. Dr. Wu was not interested in authorship when he thought the paper would only appear in a lower-tier journal but he has changed his mind. Dr. Chen does not want to grant this request because she thinks he has not done enough work to merit authorship.

- What should Dr. Chen do?
- Should Dr. Wu be a coauthor on this paper? What else should he do to merit authorship?
- How could they have avoided this misunderstanding?

CASE 3

A speech pathology researcher at a large university has developed and patented a device to help control stuttering. He transferred the patent to the university and will receive 50% of royalties. The researcher formed a startup company, with university funds, to manufacture and market the device. The university will license the device to the company. The researcher is the vice president for research at the company and owns a 20% equity interest in the company. The university's private foundation owns a 30% interest in the company and private investors own the rest. The researcher is planning to conduct a clinical trial on campus to test the device.

- Do you have any concerns about this arrangement?
- Do you have any recommendations for managing or overseeing this arrangement?

CASE 4

Parents of a child with a rare, devastating genetic disease contacted a medical geneticist at a large public university about conducting research on the disease and possibly developing a genetic test. The researcher agreed to help them. The parents established a private foundation to help fund his research and recruited other parents to provide biological samples for the study. The researcher also obtained a grant from the NIH, which ended up funding 65% of the research. The researcher was able to identify a recessive genetic mutation responsible for the disease and developed a genetic test for it. Parents could use the test to make reproductive choices. Unbeknownst to the parents, the researcher patented the genetic test and transferred the patent to his university. The researcher also formed a private company to develop and market the test. The university, company, and NIH had signed a CRADA for developing the test. The company began charging a $1,500 fee for the test and did not license other laboratories or institutions to conduct the test. The parents were very upset by this development since they had hoped that the test would be easily accessible to parents who thought they might carry the gene. The parents sued the university, the company, and the researcher. After the lawsuit was initiated, the company offered to reduce the price of the test to $500, but this did not satisfy the parents, who continued with their legal action.

- Did the researcher or university act unethically?
- How could a better outcome have been obtained?
- What do you think would have been an ideal arrangement for developing this test?

CASE 5

A large pharmaceutical company awards a $6 million contract for three years to a researcher at a university medical center to conduct a clinical trial of its new diabetes drug. The company's proposed conditions are as follows:

1. All publications and public communications concerning the research must be approved by the company.
2. The company may delay publication of data or results for up to six months.
3. The company has first rights of patenting and licensing of any discoveries.

4. The researcher will serve on the company's scientific advisory board.
   - What is the role of the university in this arrangement?
   - Should the university accept the terms as they are offered or make a counteroffer? What should the counteroffer be?

CASE 6

An industrial plant near a university is planning to give $25 million to endow a Center for Environmental Science (CES). The gift includes the following conditions:

1. The CES will have a governing board consisting of 10 members of academia and industry; five members of the board will be named by the company.
2. The governing board will have the power to appoint a director of the CES and will also approve all faculty appointments to the CES.
3. The governing board will also have the power to approve course development activities, conferences, guest lectureships, and research projects sponsored by the CES.
   - Do you see any problems with this arrangement?
   - Should the university accept this gift?

CHAPTER 6
Authorship

Authorship is a prized commodity in science, because most of the tangible rewards of academic research are based on a person's publication record. Since the 20th century, the number of authors per scientific paper has been steadily increasing. Authorship disputes are also becoming much more common. This chapter explores some of the ethical issues and problems involving authorship and describes some criteria and guidelines for authorship.

An author has been traditionally defined as someone who creates a literary text, such as a novel, a history book, or a newspaper editorial. In science, an author is someone who creates a scientific text, such as an article published in a journal, a poster presented at a meeting, a chapter in a book, or a monograph. For many years, determining authorship was a fairly simply process in science because most scientific works had, at most, a few authors, who were all involved in conducting the research and writing the text. For example, *The Sceptical Chemist* (by Robert Boyle), *Philosophiae Naturalis Principia Mathematica* (Isaac Newton), *The Origin of Species* (Charles Darwin), and *Civilization and Its Discontents* (Sigmund Freud) were all single-author works.

Determining authorship became more complicated in the second half of the 20th century, as scientists began working in larger research groups and collaborating with other researchers in other institutes and disciplines (LaFollette 1992; McLellin 1995). Collaboration increased because research problems became more complex, demanding, expensive, and interdisciplinary. A division of labor arose as people worked on different parts of research projects. Instead of a single person designing, conducting, and analyzing an experiment and writing up results, many people became involved in different parts of the process. Today, a coauthor listed on a paper may not be responsible for even writing the paper, but may simply read the final draft of the manuscript.

The number of authors on scientific papers has steadily increased. The average number of authors for all fields rose from 1.67 in 1960 to 2.58 in 1980 (Broad 1981). In biomedical research, the average number of authors per paper increased from 1.7 in 1960 to 3.1 in 1990 (Drenth 1996). In the 1980s, the average number of authors per article in medical research rose to 4.5 (LaFollette 1992). It is not at all uncommon for a paper published in biomedicine to have five or more authors, and multiple authorship is now the norm (Rennie et al. 1997). In physics, some papers may have several hundred authors. In the life sciences, 37 papers were published in 1994 that had more than 100 authors, compared with almost none with 100 authors in the 1980s (Regaldo 1995). Although some disciplines in the humanities and the social sciences have bucked this trend, multiple authorship is also becoming more common in humanistic disciplines, such as bioethics (Borry et al. 2006).

This rise in the number of authors per paper has been accompanied by a rise in disputes about authorship (Wilcox 1998). Such disputes were the most common ethical problem reported by respondents to a survey of researchers at the National Institute of Environmental Health Sciences: 35.6% of respondents had experienced or knew about authorship disputes, and 26.7% had experienced or knew about undeserved authorship (Resnik 2006). A survey of 3,247 scientists conducted by Martinson et al. (2005) found that 10% of respondents admitted to inappropriately assigning authorship in the past three years. Of the misconduct allegations that the Office of Research Integrity (ORI) received in 1997, 27% were authorship disputes that had been improperly interpreted as misconduct (Scheetz 1999). In many of these cases, a person who did not receive authorship on a paper claimed that he had been the victim of plagiarism.

The reason for authorship disputes in science is not hard to understand: People fight about what they care about, and scientists generally care about authorship. Most of the tangible rewards in academic science, such as tenure and promotion, contracts and grants, honors and prizes, and status and prestige, are based on a person's publication record. Scientists are rewarded for the quality and quantity of the publications. Scientific databases, such as the Science Citation Index, keep track of author citation records, which measure how many times an author is cited by other authors. One can increase one's citation score by publishing high-impact papers and by publishing many papers. The phrases "publish or perish" and "authorship is a meal ticket" reflect the grim realities of academic life (LaFollette 1992). Many believe that this emphasis on quantity has undermined the quality of published work (Chubin and Hackett 1990). Publication is important to a lesser extent in the private sector. Private corporations may not care whether their employees publish, and they may even discourage publication. However, one's publication record may still be important in obtaining employment in the private sector.

UNETHICAL PRACTICES RELATED TO AUTHORSHIP AND CITATION

Researchers, ethicists, and scholars have documented a number of ethically questionable practices related to authorship:

- Honorary authorship: A person is listed as an author on a paper even though he or she has not made a significant contribution to the research. One study found that 17.6% of publications in six top medical journals had authors that did not fulfill the journal's authorship criteria (Wislar et al. 2011). There are several reasons why people may be authors in name only. Sometimes a person is listed as an author as a sign of respect or gratitude. Some laboratory directors have insisted that they be listed as an author on every publication that their lab produces (Jones 2000). Sometimes individuals are named as authors as a personal or professional favor. Some researchers have even developed reciprocal arrangements for listing each other as coauthors (LaFollette 1992). Finally, a person with a high degree of prestige or notoriety may be listed as an author in order to give the publication more visibility or impact (LaFollette 1992).
- Ghost authorship: A person is not listed as an author, even though he or she has made a significant contribution, in order to hide the paper's financial connections. Some pharmaceutical companies use ghostwriters to write a manuscript, who may not be involved in planning or conducting the research. In extreme cases, even the researchers are ghosts. Pharmaceutical companies have asked physicians to be listed as honorary authors on papers in order to give the papers prestige or status. These "authors" have been involved in no aspects of planning or conducting the research or writing up the results—they are authors in name only (Flanagin et al. 1998; Jones 2000). Ghost authorship is common in industry-sponsored clinical trials. One study found that 75% of industry-initiated clinical trials had ghost authors (Gøtzsche et al. 2007). Another study found that 7.9% of articles published in six top medical journals had ghost authors (Wislar et al. 2011).

In addition to the problems noted above, many people have been denied authorship unfairly. There are several reasons why someone might prevent someone else from receiving credit for intellectual or other contributions. First, the quest for priority has been and always will be a key aspect of research: Scientists want to be the first to discover a new phenomenon or propose a new theory (Merton 1973). Many bitter battles in science have been fought over issues of priority, including the international incident over the discovery of the HIV virus involving Robert Gallo and Luc Montagnier (described in chapter 2). A researcher may be tempted to not list someone as an author or not acknowledge that person's contribution in order to achieve an edge in the contest for priority. Second, concerns about priority and credit play a key role in intellectual property rights, such as patents. To solidify their intellectual property claims, researchers may attempt to deny authorship as well as inventorship to people who have contributed to a new discovery or invention. Although we focus on authorship in this chapter, much of our discussion also applies to questions about inventions and patents. Just as a person may be listed as a coauthor on a publication, he or she could also be listed as a co-inventor on a patent application (Dreyfuss 2000). Third, although multiple authorship is becoming the norm, researchers may want to hold the number of authors to a minimum to prevent authorship from being diluted. For instance, many journals cite papers with more than two or three authors as "[first author's name] et al." If a paper has three authors, the second and third authors may have a strong interest in not allowing someone to be added as a fourth author, in order to keep their names visible.

Extreme examples of failing to grant proper authorship or credit include the following:

- Plagiarism: A person is not given proper credit or acknowledgment for his or her work. According to the standard definition, plagiarism is wrongfully representing someone else's ideas, words, images, inventions, or other creative works as one's own. Plagiarism has been and continues to be a common issue in misconduct cases investigated by the U.S. government (Steneck 1999). There are many different forms of plagiarism, not all of which are as extreme as copying a paper word for word (Goode 1993; LaFollette 1992). Although most cases of leaving someone's name off a manuscript amount to authorship disputes rather than plagiarism, scientists should be mindful that they can face a charge of plagiarism if they do not give credit or acknowledgment to people who make original and meaningful contributions to the research.

- Self-plagiarism: Researchers fail to acknowledge, disclose, or obtain permission to use material from their own previous publications. Although self-plagiarism is not as serious an ethical transgression as plagiarism, it is still an ethical problem. Although it does not involve the theft of someone else's ideas or creative works, self-plagiarism is a poor citation practice that may also involve copyright violations (LaFollette 1992). The best practice is to provide proper reference and obtain permissions (if necessary) when reusing one's previously published work.
- Citation amnesia: A person fails to cite important works in the field. As noted in chapter 3, conducting a thorough and fair review of the background literature is one of the most important steps of scientific research. It also can be useful in ensuring that people who make important contributions to the literature receive proper recognition. For many, citation is almost as important as authorship. Those who fail to cite important contributors present the reader with inaccurate and biased information and unfairly deny others the rewards of research and scholarship (LaFollette 1992; Resnik 1998a).

AUTHORSHIP CRITERIA

In light of these problems related to credit allocation in science, it is imperative that researchers discuss issues related to authorship and establish standards for authorship. We believe that authorship standards should be based on three key values: accountability, fairness, and honesty. Accountability is a key concern in authorship because it is often important to know who has made specific contributions to a project, in case questions arise. Scientists who read a paper may want to try to replicate experiments, re-analyze data, or build on the research. In some cases, a paper may come under suspicion if the data are not reproducible or errors or other problems are discovered. If a scientist has trouble reproducing a result, it is important to know who conducted or designed the relevant experiments. In many research misconduct cases, authors on the paper have tried to avoid culpability by claiming that it was someone else's fault and that they knew nothing about the problem. They have also pleaded ignorance when a paper has come under suspicion, claiming that they had nothing to do with the alleged misconduct (LaFollette 1992). This is an unacceptable situation. Authors on scientific papers need to be able to be held accountable for their part in the work and the paper as a whole (Resnik 1997).

Fairness is another key concern because people should receive appropriate recognition for their work. Credit should be given where it is due and only where it is due. It is unfair to leave someone off the authorship list for a paper who has made a significant contribution or to include someone on the list who has not made a significant contribution (Resnik 1997).

Honesty is also a key concern because it is dishonest to name someone as an author on a paper who has not made a significant contribution. Likewise, it is dishonest to not name someone as an author who has made a significant contribution. Plagiarism and ghost authorship both involve dishonesty.

In the past, many journals have used as the standard for authorship whether the person has made a "significant contribution" to the project through planning, conceptualization, or research design; providing, collecting, or recording data; analyzing or interpreting data; or writing and editing the manuscript (LaFollette 1992). We believe that this popular approach is vague and may not promote accountability, fairness, or honesty, because it would allow a person to be listed as an author as a result of planning a project, even though this person might not know how the project was actually implemented. Likewise, a person may become involved in the project at the very end and not have an important role in planning the study.

We recommend that an individual should be listed as an author on a paper only if he or she (a) has made a significant intellectual contribution to the paper; (b) has read and reviewed the paper; and (c) is prepared to publicly defend the paper (as a whole) and explain his or her role in the research (Rennie et al. 1997; Resnik 1997). People may contribute to a project in important ways without being considered an author. Important contributors can be recognized in an acknowledgments section of a publication.

Our approach is very similar to the one adopted by the International Committee of Medical Journal Editors (ICMJE):

The ICMJE recommends that authorship be based on the following 4 criteria:

Substantial contributions to the conception or design of the work; or the acquisition, analysis, or interpretation of data for the work; AND

Drafting the work or revising it critically for important intellectual content; AND

Final approval of the version to be published; AND

Agreement to be accountable for all aspects of the work in ensuring that questions related to the accuracy or integrity of any part of the work are appropriately investigated and resolved. (International Committee of Medical Journal Editors 2013)

Although we believe that the ICMJE's criteria provide useful guidelines for determining authorship on many types of scientific papers, they may not be very helpful for determining authorship on publications that do not involve the collection of data. Many papers in the humanities and social sciences, as well as theoretical papers from hard sciences, do not present any original data. These papers may review the published literature; present or interpret theories and ideas; analyze arguments, concepts, and policies; or prove mathematical theorems or develop mathematical models. In papers like these, no one may be able to claim that they designed experiments, analyzed data, and so on (Resnik and Master 2013b). When research does not involve the collection of original data, we would recommend that authorship be based on a significant intellectual contribution to the activities involved in research, such as literature review, argument analysis, mathematical modeling, and so on.

To foster accountability in authorship, we further recommend that a research article have a section at the end describing the different roles and responsibilities of the authors and contributors to a project (Rennie et al. 1997; Resnik 1997). For example, an article might say, "Joe Smith was involved in conception, data interpretation, and drafting the manuscript; Karen Shaw helped with data collection and analysis, and editing the manuscript," and so on. An increasing number of journals now require that articles submitted for publication include this type of information, and some require authors to sign a statement affirming their specific contributions to the paper. Accountability can sometimes be difficult to pin down, because it is difficult to give a complete accounting of every piece of data when a large number of researchers from different disciplines collaborate on a project. For example, when using some technologies in research, such as X-ray crystallography, different collaborators may work with only a part of the data, and no single person may be responsible for all the data. Whole-genome analysis studies and multisite clinical trials present similar concerns. A precise description of each author's contribution may help to resolve potential problems such as these.

To make sense of authorship issues, it is important to carefully describe the different roles and responsibilities in research, because these will determine who should or should not be listed as an author or as a contributor, as well as the order of authors' names. Although research roles vary considerably across disciplines and even among different projects within the same discipline, people may contribute to a project in these basic ways:

1. Defining problems
2. Proposing hypotheses
3. Summarizing the background literature
4. Designing experiments
5. Developing the methodology
6. Collecting and recording data
7. Providing data
8. Managing data
9. Analyzing data
10. Interpreting results
11. Assisting in technical aspects of research
12. Assisting in logistical aspects of research
13. Applying for a grant/obtaining funding
15. Analyzing arguments, concepts, policies, and so on
16. Proving mathematical theorems or developing mathematical models
17. Presenting or interpreting theories or ideas
18. Drafting and editing manuscripts

One person may be involved in many of these different aspects of research, although different people may perform different roles. For instance, in academic research, the principal investigator (PI) is usually a professor who proposes the hypothesis, designs the experiments, develops the methodology, writes the grant proposal, and writes the manuscript. However, the PI may use undergraduate or graduate students or postdoctoral fellows to collect and record data, review the literature, or edit the manuscript. Students and fellows may also provide assistance in other aspects of research as well. Lab assistants (or technicians) may assist with technical aspects of the experiments and are not usually listed as authors. However, lab assistants could be listed as authors if they make an important intellectual contribution in addition to their technical expertise (Resnik 1997). Statisticians may help analyze data and interpret results. Other senior colleagues, such as the laboratory director, may also help the PI by providing data from the research or by helping with experimental design, methodology, or grant writing. The laboratory director is usually a senior researcher who may or may not be the PI. The director may supervise many different projects and many different PIs.

In an academic setting, the PI is supposed to be in charge of the research, but other lines of authority and responsibility are sometimes defined (Rose and Fischer 1995). In private industry, the lines of authority and responsibility are usually more clearly defined, because private industry works on a business model rather than an academic model (Bowie 1994). The laboratory director is in charge of many different projects and many different investigators, who may be assisted by technicians or other scientists. The laboratory director reports to the company's upper-level managers. Decisions about which projects to pursue are based on market considerations, not on intellectual considerations. In the military, lines of authority and responsibility are delineated even more strictly, and decisions about funding are based on strategic considerations (Dickson 1988).

ADDITIONAL GUIDANCE ON AUTHORSHIP

In addition to the fundamental guidance on authorship discussed above, we propose the following guidelines to promote accountability, trust, and fairness in authorship:

1. To help prevent authorship disputes and misunderstanding, researchers should discuss authorship issues at the outset of the project and revisit them as necessary. For example, if the project takes a different direction, then authorship attribution and order of names may need to be reconsidered.
2. For corporate authorship, at least one person should be listed as an author. Institutions, committees, associations, task forces, and so on are listed as the sole author for a growing number of publications. Although these types of collaborations are vital to research, they can raise serious problems with accountability if they do not identify one or more people who can defend the whole paper. If a publication lists only a corporate entity as an author, then reviewers, readers, and the lay public have no idea whom to hold accountable or responsible for the project (International Committee of Medical Journal Editors 2013).
3. The order of authors should also reflect the importance of each person's role in the paper. Every publication should have a person who is the accountable author—who bears the most responsibility for the article. In some disciplines, the accountable author is listed first, with each name that follows indicating a lessening level of responsibility. The corresponding author should be the person who is responsible for drafting the paper, submitting it for publication, and responding to comments from reviewers. The accountable author and the corresponding author

are usually the same person, but they need not be. Some writers (e.g., Diguisto 1994) have proposed quantitative methods for determining authorship order, but we do not find these methods especially useful, because judgments about importance are, in large part, value judgments and cannot be easily quantified (American Psychological Association 1992; Borenstein 2011).

4. Some papers state that two or more authors made equal contributions and may be designated as co-first authors or even co-last authors (Akhabue and Lautenbach 2010). While this practice may help quell some authorship disputes by dividing up first-author credit equally, we are skeptical of this practice because it is subject to abuse. Because researchers usually do many different activities on a project of varying importance, it will seldom be the case that individuals have actually made equal contributions. To claim that two individuals made an equal contribution to a paper so they can each list the publication as a first-author paper on a curriculum vitae, when they have not really made equal contributions, is dishonest and cynical.

5. In general, all articles that result from a graduate student's thesis project should list the student as the first author. In general, graduate students should not be assigned projects where there is very little chance of publication or where publication may be many years away. We include these recommendations to avoid some of the problems of exploitation of subordinates that unfortunately occur in research, which we discussed in chapter 4.

6. To the extent that it is possible, papers should clearly state the contributions of different authors and should acknowledge all contributors. This policy encourages both accountability and fairness in that it provides readers with some idea of who is most responsible for different aspects of the paper (*Nature* 1999). Some writers have argued that it is time to do away with the outmoded category of "author" in scientific research and replace it with a different system of credit allocation that simply details how different people have contributed to the project (Rennie et al. 1997; Resnik 1997). We are sympathetic to this proposal but also recognize the difficulty of overcoming long-standing traditions and institutional personnel policies that place a heavy emphasis on authorship.

7. Many of these guidelines also apply to the concept of inventorship. Inventors, like authors, receive credit for their work and can be held accountable. It is also important to promote accountability, trust, and fairness when collaborations result in an invention (Dreyfuss 2000).

QUESTIONS FOR DISCUSSION

1. Why is authorship an important topic in research ethics?
2. How does your laboratory or research group decide authorship issues?
3. Have you ever been an author on a paper? If so, was authorship handled properly?
4. Do you know of any cases in which someone was named as an author on a paper even though he or she did not make a significant contribution?
5. Do you know of any cases where someone was not named as an author on a paper even though he or she did make a significant contribution?
6. What can you do if you do not agree with the authorship on a paper?
7. Do you think it is fair for a scientist to insist that he or she be named as an author on every paper produced by his or her laboratory?
8. Do you have any criticism of our proposed criteria for determining authorship? What about the ICMJE criteria?
9. What do you think of the idea of stating that two people contributed equally to a research project? Do you think the idea of naming co-first authors makes sense?
10. What do you think of the idea of eliminating the authorship category in favor of a designation that describes research roles more precisely, such as "data collector," "data analyzer," and so forth?

CASES FOR DISCUSSION

CASE 1

A graduate student was studying at a university where his faculty mentor is also a full-time employee of the affiliated hospital. He and his mentor discovered some previously unknown adverse effects from a major environmental airborne toxin, and the media covered the story. The mentor then died suddenly of a heart attack. They had a manuscript already written and about to be submitted for publication in a prestigious journal. The chair of the department, who worked in a closely related area, became the new student's mentor. She took the manuscript and put her name as the senior author (last) and eliminated the name of the deceased. She had no involvement in the project prior to the death of the former mentor. The paper was published after minor revision.

- What should the student do?
- What should the mentor do?

CASE 2

Ms. Pedroia is a technician working in Dr. Wainwright's cell biology lab. Ms. Pedroia has isolated proteins for Dr. Wainwright in the past and has become very skilled at these techniques. Dr. Wainwright is working on a project on protein QP, which is thought to play a role in programmed cell death. Dr. Wainwright asks Ms. Pedroia to isolate protein QP, so they can study its role in programmed cell death. Ms. Pedroia performs the experiments and produces excellent work. Dr. Wainwright circulates a draft of a paper on the protein that includes data from experiments performed by Ms. Pedroia as well as data from two graduate students and a postdoctoral student. The paper lists the postdoctoral student as first author, followed by the graduate students, and then Dr. Wainwright. Ms. Pedroia is mentioned in the acknowledgments but not named as an author. Ms. Pedroia asks Dr. Wainwright if she can be listed as an author because she isolated the protein used in the study. Dr. Wainwright tells her, "You're just a technician performing technical work. You don't need to be listed as an author. The salary you receive should be reward enough."

- What do you think of Dr. Wainwright's attitude toward listing technicians as authors? Is this inappropriate or unethical? Do you know other scientists who take a similar attitude?
- Should Ms. Pedroia be listed as an author? What additional information do you need to make this determination?
- What can Ms. Pedroia do?

CASE 3

Dr. Thomas published a review article about recent developments in the psychology of moral reasoning and judgment. In the article, he mentioned his own work prominently but failed to mention the work of several other researchers who have made key contributions to the field. Dr. Thomas is clearly one of the most important researchers in the field, and he has done some important work. But he also has some long-running feuds with some of the other prominent researchers in the field, based in part on fundamental disagreements. In his review article, in several instances he cited his own work instead of giving proper credit to colleagues who had published their articles before his.

- Is this plagiarism?
- Is it unethical?

CASE 4

Drs. Clearheart and Wing are studying socioeconomic factors related to incarceration. They recently read a paper published by Drs. Langford and Sulu on the relationship between juvenile incarceration and the mother's age at birth. Clearheart and Wing believe that they may be able to incorporate the supporting data obtained by Langford and Sulu in their analysis, so they send them an email asking them to share the data used to support their publication. A note accompanying the publication said that supporting data were available upon request. Langford and Sulu agree to send Clearheart and Wing the supporting data, provided that Clearheart and Wing list them as authors on any publications that use the data. Dr. Wing is uncomfortable with agreeing to this request, because he believes that one should do more than just provide data to be an author. Dr. Clearheart wants to honor their request. "Our publication will be much stronger," he says, "if we incorporate their data into our analysis."

- What should they do?
- Is it ethical to name someone as an author just for providing data?
- Is it ethical to only share data in exchange for authorship?
- Does the source of funding for Langford and Sulu make a difference to these issues?

CASE 5

Three economists, Stroud, Jones, and Wicket, published a paper describing a mathematical model for representing collective bargaining. The following year, Stroud and two other authors, Weinberg and Smith, published a paper that applied the model to a collective bargaining dispute between a teachers' union and a school district. The paper included two paragraphs that were identical, word for word, to two paragraphs in the paper published by Stroud, Jones, and Wicket. The two paragraphs in the paper by Stroud, Weinberg, and Smith did not mention or even cite the paper by Stroud, Jones, and Wicket.

- Is this unethical?
- Is this plagiarism? Self-plagiarism? A possible copyright violation?

CASE 6

Dr. Gumshoe is a family physician specialist conducting a clinical trial on a new treatment for foot wounds for people with diabetes. The treatment is a cream that she developed. Although all of the compounds in the cream have been approved by the U.S. Food and Drug Administration (FDA), the treatment itself has not. The FDA has classified it as an investigational combination therapy. Dr. Gumshoe has completed the clinical trial, which has demonstrated that the new treatment is twice as effective as current therapy for diabetic foot wounds. She is getting ready to publish a paper and needs to decide (a) who should be an author and (b) the order of authorship. The following people have worked on the project:

Dr. Gumshoe developed the cream, designed the experiments, interpreted the data, and wrote the paper.

Dr. Wong is a pharmacist who helped Dr. Gumshoe develop the cream, interpret the data, and edit the paper.

Dr. Sabrunama is a biostatistician who helped to design the experiments and analyze and interpret the data; he read the paper but did not edit it for content.

Ms. Stetson is a nurse who provided treatment to patients in the study and collected data; she read the paper but did not edit it for content.

Ms. Williams is a medical student who provided treatment to patients in the study and collected data; she read the paper but did not edit it for content.

Mr. Gumshoe is Dr. Gumshoe's husband. He has provided legal assistance to Dr. Gumshoe concerning her FDA and institutional review board applications and patents on the treatment. He read the paper and edited it for style and grammar.

Mr. Jensen is a pharmacy technician who works for Dr. Wong and helped to prepare the treatment.

Dr. Chu is a colleague of Dr. Gumshoe's. He has discussed the project with her several times over lunch. He encouraged her to initiate the clinical trial and has given her critical feedback.

Dr. Rogers is a diabetic foot specialist. He provided Dr. Gumshoe with tissue samples and data that she used in her study.

- Who should be an author?
- Who should receive an acknowledgment?
- What should be the authorship order?

CASE 7

Ms. Wilson and Mr. O'Brien are graduate students who have been working in Dr. Klein's neuroscience laboratory at Big University on a study of Parkinson's disease in a mouse model. Two technicians, Ms. June and Mr. Chin, are also working on the project. Dr. Klein initially promised that both students would receive equal authorship credit on a paper describing the research, based on their equal work. Mr. O'Brien's name would go first, followed by Ms. Wilson, Mr. Chin, Ms. June and Dr. Klein. An asterisk would indicate that Mr. O'Brien and Ms. Wilson contributed equally to the research. Mr. O'Brien decided to leave the laboratory in order to enroll in a veterinary medicine program, but he still maintained contact with Dr. Klein and wanted to remain on the paper. In reviewing the data, Dr. Klein discovered that there were some problems with the research and that some of the experiments needed to be repeated. Ms. Wilson conducted these experiments. Based on the additional work that she did, Dr. Klein decided that Ms. Wilson's name should go first on the manuscript, although there would still be an asterisk indicating that Ms. Wilson and Mr. O'Brien contributed equally to the research. Dr. Klein circulated a draft of the manuscript to members of the team with new authorship designations. Mr. O'Brien was very upset about this change, claiming that Dr. Klein had broken his promise. He contacted the ethics office at Big University about this issue.

- Whose name should go first?
- Does Dr. Klein have an obligation to keep his promise to Mr. O'Brien?
- Should the paper state that Mr. O'Brien and Ms. Wilson contributed equally?

CASE 8

Mr. Krump is a physics Ph.D. student specializing in nanomaterials and working under the direction of Dr. Lloyd at University K. During the course of his research, Mr. Krump realizes that he needs to collaborate with Dr. Pester at University L to access some equipment that is not available at University K. Mr. Krump ends up spending most of his time at University L working with Dr. Pester, and after a year he is ready to present some of his results at a professional meeting. He prepares an abstract to submit to the meeting with this authorship order: Krump, Driver (a technician who provided considerable help with developing and conducting experiments), Pester, and Lloyd. Dr. Pester is upset because he was not named as the last (senior) author. He argues that since he was primarily responsible for supervising most of the work done for the project, his name should go last. Dr. Lloyd argues that he should go last because he is Mr. Krump's Ph.D. director at University K. Although most of the experiments were done at University L, the work as a whole is in support of a Ph.D. at University K.

- Who should be the last author on this abstract?
- Would it make sense to name co-senior authors?

CHAPTER 7

Publication and Peer Review

This chapter provides a historical overview of scientific publication and peer review and describes the current practices of scientific journals and granting agencies. It also examines a number of different ethical issues and concerns that arise in publication and peer review, such as quality control, confidentiality, fairness, bias, electronic publication, wasteful publication, duplicate publication, publishing controversial research, and editorial independence. The chapter also addresses the ethical responsibilities of reviewers and concludes with a discussion of the relationship between researchers and the media.

A BRIEF HISTORY OF SCIENTIFIC PUBLICATION AND PEER REVIEW

Throughout history, advances in communication technologies have helped to accelerate the progress of science (Lucky 2000). Written language was the first important innovation in communication that helped promote the growth of science. The Egyptians used hieroglyphics as early as 3000 B.C., and by 1700 B.C. the Phoenicians had developed an alphabet that became the basis of the Roman alphabet. With the invention of writing, human beings were able to record their observations and events as well as their ideas. The Egyptians and Babylonians, for example, made detailed observations of the movements of constellations, planets, and the moon in the night sky, as well as the position of the sun in daytime. Ancient Greek and Roman scientists communicated mostly through direct conversations and occasionally through letters. Philosopher-scientists, such as Pythagoras, Hippocrates, Plato, Aristotle, Euclid, Hero, Ptolemy, and Archimedes, discussed their ideas with students and colleagues in their respective schools, academies, and lyceums. Although these scientists also published some influential books, such as Euclid's *Elements*, Plato's *Republic*, and Ptolemy's *Almagest*, books were very rare because they had to be copied by hand onto papyrus rolls.

Egypt, especially the city of Alexandria, was the cultural province of Greece and later Rome. The Roman Empire built the largest network of roads and bridges in the world, which increased commercial and scientific communication between the Far East and Middle East and the West. From about 40 B.C. to 640 A.D., most of the world's recorded scientific knowledge rested in the great library of Alexandria. Invading forces burned the library three times, in 269 A.D., 415 A.D., and 640 A.D. Each time the library burned, scholars rushed to save books from being lost forever. To people in the modern world, the idea of there being only a single copy of a book that, if lost, is lost forever, is almost inconceivable (Ronan 1982). During Europe's Dark Ages (600–1000 A.D.), Islamic science and philosophy flourished. Islamic scholars translated Greek texts into Arabic and made significant contributions to mathematics, physics, astronomy, medicine, and philosophy. During the 13th century A.D., European scholars translated Islamic texts into European languages. The infusion of knowledge from the Islamic world helped to stimulate European science and philosophy (Al-Khalili 2012).

Aside from the development of written language, the invention of the printing press during the 1400s by the German goldsmith Johannes Gutenberg was the single most important event in the history of scientific communication. The Chinese had developed paper in the 2nd century A.D. By the 9th century, they had printed books using block print and woodcuttings. These inventions were brought to the Western world through trade with Arabic/Islamic countries. Gutenberg added to these established printing technologies a key innovation, movable type, which allowed the printer to quickly change the letters of the printing template. In 1450 Gutenberg established a printing shop and began to print the first works using his press, which included sacred texts such as the Bible (1454) and prayer books, grammar books, and bureaucratic documents. The selection of books soon expanded to include guidebooks, maps, how-to books, calendars, and currency exchange tables. In 1543, two influential and widely distributed scientific works also appeared in print: Andreas Vesalius's *On the Fabric of the Human Body* and Nicolas Copernicus's *The Revolutions of the Heavenly Bodies*. During the 16th century many important scientific and technical books, often originally written in Latin or Greek, were translated into vernacular and printed works (Burke 1995).

The printing press increased the rapidity and quantity of scientific communication like no other invention before or since (Lucky 2000). It also helped transform Europe from a medieval to a modern culture and thus helped stimulate the Scientific Revolution. The printing press helped transform Europe from a society based on oral tradition and memory to a literate society based on permanent, shared records and writing. People learned to read and developed a passion for books and learning. The Catholic Church lost control of the interpretation of the Bible when this work was translated into the vernacular, and people began fashioning their own interpretations of what they read, an event that helped spur the Protestant Reformation. In 1517, Martin Luther printed copies of his *Ninety-Five Theses* criticizing the church and nailed them to a bulletin board in his own church in Wittenberg, Germany. As others printed copies, Luther's complaints about indulgences, corruption, and paganism spread all over Europe in less than a month (Burke 1995).

By the 1600s, scientific books were common items in libraries throughout the world. But because it took several years to research, write, and publish a book, more rapid communication was needed as well. Scientists continued to correspond within letters, of course. Indeed, the letters of Descartes, Galileo, Newton, Boyle, and Harvey are considered to be key documents in the history of science. An important step toward more rapid and more public communication took place in 1665, when the world's first two scientific journals, *The Philosophical Transactions of the Royal Society of London* and the *Journal des Sçavans*, were first published. The first scientific association, the Royal Society of London, was a private corporation formed in 1662 to support scientific research and the exchange of ideas. Its journal is still published today. The world's second scientific society, the Paris Academy of Sciences, was formed in 1666 as an organization sponsored by the French government. By the 1800s, many other scientific associations and scientific journals had arisen (Meadows 1992).

The advantage of scientific journals is that they provided rapid communication of ideas, data, and results. Journals can also print a high volume of material. However, journals face the problem of quality control. The Royal Society addressed this issue in 1752, when it started evaluating and reviewing manuscripts submitted to its journal (Kronic 1990). It formalized the peer-review process in the 1830s. The Royal Society took this step because its members became concerned about the quality of papers that were published in the journal. Some of the papers it published had included highly speculative and rambling essays, as well as works of fiction (LaFollette 1992). Soon other journals followed this example, and the peer-review system began to take shape.

Other important innovations in communication technologies included the telegraph (1837), transatlantic telegraph (1858), telephone (1876), phonograph (1877), radio (1894), and television (1925–1933). Developments in transportation also enhanced scientific communication, because printed materials still must be transported in order to disseminate them widely. Important developments in transportation included the steam locomotive (1804), transcontinental railways (1869), the automobile (1859–1867), and the airplane (1903) (Williams 1987).

After the printing press, the computer (1946) is arguably the second most important invention relating to scientific communication. Computers allow researchers to collect, store, transmit, process, and analyze information in digital form. Computers are also the key technology in the Internet, which combines computers and other communication technologies, such as telephone lines, cable lines, and satellite transmitters, to form an information network. The Internet allows researchers to publish scientific information instantaneously and distribute it to an unlimited audience via electronic mail, discussion boards, and web pages. The Internet also allows scientists to instantly search scientific databases for articles and information (Lucky 2000). It is like having a library, newspaper, shopping catalog, magazine, billboard, museum, atlas, theater, and radio station all accessible through a computer terminal (Graham 1999). Although the Internet is a monumental leap forward in the rapidity and quantity of scientific communication, it also poses tremendous problems relating to quality control, because anyone can publish anything on the Internet (Resnik 1998b).

THE CURRENT PEER-REVIEW SYSTEM

Although peer review had its origins in scientific publishing in the 18th century, it was not institutionalized until the 20th century, when it began to be used to legitimize specific projects that required the expenditure of large sums of public funds (Burnham 1990). In 1937, peer review for awarding grants from the National Cancer Institute (NCI) was made into a public law. Today, all major federal funding agencies, such as the National Institutes of Health (NIH), the National Science Foundation (NSF), the Department of Energy (DOE), the Environmental Protection Agency (EPA), and the National Endowment for the Humanities (NEH), use peer review to make decisions on funding awards.

Peer review brought together two potentially conflicting concepts—expertise and objectivity (Shamoo 1993). The need for peer review of public funds arose in order to provide a mechanism of quality control and to prevent favoritism, the "old boy network," and fraud in allocating public money. The system was implemented in order to make objective decisions pertaining to the quality of grant proposals. Peer review arose in scientific publication in order to evaluate the quality of manuscripts submitted for publication and to provide a quality control mechanism for science. Another advantage of peer review is that it is less centralized and bureaucratic than other processes one might use to fund research (LaFollette 1994b). Scientists, not politicians or bureaucrats, control peer review. On the other hand, peer review also allows for a certain amount of government oversight, and thus it provides a venue for public participation in the setting of funding priorities (Jasanoff 1990).

There are numerous types of peer-review processes developed for various purposes. In this chapter, we consider three types of peer review of government contracts and grants, scientific publications, and tenure and promotion decisions.

GOVERNMENT CONTRACTS AND GRANTS

Peer review is frequently used to award research grants and contracts. Government grants provide public money to fund a large portion of research across the country. This is one area of peer review under direct public scrutiny where citizens can raise issues of fairness, equity, justice, and public accountability. Many private organizations, such as private foundations, also use peer review to award grants. A funding agency will usually make a public announcement for a request for applications (RFA) or request for proposals (RFP). The announcement will describe the area of interest where the agency is seeking proposals or applications, as well as the criteria for making an award. The investigators usually come up with an idea for a research project that meets the conditions of the RFA or RFP.

Contracts operate a little differently. When an organization awards a contract, it usually has a specific type of research in mind. It will usually publicly announce that it is planning to award a contract for the research, and research organizations can submit applications. A contract may or may not go through peer review. Even when contracts undergo peer review, it is selective and does not conform to the usual "independent" peer review used to evaluate grant proposals. Because contracts do not conform to the standards set by independent peer review, one may question the current practices in granting contracts in science, but we do not explore that issue here. We concentrate here on the peer-review standards for grants.

In the peer-review process for government agencies, the first steps are the selection of peers and the definition of "peers." The U.S. General Accounting Office (the forerunner of the current Government Accountability Office, GAO) report of peer review provides a thorough evaluation of this process. The selection of peer reviewers differs among the NIH, the NSF, and the NEH (U.S. General Accounting Office 1994). Further, the hierarchy of peer-review structure and its impact also differ at the three agencies. NIH has an initial peer review at the proposal's study section level (it has more than 100 study sections). These study sections belong officially to the Center for Scientific Review (CSR), which reports directly to the NIH director and not to each institute within NIH. The independence of the CSR from actual program managers at each institute preserves the integrity of the review process. However, in special cases, institutes can construct their own study sections, especially for large program projects and center grants. A study section usually consists of 18–20 members. Its decisions are not final, because NIH advisory councils have the final authority. However, the councils usually follow the study section ratings. The executive secretary of each study section is the one who recommends new members for the study section, at the approval of senior administrators. The executive secretary keeps a large list of potential study section members, based on discipline, knowledge, gender, age, and so forth. The executive secretary is usually a career staff member of the NIH with an M.D. or Ph.D. degree. The NIH uses nearly 20,000 reviewers annually (National Institutes of Health 2007b).

At the NSF, most of the initial peer review occurs electronically, via a secure website, followed by a meeting of a panel of 8–12 members who review the comments on the website. The panels are headed by NSF program directors, who are NSF career employees with advanced degrees. Each program director has the authority to select panel members and send materials to reviewers. Each program director also keeps a large list of potential reviewers based on discipline, publications, gender, race, age, and knowledge. NSF uses over 60,000 reviewers annually (U.S. General Accounting Office 1994).

At the NEH there is only one peer-review system, which is based on standing panels of about five members, who are selected from a large list based on qualification similar to the criteria used by NIH and NSF. At times, NEH program managers solicit evaluation from external reviewers to supplement the panel's deliberations. Annually, the NEH uses about 1,000 scholars for this review process (GAO 1994).

In evaluating proposals, reviewers at government agencies consider and address a number of different criteria:

1. The scientific or scholarly significance of the proposal
2. The proposed methodology
3. The qualifications of the principal investigator (PI) and other participants
4. Prior research or data that support the proposal
5. The level of institutional support and resources
6. The appropriateness of the budget request
7. Dissemination plans
8. Compliance with federal regulations
9. The proposal's potential social impact
10. The social impact of the research

Reviewers take these factors into account and rate proposals based on a relative point scale. The NIH uses comparative merit scores based on the scores of several previous review cycles. These comparative scores are given as percentile scores from lowest (0 percentile) to highest (100 percentile). The NSF allows each program to develop its own scoring method, but each program uses the same scoring method for all proposals it reviews. NSF criteria for scoring are similar to those of NIH, except there is a larger variation in scoring since most scoring is done by mail. For both the NIH and NSF, there is a good relationship between ratings and funding decisions. However, funding decisions are also greatly influenced by the program or project managers. The NSF's program directors have a much greater ability to bypass the scores in order to expand opportunities for women, minorities, and geographic areas and to initiate what they think are new and innovative projects. The NEH panels review proposals beforehand, deliberate at their meeting, and then score each proposal. The NEH's criteria for scoring are similar to those of the NIH and the NSF.

Private foundations and private corporations follow whatever review process they deem suitable for their purpose, and many use methods that evaluate proposals on ethnic, political, or religious grounds. Many private foundations, such as the Howard Hughes Medical Institute and the American Heart Association, use methods for awarding funds very similar to the peer-review mechanisms employed by government agencies. However, there is very little public scrutiny of their decision-making process other than what little is prescribed by the Internal Revenue Service (IRS) for nonprofit status. Although these foundations are philanthropic and public service institutions that contribute to the advancement of knowledge, most are indirectly subsidized by taxpayers because they are classified by the IRS as nonprofit (501(c)(3)) organizations, which are tax-exempt. One could argue that these organizations should be held more publicly accountable if they receive tax breaks.

Most private and public organizations that award research grants now use secure websites, email, and other electronic communications for submitting, reviewing, and overseeing grant proposals. Advances in information technology will continue to help improve the efficiency of the process.

JOURNALS

Although the concept of peer review for publication has its origins in the 18th century, in the 20th century peer review evolved into a method for controlling quality of publications as well as providing a stamp of approval by the established peers in a given field. The peer review of manuscripts varies from journal to journal, although the usual procedure has the editor-in-chief (or an associate if it is a large publication) who selects two or more reviewers, often experts in the field, to review each manuscript. A few editorial offices of journals that receive a large volume of manuscripts, such as *Science, Nature,* and the *New England Journal of Medicine,* screen papers for quality and suitability beforehand to select only a small percentage of manuscripts to send to reviewers. Acceptance rates at journals vary from less than 5% at the high-impact publications, such as *Science* and *Nature,* to higher percentages, depending on the journal.

Reviewers are given guidelines on reviewing the paper, but in reality reviewers are like jurors in courts: They can ignore the guidelines and base their opinion on whatever factors they deem to be appropriate. Most reviewers, however, evaluate manuscripts based on the following criteria:

1. Appropriateness of the topic for the journal
2. Originality of the research
3. The significance of the research
4. Strength of the conclusions, results, or interpretations as supported by the data, evidence, or arguments
5. The validity of the research methods and the research design, given the research goals or aims
6. The quality of the writing

Reviewers may recommend the following statuses for a manuscript:

- Accepted as is
- Accepted following minor revisions
- Accepted following major revisions
- Rejected, but encouraged to resubmit with revisions
- Rejected

Usually, if both reviewers highly recommend the acceptance or the rejection of the manuscript, the editor-in-chief follows that recommendation. However, when the reviewers are lukewarm in acceptance or rejection, or if the reviewers conflict in opinion, the editor usually has some latitude in making the decision. Some editors may simply accept or reject a paper, whereas others may send it to another reviewer for deciding between conflicting opinions. Of course, editors may also decide, in some rare cases, that the reviewers are completely mistaken and accept a paper that reviewers have rejected, or vice versa (LaFollette 1992).

High-profile cases of misconduct in published research, such as the Hwang stem cell case discussed in chapter 2, have caused some journals, such as *Science* and *Nature*, to rethink their misconduct policies. *Science*, for example, has decided to give additional scrutiny to high-impact papers. Despite the increased attention to issues of scientific misconduct, a survey (Redman and Merz 2006) found that few of the top 50 highest impact journals have adopted policies for dealing with misconduct. Bosch et al. (2012) examined 399 top biomedical journals and found that only 35.1% had publicly available definitions of misconduct and 44.9% had publicly available procedures for dealing with misconduct. Resnik et al. (2010) found that having a misconduct policy is positively associated with the impact factor of the journal.

PROMOTION AND TENURE

In public and private academic and research institutions, personnel decisions such as appointment, promotion, and tenure are based on committee recommendations. The criteria followed in making these personnel decisions vary considerably among community colleges, small colleges, local universities, research universities, industrial research organizations, and government laboratories. Although small colleges and community colleges emphasize a person's contributions to teaching, advising, or service to the institution, most of the other institutions place considerable emphasis on a person's research record, that is, the quantity and quality of publications and presentations, and the person's success in obtaining contracts or grants or patents. The committee members as well as relevant administrators are in essence conducting an internal peer review of the candidate's past performance and potential contributions. Due to limited and shrinking funds in the past decade, university administrators have overemphasized the amount of dollars raised by the investigator in promotion criteria. The committees also solicit reviews of publications and contracts/grants from established researchers/scholars from outside the institution. The input of internal and external peer reviewers is crucial to the personnel decisions. If the committee recommends a candidate for tenure, for example, then other administrators and committees will usually follow this recommendation. Because most institutions emphasize research over teaching, advising, and service, individuals who are seeking tenure or promotion often face difficult choices in balancing their commitments in these different areas.

The discussion of mentoring in chapter 4 notes that one way to improve mentoring is to ensure that researchers are adequately rewarded for high-quality mentoring. We recommend that mentoring play a key role in personnel decisions. Many commentators have also noted that the pressure to publish contributes to a variety of ethical problems in science, such as plagiarism, fraud, undeserved authorship, and careless errors (National Academy of Sciences 1992). To address these pressures to publish, it is important to consider ways of reforming the tenure and promotion system. One key assumption that needs to be examined is the idea that, for publication, "more is better." The emphasis on the quantity of publications, as opposed to quality, is a key factor in the pressure to publish. To address this issue, some universities have decided to review only a select number of publications and to focus on the quality of the candidate's work.

PROBLEMS WITH PEER REVIEW

The idea of peer review makes a great deal of sense. Indeed, peer review is regarded by many philosophers of science as a key pillar of the scientific method because it promotes objectivity and repeatability (Haack 2003; Kitcher 1993). Science can be "self-correcting" because scientists review and criticize research methods, designs, and conclusions and repeat experiments and tests. Indeed, it is hard to imagine how science could make progress without something like a peer-review system (Abby et al. 1994; Smith 2006). The peer-review system has come under severe criticism in recent years. In this section, we discuss some ethical and epistemological problems with peer review. Our negative comments about some aspects of the system should not be taken as a condemnation of the system as a whole or of individuals who serve as reviewers. On the contrary, the peer-review system is essential to scientific progress, and the overwhelming majority of individuals involved in peer review strive to do their very best. Some of the problems are described below.

BIAS

Numerous scholars have provided evidence that peer reviewers have significant biases (Bower 1991; Chubin and Hackett 1990; Cole and Cole 1981; Cole et al. 1978; Fletcher and Fletcher 1997; Oxman et al. 1991; Roy 1993; Shamoo 1993, 1994a). Some of the biases that can affect peer review include theoretical, conceptual, and methodological disagreements; professional rivalries; institutional, geographic, racial, and gender biases; and personal feuds (Garfunkel et al. 1994; Godlee 2000; Hull 1988; Resnik 2011; Ross 2006). Resnik et al. (2008) surveyed 283 researchers at the National Institutes of Environmental Health Sciences (NIEHS) concerning their perceptions of problems with the peer-review process and found that 50.5% had experienced reviewer bias sometime during their careers.

Because editors and grant review panels may reject papers or research proposals based on one negative review, biases can profoundly affect the peer-review process. As noted above, most scientific journals assign only two or three reviewers to a given paper. Although a peer-review panel includes many reviewers, usually only a few people are assigned as primary reviewers for a given proposal. Other panel members will not read the proposal very closely and will not be asked to make extensive comments. Because these panels rely heavily on primary reviewers, it may take only a single biased primary reviewer to eliminate a grant proposal.

Bias is especially pronounced in the realm of controversial research (Barber 1961; Chalmers et al. 1990; Godlee 2000). Controversial research does not fit neatly into well-established research traditions, norms, or paradigms. It is what the famous historian of science Thomas Kuhn (1970) dubbed "revolutionary science" (in contrast with "normal science"). Research can be controversial for a number of reasons: It may be highly creative or innovative, it may challenge previously held theories, or it may be interdisciplinary. Interdisciplinary work provides an additional challenge for reviewers because reviewers may come from different disciplines with different standards for review, and no single reviewer may have all the education or training required to give an overall evaluation of an interdisciplinary project.

Because reviewers often are established researchers with theoretical and professional commitments, they may be very resistant to new, original, or highly innovative ideas or ideas that challenge their own work. Historians of science have understood this phenomenon for many years. For example, Kuhn (1970) notes that quantum mechanics was not fully accepted, even by Einstein, until the old generation of Newtonian physicists died off. Although research carried out within specific disciplinary parameters (i.e., "normal" science) plays a very important role in the overall progress of science, the most important advances in science occur through controversial or "revolutionary" science (Kuhn 1970; Shamoo 1994a). History provides us with many examples of important theories that were resisted and ridiculed by established researchers, such as Gregor Mendel's laws of inheritance, Barbara McClintock's gene-jumping hypothesis, Peter Mitchell's chemiosmotic theory, and Alfred Wegener's continental drift hypothesis.

To provide objective and reliable assessments of controversial research, journal editors and review panel leaders should be willing to do what it takes to "open the doors" to new and novel work. If they close these doors, then they are exerting a form of censorship that is not especially helpful to science or to society. What it takes to open the door to controversial research may vary from case to case, but we suggest that editors and review panel leaders should always try to understand controversial research within its context. For instance, if an editor recognizes that a paper is likely to be controversial, he or she should not automatically reject the paper based on one negative review but should seek other reviews and give the paper a sympathetic reading.

The issue of publishing controversial research reveals an important flaw in the idea of quality control: If a journal tries to ensure that all articles meet specified standards related to quality, then it may not publish some controversial (but good and important) studies. One way to ensure that controversial ideas are not ignored is to publish a larger quantity of articles with less control over quality. Thus, the scientific community faces a dilemma of quality versus quantity. A partial solution to this dilemma is to increase the number of journals as well as the number of ways to disseminate information, to allow outlets for controversial studies. The advent of Internet publishing has increased the quantity of published material without a proportional increase in the cost of publication, which allows researchers to publish more data and results. It will still be difficult to get controversial work published in the top, peer-reviewed journals, but controversial work can still be published in mid-range to lower-range journals, in web-based journals, and so forth (Bingham 2000).

UNRELIABILITY

Two problems undermine the reliability of peer review: failure of reviewers to agree about the quality work and failure of reviewers to catch errors or other problems. Evidence shows that peer reviews often disagree about the quality of submitted work (Fletcher and Fletcher 1997). One study found that reviewers agree on their overall recommendation less than half the time (Kravitz et al. 2010). There is considerable evidence that the peer-review process may not catch even simple mistakes and that it is certainly not effective at detecting plagiarism and fraud (Goodman 1994; LaFollette 1992; Peters and Ceci 1982). From our own experience, we have come across many published papers that still have obvious and nontrivial mistakes. Peer review is not good at detecting these partly because reviewers usually do not have access to all the materials they would need to detect fraud, such as the original data, protocols, and standard operating procedures. Some journals have begun to use information technology to detect fraud. For example, statisticians have developed computer programs that can determine whether a dataset has probably been fabricated or falsified. A fabricated or falsified dataset will usually lack the random variation that is found in a genuine dataset, because human beings tend to follow patterns when they choose numbers. However, a very astute perpetrator of fraud could evade these programs with a program that introduces random variation into fabricated or falsified data! One computer program that is impossible to evade can detect plagiarism. The program compares submitted papers with published papers for degrees of similarity. If two papers are very similar, or they have similar sections, they can be flagged as potential plagiarism. There is evidence that peer review often does not improve the quality of published work. Some studies have shown that peer review may not be a very effective gate-keeping mechanism, because most articles rejected by more prestigious journals are eventually published elsewhere (Lock 1991). Studies have also shown that peer review is effective in improving the quality of published articles even if does not make articles perfect (Callahan 1998; Goodman 1994).

LACK OF FAIRNESS

As discussed above, the decisions of individual reviewers, editors, and panel leaders can control the outcomes of peer review. A great deal often depends on who is selected to review an article or proposal and on how the reviewers' assessments are interpreted. The system is designed in such a way that it is very easy for reviewers to affect outcomes in order to help someone they know and like or to hinder someone they don't know or like. For example, an editor's biased choice of reviewers can have an impact on the review outcome.

Many factors can give unfair advantages (or disadvantages) to the authors of manuscripts. Factors such as the author's name and institutional affiliation affect the judgments of editors and reviewers, who are more likely to give favorable reviews to well-respected authors from prestigious institutions than to unknown authors from less prestigious institutions (Garfunkel et al. 1994; LaFollette 1992). Most scientific journals currently use a single-blind system, where authors do not know the identities of reviewers, but reviewers know the identities of the authors.

Many journals ask authors to suggest potential reviewers or to name individuals who should not serve as reviewers. The journals may use these reviewers, select their own, or use some combination of author-suggested and journal reviewers. The Internet journal *BioMed Central* (BMC) requires that an author suggest four reviewers. The editor can chose from his roster and from the author-suggested reviewers. All reviews are published alongside the paper, if accepted. A study by Wager et al. (2006) found that author-suggested reviewers were more likely to recommend acceptance than were editor-chosen reviewers. However, excluding some differences in the overall recommendation, both sets of reviewers offered similar recommendations for improvement and gave reviews of similar quality.

Concerning fairness in grant review, there is evidence that people who know members of the review panels and who know how the process works are much more likely to have their grants approved than are people who lack this inside information (Shamoo 1993). Some studies have shown that the peer-review system may give favorable treatment to researchers from large or more prestigious institutions and that it may disfavor researchers from certain geographic areas. Men also get higher grant awards than do women (Agnew 1999a, 1999b; Marshall 1997a). Thus, something like an "old boys network" exists in peer review (Armstrong 1997; Chubin and Hackett 1990; Glantz and Bero 1994; Godlee 2000; Marshall 1997a).

Fairness has become such an important issue in peer review partly because scientific resources and rewards, such as grants and publications, are scarce. When rewards are scarce, questions about how to distribute rewards fairly are paramount. Not every paper will be published in a top journal, and not every grant will be funded. Indeed, many top journals have acceptance rates of 10% or less (LaFollette 1992). After nearly doubling in five years, the NIH budget has leveled off and has begun to decline when inflation is taken into account. Recent budgetary restrictions, known as sequestration, have eroded the NIH's budget. At one time the NIH funded about 30% of proposals but that number dropped to 14% in 2013 (Gross et al. 1999; Malakoff and Marshall 1999; National Institutes of Health 2007a, 2007b, 2013). Other agencies, such as the NSF, have not kept pace with NIH in recent years and tend to fund an even lower percentage of proposals. Some administrations with strong ideological views have attempted to influence the selection of peer reviewers (Ferber 2002).

The selection of peers to review grant proposals can profoundly affect the review process. Glantz and Bero (1994) showed that the professional interests of reviewers play a critical role in their level of enthusiasm for a grant proposal, which affects its score. The overall effect of reviewer selection is that it gives an unfair advantage to applicants who know the professional interests of potential reviewers. These applicants are likely to be those people who know the potential reviewers—the "old boys network."

The requirement of preliminary data can create an unfair disadvantage to beginning investigators or those who lack sufficient funding. Even though no federal agencies officially require preliminary data, the GAO report on peer review (U.S. General Accounting Office 1994) includes testimony from investigators who said that preliminary data are an essential component of a new grant application. Even more troubling for new investigators is where to obtain funding for their preliminary data. If investigators already have funding for another project, they must funnel some of that funding to obtain preliminary data for a new project. There are very few resources to produce truly preliminary data. Therefore, this policy pushes investigators into "theft" of funding from one project to another, an unethical zone of behavior that could manifest elsewhere. Lack of funding for preliminary data also encourages investigators to "stretch the truth" on grant applications by overestimating the significance of their preliminary work (Grinnell 1992; LaFollette 1992). Recent survey data confirm such claims (Anderson et al. 2007).

Those who are involved in the peer-review process, especially members of advisory councils, can also gain unfair "insider information" relating to how the process works, what types of proposals agencies would like to fund, what it takes to write convincing applications, and so on. In securities trading, financial institutions or individuals can go to jail for using "insider information" for economic gains. In science, those with insider information are not punished but are free to use it and gain greater chances for funding for their projects. For example, evidence shows that NIH's members of the advisory councils (past, present, and nominated) are twice as likely to have their research grant applications funded compared with the rest of the scientific investigators, despite the fact that their merit scores by the study sections were no different (Shamoo 1993). According to the GAO (U.S. General Accounting Office 1994), 97% of NSF applicants who were successful in obtaining funding had been reviewers in the last five years. One may partly explain these results by arguing that insiders are more likely to obtain funding because they have better expertise, a better understanding of peer review, or better knowledge of research or methods. While we do not deny this point, we doubt that these factors can completely explain these results because the study just cited that the merit scores were no different. We believe it is likely that funding decisions are often influenced by access to the right people with the relevant insider information.

OTHER PROBLEMS WITH PEER REVIEW

Peer review has other ethical and scientific problems in addition to those discussed above. In addition to bias, problems identified by respondents to the survey conducted by Resnik et al. (2008) included the following: the reviewer was incompetent (61.8%), the reviewer required unnecessary references to his or her publications (22.7%), the reviewer comments included personal attacks (17.7%), the reviewer delayed the review so he or she could publish an article on the same topic (9.6%), the reviewer breached confidentiality (6.8%), and the reviewer used ideas, data, or methods without permission (4.5%). Other commentators have noted that conflict of interest (COI) is also a common problem in peer review, but we know of no data concerning the prevalence of these problems (Lawrence 2003; Mulligan 2005; Smith 2006b).

It is important to also realize, as noted in chapter 3, that political factors often play a significant role in government research-funding decisions. Congress establishes the overall level of research funding for different agencies (NIH, NSF, etc.) and influences funding priorities within those agencies. Patient advocacy groups, nonprofit groups, and industry representatives also influence funding priorities (Resnik 2009). Usually, these influences operate at a general level and do not affect particular funding decisions. However, as also noted in chapter 3, politicians and interest groups have attempted to interfere with the peer-review process. Although the public has a right to hold scientific funding agencies accountable for how they spend money, meddling in the peer-review process threatens the objectivity of research and can have a chilling impact on scientists, who may decide not to conduct controversial research in order to avoid political pressures (Kempner 2008).

Although the peer-review system is far from perfect, it does work very well for the vast majority of papers and grant proposals. Moreover, it is hard to imagine any reasonable alternative to peer review. Without peer review, researchers would have no way to control the quality of articles or funded research or to promote objective, reliable research—there would be no way to separate the wheat from the chaff. From its inception in 1752, peer review was never meant to be infallible. As Knoll (1990, p. 1331) states: "We tend to forget that just because peer review reviews scientific work does not mean that it is itself a scientific process."

However, the fact that we have no reasonable alternatives to peer review does not mean that we cannot or should not make an effort to improve the current system. It is important to conduct more research on how the current system works (or fails to work) and to experiment with different peer-review practices. To its credit, the NIH is considering ways to reform its system of grant review, such as awarding longer grant periods, reviewing grants retrospectively, inviting public participation in study sections, relaxing pressures to produce preliminary data, and finding ways to fund controversial research (Marshall 1997a; National Institutes of Health 2007b; Zurer 1993).

Journals have also considered ways to reform the peer-review system. One of these reforms is using a double-blind peer-review system, where reviewers do not know the identities of authors. There has been some debate about the strengths and weaknesses of double-blinded peer review. Studies have shown that more than half the time reviewers can still identify authors even when they are not given the authors' names or institutional affiliations (Rooyen et al. 1998). The effects of blinding on the quality of peer review are not clear. Some studies have shown that masking the identities of authors improves peer review (Blank 1991; McNutt et al. 1990), while other studies indicate that it does not (Justice et al. 1998; Laband and Piette 1994; Rooyen et al. 1998). Rooyen et al. (1998) examined 1,051 full articles published in 1984 in 28 economic journals. They then compared the citations of these articles in the following five years, 1985–1989. They found that papers from journals using double-blind peer review were cited more often than were papers from journals using single-blind review. These results suggest that the quality of published papers that have double-blind reviews is better on average than that of papers published that have single-blind review, although this may be due to the fact that journals that use double-blind review tend to be better than those that use single-blind review. Even if the evidence does not show that masking the identities of authors improves the quality of peer review, one can still argue that this practice is important in promoting the confidence, fairness, and integrity of peer review.

Some journals have experimented with open (unblinded, unmasked) review. The main argument for open review is that it should improve the quality and integrity of review. If reviewers know that their identities can be discovered and made public, they will be more likely to give careful, responsible, and ethical reviews (Davidoff 1998; DeBakey 1990; Godlee 2002). However, one can argue that if reviewer identities are not anonymous, then reviewers may be less likely to be critical or unbiased, because they may fear repercussions from authors (LaFollette 1992). It might be especially difficult, for example, for a younger researcher to offer candid criticism to an established researcher, because the younger researcher might fear for repercussions to his career. Also, some experts may not want to serve as reviewers in an unmasked system. Some studies have shown that unmasking the reviewers may not improve the quality of peer review (Godlee et al. 1998; Rooyen et al. 1998). Walsh et al. (2000) published a randomized trial comparing single-blind to open review, and reviewers who had their identities shared with the authors produced better reviews, were more courteous, took longer to complete the review, and were more likely to recommend publication than reviewers who remained anonymous.

Another recent innovation by a number of journals is the concept of "target articles with open commentary." In this practice, authors submit an article for publication, which is peer reviewed. If the editors decide to publish the article and think it will generate interesting discussion, they then solicit or invite commentaries to be published along with the article. They may also use email discussion boards to allow further debate (Bingham 2000). The advantage of this system is that it combines the virtues of quality control (blinded peer review) with the virtues of openness, diversity, and accessibility. We encourage journals and researchers to experiment with other innovations in peer review.

A challenge for journals and granting agencies is to find ways to give a fair review to creative and controversial projects or papers, as discussed above. Because science often makes progress through creative or unconventional leaps, it is important to test innovative or controversial ideas. Because a few of these ideas may bear fruit, editors and granting agencies may be willing to take some risks in order to reap potentially high rewards. Because these controversial projects may use unorthodox methods, it may be necessary to modify the normal peer-review process somewhat to accommodate these proposals. For example, granting agencies could loosen their informal requirements of prior work as well as their demands to produce results within certain deadlines. To ensure that research is still of high quality, agencies could perform more frequent site visits and data audits.

ETHICAL DUTIES IN PEER REVIEW

Evidence suggests that reviewers have acted unethically during the peer-review process by violating confidentiality, stealing ideas, and so on (Dalton 2001; Lawrence 2003; Resnik et al. 2008). The Committee on Publication Ethics (2013) has developed some ethical guidelines for reviewers and editors, and various granting agencies have their own rules and policies for peer review. In this section, we briefly describe some ethical duties of editors, panel directors, reviewers, and others involved in peer review and give a brief rationale for these duties. Some of these are discussed below.

Confidentiality

Everyone involved in the peer-review process should maintain the confidentiality of materials being reviewed. Papers submitted for publication or grant proposals often contain data, results, ideas, and methods that have not been previously published. This material belongs to those who are submitting the paper or proposal, and it is privileged information. If a reviewer discusses a paper still in the review process with an outside party, then that outside party could use that information to his or her advantage, for example, to steal the ideas or results or to get a jump on the competition. The whole system of peer review would collapse if those who submit papers or proposals could not trust that their work will remain confidential (Godlee 2000; LaFollette 1992). Most granting agencies and journals now require reviewers to agree to treat all materials that they review as confidential, and some even require reviewers to destroy papers or proposals after they complete their review. Some researchers share review materials with postdoctoral fellows or students to teach them how to review a paper or proposal, and some asked fellows or students to help them with the review. While this practice has some value, researchers should not share reviews with others without permission from the editors.

Respect for Intellectual Property

The ideas, data, methods, results, and other aspects of a paper or proposal submitted for review should be treated as the intellectual property of the authors or PIs. Those involved in the process should therefore not use any of this property without the explicit permission of the authors or PIs (Godlee 2000). Many scientists can attest to having their ideas stolen during peer review (Resnik et al. 2008). One common scenario is as follows: Researchers submit a paper to a journal. The journal takes a long time to make a decision on the paper and then finally rejects the paper. In the meantime, another research team publishes a paper on the exact same problem using identical methods with almost identical results. Is this sheer coincidence or theft? Most researchers will not be able to prove that their ideas have been stolen, but they will remain suspicious. However, many researchers are so wary of this problem that they will omit important information from papers in order to prevent others from stealing their work before it is published (Grinnell 1992; LaFollette 1992). It almost goes without saying that the peer-review system could not function if authors or PIs could not trust that their work would be protected from theft.

Addressing Conflicts of Interest

If reviewers or editors have a personal, professional, or financial interest that may undermine their ability to give a fair and unbiased review, then they should declare that conflict to the relevant parties, such as editors or panel leaders (Godlee 2000; Resnik 1998b; Shamoo 1994a). One very common type of conflict of interest in peer review is when the reviewers have relationships with authors or PIs, who may be current or former students, colleagues at the same institution, or bitter rivals. Another common type of conflict of interest is when the reviewers have financial interests related to the work they are reviewing, such as stock in the company sponsoring the research or a competitor. It is important to disclose these conflicts and some should be avoided altogether, such as reviewing the work of a current or former student or a colleague at the same institution. Many granting agencies and journals now require reviewers to disclose conflicts of interest. Chapter 9 discusses conflicts of interest in depth.

Punctuality

Reviewers should complete their reviews within the stated deadlines, especially for papers submitted for publication. If reviewers cannot complete the review by the deadline, they should not accept the assignment and may recommend someone else (LaFollette 1992). Scientific research occurs at a very rapid pace. Slow reviews can have adverse effects on the careers of researchers: One research team may be "beaten to the punch" by a different research team while they wait for their work to be reviewed. In research related to public policy or current events, much of the material in a paper submitted for publication may go out of date if the paper is not published on time. Researchers may fail to get tenure, promotion, or a good rating if they have some major papers that have not been reviewed in a timely fashion. Although the length of review varies from journal to journal, most have a decision within three months of submission, and many have a decision in less than three months. Email correspondence and electronic submission systems have greatly increased the speed of review. Authors should not hesitate to contact editors if they are concerned about the status of a manuscript or its stage in the review process.

Professionalism

Reviewers should conduct careful, thorough, critical, and responsible reviews of papers or proposals. Reviewers should not offer to review a paper or proposal if they lack the expertise to make an informed judgment about its quality. In writing comments, reviewers should avoid insults, personal attacks, and other unprofessional remarks and make every effort to provide authors or PIs with useful comments for improving the manuscript or proposal (LaFollette 1992; Resnik 1998b). Although senior researchers can develop some understanding of the peer-review process and learn to accept harsh and irresponsible criticism, beginning researchers and graduate students may have an especially difficult time dealing with unprofessional reviews of their work. Insults can undermine a person's self-confidence and trust in his or her colleagues.

OTHER ISSUES IN SCIENTIFIC PUBLICATION

Wasteful and Duplicative Publication

Some scientists publish papers according to the least publishable unit (LPU), or the smallest paper that can be accepted for publication. Scientists may do this to increase the quantity of their publications, because one study can be divided into several publications. Many commentators have criticized this practice as wasteful and irresponsible (Huth 2000; Jones 2000). We concur with this assessment and encourage researchers not to divide substantial papers into LPUs. However, we recognize that there are sometimes advantages to dividing larger papers into smaller parts, because a large paper may cover too many topics or take up too much room in a journal. Authors should divide papers to improve the quality and clarity of their arguments and analysis, not to increase the quantity of their publications.

The practice of duplicative publication (a form of self-plagiarism) has also been criticized (Huth 2000). For example, some researchers have published the exact same paper in different journals without telling the editors. Others have published papers substantially similar to papers they have published elsewhere (LaFollette 1992). Duplicative publication is unethical because it is wasteful and deceptive: Most journals expect that papers submitted for publication have not already been published, even as a different but substantially similar work. Most journals ask authors to certify that the manuscript is original and has not been previously published, and many also use computer programs to compare submitted articles to published ones to check for plagiarism and self-plagiarism (Butler 2010). Some types of duplicative publication are warranted, however, because they may serve important educational purposes, for example, when papers are published in a different language or for a completely different audience. If an older paper has historical significance, it may be appropriately republished so that the current generation of researchers can become familiar with it. In all of these cases where duplicative publication is appropriate, the editors should clearly reference the original work.

Multiple Submissions

Most journals forbid multiple submissions, and most require authors to certify that their manuscripts are not under submission elsewhere (LaFollette 1992). There seem to be two reasons for this practice. The first is to save resources: If a journal is going to go to the trouble to review a paper, then it does not want the paper snatched up by another journal. The second is to avoid disputes among journals: Journal editors do not want to have to negotiate with other journals or authors for the rights to publish papers. On the other hand, the rest of the publishing world does not follow this exclusive submission policy. Law journals, poetry journals, magazines, newspapers, and commercial and academic presses allow multiple submissions. Indeed, one could argue that the peer-review process would be improved if journals did not require exclusive submissions, because this would force journals to compete for papers and to improve the quality and punctuality of the review process. Established researchers who can afford to wait can often choose among competing journals, even if they only submit a paper to one journal at a time. If researchers submit a paper to a journal and decide that they do not want to make changes recommended by the reviewers, then they can submit the paper to another journal.

Editorial Independence

Many journals are sponsored by professional organizations. For example, the American Association for the Advancement of Science sponsors *Science*, the American Medical Association sponsors the *Journal of the American Medical Association* (JAMA), and the Federation of American Societies for Experimental Biology sponsors the *FASEB Journal*. Other journals, such as the *Proceedings of the National Academy of Sciences of the USA* (PNAS) and the *Journal of the National Cancer Institute*, are sponsored by government or para-governmental organizations. Some journals are sponsored by private think tanks, such as the *Hastings Center Report* and the *Cato Policy Report*. Other journals are sponsored by religious, political, or business organizations. Some are completely independent and have no sponsors.

For those journals that have official sponsors, problems relating to editorial independence sometimes arise. In one recent example, it appears that the American Medical Association fired *JAMA*'s editor George Lundberg after he decided to publish a controversial study on sexual practices and perceptions among adolescents (Fletcher and Fletcher 1999). We strongly support the idea of editorial independence as vital to the peer-review process and the progress and integrity of research. However, we also recognize that private organizations have a right to control the materials they publish. A Jewish organization, for example, has no obligation to publish anti-Semitic writings. One way to settle these conflicts is for organizations that sponsor specific publications to publicly state the editorial goals of those publications. This will allow readers and prospective authors to understand a journal's particular editorial bent and to plan accordingly. If authors realize that their work goes against the stated aims of the journal, they may submit their work elsewhere.

Controversial Research

We have already discussed questions related to reviewing controversial research, but ethical dilemmas can also arise even when the reviewers agree on the merits of a controversial paper. The editors may still have some reservations about publishing the paper even when the reviewers recommend publication as a result of the potential social or political implications of the research. For example, in 1998 *Science* and *PNAS* both published papers on human embryonic stem cells. Many people oppose research on embryonic stem cells because it involves the destruction of human embryos, but these journals decided to publish these papers to promote progress in these important new areas of research and to help stimulate public debate on the topic (Miller and Bloom 1998). Other areas of research that have generated a great deal of public debate (and at times acrimony) include cloning, human intelligence, genetic factors in crime, sexuality, and global warming. Although we recognize that editors must consider the social, security, or political implications of articles, their primary obligation is to publish new findings and stimulate debate, not to protect society from "harmful" or "dangerous" research. Only a few decades ago Alfred Kinsey and his colleagues had difficulty publishing their research on human sexuality because of its controversial nature. Indeed, much of this research was conducted with private money and published with private support.

Research Raising Security Issues

The specter of terrorism looms over the 21st century. Terrorists have killed thousands of people, destroyed major buildings such as the World Trade Center in New York, and disrupted commerce and trade. Terrorist groups have used biological and chemical weapons and continue to seek other weapons of mass destruction, including nuclear weapons. Given the significance of this threat to national and international security, it is incumbent on all people, including scientists, to help prevent, discourage, mitigate, or respond to terrorism. We discuss issues pertaining to the publication of research with security implications in more depth in chapter 12.

Electronic Publication

Most publications now publish in both paper and electronic form. Some journals are now entirely in electronic form, and almost all journals publish article abstracts in electronic databases. Most books are also now available online. It is likely that these trends will continue and that one day almost any article, book chapter, or book will be available in some form through the Internet and electronic databases and bibliographies. Internet information services, such as Google Scholar, Blackwell, Informaworld, and Springer, have already made tremendous strides in this direction. Given their high costs, printed journals may soon become obsolete (Butler 1999a).

Electronic publication offers many important benefits to researchers. It can allow more rapid review and publication. It can increase access to publication for those who do not have access to regular print journals. Researchers can more easily search for specific articles, topics, or authors with a search engine, which can locate in less than a second a document that may have taken a month to find using older methods. Electronic publication also increases the quantity of published material and reduces the cost.

Since 2001, an increasing number of journals have begun to publish articles via an open-access system. By 2011, 11% scientific articles were published via open access (Van Noorden 2013). Under the traditional publishing arrangement, authors transfer their copyrights to the publisher, and the publisher charges a fee for access to the articles. Publishers earn their revenue, under this system by selling copies of the journal or access to articles. Under the open-access system, authors pay a fee upfront to publish their articles, which are then made available to readers free of charge (Schroter et al. 2005). The publishers derive income not from selling products or access to articles, but from fees paid by authors. The Public Library of Science (PLoS), a private nonprofit organization, now publishes many Internet open-access scientific and medical journals. Many high-impact journals, such as the *New England Journal of Medicine* and *Journal of the American Medical Association*, also publish selected articles on an open-access basis.

The chief advantages of an open-access system are that it promotes openness and the dissemination of knowledge, and it allows researchers who cannot afford to purchase articles, such as researchers from developing countries, to have access. In 2005, the NIH adopted an open-access policy (Schroter et al. 2005). The NIH now requires that all of the articles that are funded by NIH are available to the public for free on its website. The rationale for this policy is that since the public has already funded the research, it should not have to pay a second time for access. Publishers have objected that this policy will put them out of business by undercutting the fees they charge to access NIH-funded articles (Kaiser 2004). It remains to be seen whether the traditional publishing model can survive in the electronic age.

Despite all of these advantages, electronic publication also has some disadvantages. A problem with open access is that it can be very costly to finance, with some journals needing to charge authors several thousand dollars to publish an article. Open-access fees range from less than a hundred dollars to five thousand dollars. PLoS journals generally charge around $1,500 to publish an article (Van Noorden 2013). Researchers from developing countries or small institutions may not be able to afford to pay these fees. Some journals waive or reduce publishing fees in some circumstances.

Another problem is quality control: how to tell the difference between good science, bad science, pseudoscience, and fraudulent science. Before electronic publication, researchers could rely on the reputation of the journal to help them make judgments about the quality of published material, a method still useful today. However, as more and more electronic articles are published outside of well-established journals, it will become much more difficult to rely on journal reputation. Also, many articles are published directly on web pages, without any supervision by journal editors.

The problems raised by for-profit electronic journals illustrate the concerns about quality control. Many journals have sprung up in the last ten years that offer to publish articles on an open-access basis for a fee (usually several thousand dollars). These journals aim to make a profit—some have profit margins of 20–30%—so they encourage authors to submit and promise quick review. Some share profits with reviewers and editors, and some provide authors who make referrals with monetary awards. For-profit publishers generated $9.4 billion in revenues in 2011. Critics have argued that these journals exhibit very little control over the quality of the research they publish and basically rubberstamp submissions in order to generate fees (Van Noorden 2013). Even reputable open-access journals, such as those published by PLoS, have a 70% acceptance rate, as compared to traditional, top-tier journals, which may have an acceptance rate of 10% or less (Van Noorden 2013).

Science and the Media

Many scientific discoveries and results have a significant bearing on public health and safety, education, the economy, international relations, criminal justice, politics, and the environment. These research findings are newsworthy in two different ways: First, they are events that the public should know about; second, they are events that many people find intrinsically interesting. For many years, scientific discoveries and results have been reported in newspapers and magazines and on radio and television. Science is also discussed in popular fiction and movies. In chapter 12, we discuss researchers' social responsibilities concerning communications with the media in more detail. Here we focus on a particular issue or prior publication in the media or "press conference" science.

The controversy over cold fusion illustrates this problem. According to standard theories of fusion, fusion can only occur at the extraordinarily high temperatures and pressures found in the center of stars. On March 23, 1989, Stanley Pons, the chairman of the chemistry department at the University of Utah, and Martin Fleischmann, a chemistry professor at Southampton University, announced at a press conference in Salt Lake City, Utah, that they had produced nuclear fusion at room temperatures by using equipment available in most high school chemistry laboratories. They had not yet submitted their work to a peer-reviewed journal. Researchers around the world rushed to try to replicate these results, but the Utah press release did not provide adequate information to do this. Pons and Fleischmann made their announcement to ensure that they would not be scooped by other research groups in the race for priority and to protect their pending patent claims. Once other researchers failed to replicate their work, mainstream physicists came to regard their work as careless, irresponsible, or even fraudulent. Although cold fusion research continues to this day, and Pons, Fleischmann, and others continue to publish results, the cold fusion community has become isolated from the traditional fusion community (Beaudette 2000; Chubb 2000; Resnik 1998a).

In retrospect, one wonders whether this press conference actually hindered the cause of cold fusion by calling too much attention to the subject before the work was adequately peer reviewed. If the work had been published in a low-profile physics journal and others with an interest in the subject had reviewed the work in an orderly fashion, then cold fusion research could still have been regarded as controversial but not irresponsible or fraudulent. Fleischmann (2000) considered this option and favored delayed publication in an obscure journal. Thus, this press conference may have hindered the progress of science. Another problem with this prior publication in the media is that it wasted valuable resources as researchers scrambled to replicate the results with insufficient information. This probably would not have happened if this research had been published in a peer-reviewed journal first.

The whole cold fusion episode also undermined the public's trust in science in that the researchers made extraordinary claims in their press conference that have not been verified. This makes scientists look foolish or incompetent. Other types of press conference science have the potential to do much more damage to science's public image as well as to the public. Premature announcements of research on diseases or new medical treatments can have adverse effects on public health and safety (Altman 1995). For example, if researchers announce in a press release that they have discovered that a blood pressure medication has some serious drug interactions, then patients may stop taking the medication, and some may have a hypertensive crisis as a result. If this claim has not been peer reviewed and turns out to be false, then the press conference will have resulted in unnecessary harm to patients. However, if researchers have very good evidence, and they feel that it is important for the public to know their results as soon as possible, then they may choose not to wait for their work to go through the peer-review process, because a delay of several months could result in unnecessary loss of life or injury.

To deal with issues relating to prior publication in the media, many journals have adopted policies requiring authors to certify that they have not discussed their work with the media before submitting it for publication (LaFollette 1992). Many journals also forbid authors from prior publication of their works on web pages as a condition of acceptance, though some make an exception for research involving significant health or safety issues that need to be communicated to the public immediately. Top journals, such as *Science, Nature, JAMA*, and the *New England Journal of Medicine*, have adopted embargo policies for science journalists (Marshall 1998). These policies allow reporters to have a sneak preview of articles prior to publication on the understanding that the reporters will not disclose the information to the public until the article is published. These policies allow reporters to have early access to newsworthy stories, and it allows journals to ensure that communications with the media do not undermine peer review and that scientists get adequate publicity. Although embargo policies often work well, confusion can arise regarding the status of work presented at scientific meetings: If a reporter working on an embargoed story learns about the story at a scientific meeting, would she break the embargo to cover the story at the meeting? A similar confusion can arise with journals' own prior publication policies: Does presenting results at a scientific meeting count as prior publication?

QUESTIONS FOR DISCUSSION

1. What are the purposes of peer review?
2. Do you think peer review is effective?

3. What suggestions would you make to improve the current manuscript review process for journal publication?
4. What is your personal experience or your colleagues' or mentor's experience with peer review?
5. How would you promote ethical practices among your colleagues regarding peer review?
6. Do you think researchers should disseminate their findings in the media? How and why?
7. Do you think the peer review of government-funded research can or should be completely free from political or other "extra-scientific" influences?

CASES FOR DISCUSSION

CASE 1

Dr. Little is a stem cell biologist at a large university. His research focuses on chemical signaling involved in bone marrow stem cell differentiation. Dr. Little receives a paper to review for a prestigious journal. The paper investigates the role of protein Q in a signaling pathway related to the differentiation of bone marrow stem cells. Dr. Little is familiar with this type of research and was already planning to conduct a study similar to the one reported in the paper. Dr. Little decides to initiate the study he was already planning to conduct. He also delays his review of the paper to give his team time to conduct the experiments. After three months, Dr. Little submits his review. He recommends that the paper be revised and resubmitted. His main critique of the paper is that it needs additional data from other experiments to validate the techniques used to study protein Q's interactions. Dr. Little submits a paper on protein Q's role in bone marrow stem cell differentiation to a different journal. Dr. Little's paper is accepted and published. The paper that Dr. Little was reviewing is eventually published, but Dr. Little receives top billing for elucidating the role of protein Q in bone marrow stem cell differentiation and the other paper becomes a mere footnote.

- Did Dr. Little act unethically?
- Should Dr. Little have reviewed the paper?
- Should he have informed the journal editor that he had a conflict of interest?
- How should the journal editor respond to the disclosure of a possible conflict of interest, especially if Dr. Little is one of a few people in the world who is qualified to review the paper?
- Should the editor have prompted Dr. Little to turn in his review earlier?
- What do you think of Dr. Little's recommendation that the paper provide additional data?

CASE 2

Dr. Miller is an experimental psychologist studying the impact of recreational drugs (marijuana, cocaine, etc.) on learning in laboratory animals. She receives a paper to review from a journal and gives it to Dr. Barista, a postdoctoral fellow, to review. She asks Dr. Barista to read the paper and provide comments, as this would be a good learning experience. Dr. Barista writes a thoughtful review of the paper (two single-spaced typed pages) and sends it to Dr. Miller. Dr. Miller reads the review, adds a few sentences of her own, and sends it to the journal. Dr. Miller presents the review as her own work and does not tell the journal about Dr. Barista's contribution.

- Did Dr. Miller act unethically?
- Should she have given credit to Dr. Barista?
- Did Dr. Miller commit plagiarism?
- Should she have asked the journal for permission to send the paper to Dr. Barista?

CASE 3

Shelly Trooper is a graduate student in a public health program at a university. She is working on a doctoral dissertation on the role of low-cost, public health clinics in providing medical care in Appalachia. She presented some of her findings at a national public health conference. She received a great deal of positive feedback at the conference and her advisor, Dr. Schrumer, said that her work was publishable. He encouraged her to submit a short paper for publication in a middle-tier journal. Ms. Trooper drafted a paper and submitted it to the journal, but she never showed it to Dr. Schrumer. After three months, she learned that her paper was rejected. The comments she received from one reviewer were devastating to her. The reviewer said that "an undergraduate student could have written a better paper," "the paper is confused and rambling," "the author has no business doing public health research and should consider another career," and "I can't believe I wasted my time reading this garbage." Ms. Trooper is very distraught and is considering quitting the program.

- Did the reviewer act unethically and unprofessionally?
- Should Dr. Schrumer have encouraged Ms. Trooper to allow him to comment on the paper before sending it to the journal?
- Did the editors of the journal have a responsibility to delete these offensive remarks from the reviewer comments before sending them to Ms. Trooper?

CASE 4

A very busy researcher is also a member of an NIH study section. He received 15 proposals to review in four weeks. He is the primary or secondary reviewer for six proposals. The primary and secondary reviewers are supposed to prepare a report about each proposal. Also, all reviewers are supposed to read all of the proposals. The researcher delayed reading the material until the night before the meeting. He read thoroughly two of the six proposals where he was the primary/secondary reviewer and prepared reports. Lacking in time, he skimmed the other five proposals and wrote reports laden with generalized statements of praise or criticism. He never read the other nine proposals.

- What should he do?
- What would you have done?

The same busy researcher received the same 15 grant proposals to review in four weeks. He gave 10 of them (five for which he was primary/secondary reviewer and five others) to his most senior postdoctoral fellow to read and comment on. During the study section deliberation four weeks later, the chairman of the study section realized that the researcher had never read those five proposals, because he was not able to discuss them.

- What should the reviewer do?
- What should the reviewer have done?
- What should the chairman of the study section do?

CASE 5

A senior scientist at a major East Coast medical school was also a member of the grant review board for a large medical foundation. He was also a member of an NIH study section. During foundation review deliberations of a grant proposal from a relatively junior scientist, he stated, "We just turned down his NIH research proposal, which was basically on the same topic." However, the outside reviewers recommended this proposal be funded by the foundation. Prior to the senior scientist's comments, the discussions were moving in favor of funding. After his comments, the entire discussion became negative, and the proposal ultimately was not funded.

- What should the senior scientist have done?
- What should the junior scientist do if she hears what happened?
- What should the chairman of the review group at the foundation have done?

CASE 6

An associate professor in a university is also on the editorial board of a major journal in her field. She receives a paper to review in her field. While reading the manuscript, she recognizes that the paper's researcher is on the path to discovering an important peptide that the professor's close friend is also pursuing. She calls her close friend and discusses her friend's project and how he is progressing with it. She never mentions that she is reviewing the submitted paper. But at the end of their conversation, she informs her friend, "If I were you, I would hurry up and submit the work quickly before someone else beats you to it." She repeats the same sentence twice and adds, "I would recommend that you send it as a short communication so that it can be published shortly." The associate professor then mails her review paper three months later. She recommends acceptance with major modifications and few additional experiments.

- What should the associate professor have done?
- What should her close friend have done?
- What should the author of the submitted paper do if he hears about it?

CASE 7

An editor of a journal receives a controversial paper in the field questioning the existing paradigm. The editor knows that if he sends the manuscript to two experts on his editorial board, they will most likely reject it. He sends the manuscript for review anyway, and he also sends it to an outside third reviewer who is neutral on the subject. To his surprise, one of the two editorial board members recommended acceptance, while the other recommended rejection. The outside third reviewer also recommended acceptance. The editor decided to accept the paper but felt obligated to call the reviewer who recommended the paper to be rejected and inform him of his decision. The purpose of the call was to keep editorial board members happy and content. The editorial board member informed the editor that if he accepts this piece of garbage, she would resign from the board.

- What should the editor have done? And do?
- What should the two editorial board members have done?
- What should the author do if she hears about it?

CASE 8

An editor of a major ethics journal receives a paper dealing with a controversial topic on the use of human subjects in research. The paper deals with surveying the open literature for questionable ethical practices toward a vulnerable population. The editor mails the article to several reviewers, among them two researchers whose own work was part of the survey. These two reviewers are not members of the editorial board, so they were ad hoc reviewers for this paper. The instructions from the editor clearly state that the paper is a privileged communication. The two ad hoc reviewers copy the manuscript and mail it to about two dozen researchers whose work is mentioned in the paper. After three months, the paper is accepted based on the other reviewers' comments, because the two ad hoc reviewers never mailed back their reviews. The author receives the page proofs, makes a few corrections, and mails it back to the production office. A few weeks later, the editor calls the author to inform him that the paper will not be published because of a threat of a libel lawsuit from "some researchers" cited in the paper. She tells the author that the publisher does not have the resources to fight a lawsuit.

- What should the editor do or have done?
- What should the ad hoc reviewers have done?
- What should the author do?

CASE 9

A university's promotion and tenure committee is deliberating on the promotion of an assistant professor to an associate professor with tenure. This is a crucial step in a faculty member's career. The assistant professor's package before the committee contains six strong letters of recommendation (three from inside and three from outside the university), a strong curriculum vita that includes 30 papers in peer-reviewed journals, an R01 grant for $1 million for five years, and a good but not exemplary teaching record. The letter from the chair of the department is supportive but not glowing. The department chair's concerns are legitimate in that this faculty member is not a "good" citizen and is hard to manage. He resists any additional duties that are not related to research. The department chair wants the committee to turn him down so she will be off the hook. She took additional informal steps to stop his promotion, including talking to the chair of the committee and two of its members about her concerns.

- What should the department head do or have done?
- What should the chair and members of the promotion and tenure committee have done and do?
- What should the faculty member do if his promotion is turned down? If he hears about why?

CASE 10

Three authors submit a paper on superconductivity theory to a prestigious journal. They become irritated when the journal does not make a decision after four months. Finally, after six months, the journal decides to reject their manuscript. The journal does not provide them with any substantial comments and says that there was a delay in getting a review back from the second reviewer. The editor recommends that they try to publish their paper elsewhere. The next month, a paper comes out in a different journal that is suspiciously similar to their paper. The theory described by the paper is very similar to one they developed, with a few modifications. The paper uses several sentences in the discussion section that bear a strong resemblance to sentences from their paper. It also draws similar conclusions.

- What might have happened in this case?
- Can you find fault with the conduct of the editor or reviewer(s)?
- What should the authors do now?

CHAPTER 8
Intellectual Property

This chapter discusses the history of intellectual property (IP) and its ethical and legal foundations. It provides an overview of the U.S. IP system and discusses patents, copyrights, trademarks, trade secrets, and ownership of research data. The chapter also examines some key pieces of IP legislation and IP cases and discusses some ethical controversies, such as patents on biological materials.

HISTORY AND OVERVIEW OF INTELLECTUAL PROPERTY

In previous chapters in this book we have mentioned IP when discussing research misconduct, data sharing, and collaborations with industry. In this chapter, we discuss IP issues in more depth. The material covered in this chapter will also be useful in understanding conflicts of interest.

When most people think of their property, they imagine their house, their land, their car, their book collection—something that they can touch, see, feel, hear, smell, or taste. Many of the property rights that people have pertain to tangible objects located in time and space. But people also claim to own things that are not located in any particular time or space, such as a song, a poem, the coding for computer software, a play, a formula, or any intangible invention. These kinds of intangible things that we claim to own are known as IP (Foster and Shook 1993). In general, property rights are collections of rights to control something, such as a house. Someone who owns a house has a right to sell, rent, modify, paint, use, or tear down the house. People who have IP have rights to control

Nothing in this chapter should be taken as legal advice. Engaging an IP attorney is recommended in the event of contemplating issues related to patents, copyrights, or trademarks.

intangible objects that are products of human intellect (Garner 1999). For instance, if you own the copyright to a play, you are granted the right to prevent other people from performing the play without your permission. You also have the right to sell your copyright on the play.

Modern property right laws have their basis in Roman laws, which influenced the development of legal systems in Europe and the United States. Nations recognized property before the advent of the Roman Empire—Jewish laws dating to the time of Moses's address regarding property issues, for example—but the Romans developed what was at that time the world's most comprehensive and precise legal system. The U.S. Constitution draws heavily on the property rights theories of the 18th-century English philosopher John Locke.

Although the Western world has recognized property for thousands of years, IP is a more recent development. While ancient Greek and Roman authors and inventors were concerned about receiving proper credit for their discoveries, the Greeks and Romans did not have IP laws per se. Although the origins of patents are obscure, some of the world's first patents were granted in England in the 1400s when the monarchy granted privileges, known as letters patent, to manufacturers and traders. King Henry VI granted the first known English patent in 1449 to John of Utynam for a method of making stained glass. During the next 200 years, patents became a routine part of commerce and industry in England, although disputes arose concerning the length of the patent period and the conditions for patenting (Foster and Shook 1993).

The steam engine (1769) was probably the single most important patent awarded by the British government. This invention helped to provide additional justification for patents and served as a model of science–industry collaboration. James Watt (1736–1819) developed a more efficient version of the steam engine, which had been developed by Thomas Newcomen and Thomas Savery. He was awarded a patent in 1769 titled "A New Method of Lessening the Consumption of Steam and Fuel in Fire Engines." Watt collaborated with the entrepreneurs John Roebuck and Matthew Boulton. Roebuck made two-thirds of the initial investment required to develop the steam engine but went bankrupt. Boulton acquired Roebuck's share of the patent. Watt's steam engine was useful in draining mines and later was used for machinery in factories. Watt and Boulton made large profits by selling the steam engine. The product was the outcome of creativity coupled with private investment and marketing (Burke 1995).

The need for copyright coincides with the development of the printing press in the 1500s. Before the printing press, copying of books and author's writings was rare, and most people were illiterate. Books and other documents were copied laboriously by hand in Europe. Because it took so much effort to copy a book, the problem of unauthorized copies did not arise often. After the printing press was invented, it was possible to make thousands of copies with relative ease, and literacy increased. The question naturally arose as to who would control the making and selling of these copies and also whether "unauthorized" copies would be allowed. Thus, the idea of a "copyright" was developed in 18th-century England as a way of giving authors and publishers some control over printed works. In 1710, the English Parliament passed a statute granting copyright protection to books and other writings. Prior to this statute, copyrights were protected by common law (Miller and Davis 2011).

The first U.S. patent was awarded in 1641 to the Massachusetts Bay Colony for the production of salt. The framers of the U.S. Constitution were aware of the scientific and technical developments that were occurring before their eyes and the need to grant IP rights to authors and inventors to encourage the advancement of science, technology, industry, and the practical arts. One of the primary authors of the Constitution, Thomas Jefferson, was himself an author and inventor. Benjamin Franklin, who helped draft the Constitution and the Declaration of Independence, was both a statesman and a prolific inventor whose inventions included the harmonica and the lightning rod. Given their familiarity with science and technology and their appreciation of the importance of free enterprise and commerce, it should come as no surprise that the founding fathers included a provision about IP rights in the U.S. Constitution. Article 1, Section 8, provides the basis for IP laws in the United States when it states that Congress shall have the power "to promote the progress of science and useful arts, by securing for limited times to authors and inventors the exclusive right to their respective writings and discoveries." In 1790, Congress enacted the first patent and copyright laws, long before the U.S. Patent and Trademark Office was officially established in 1836. The patent laws have been amended numerous times (Miller and Davis 2011). Congress also enacted laws establishing the U.S. Copyright Office. These laws have also been revised several times, with the most significant revision occurring in 1976 (Miller and Davis 2011).

During the 1800s, science–industry and government–industry collaborations continued to bear fruit (see the discussion in chapter 5). By the end of the century, many companies had their own laboratories and employed scientists, engineers, and technicians. The great master of invention, Thomas Edison, obtained thousands of patents from his private laboratory in Menlo Park, New Jersey, including those for the electric light bulb (1879), the phonograph (1877), the stock ticker, and the duplex repeating telegraph (Burke 1995). In the 20th century, many new science–industry and government–industry collaborations produced more inventions and discoveries, such as the automobile, the airplane, plastics, synthetic fabrics, and computers. In most of these cases, governments funded the basic research that laid the foundations for practical applications and commercial products (Dickson 1995).

There are some international treaties pertaining to IP. The first international IP treaty was the Paris Convention of 1883, which was adopted by 20 countries initially and has been adopted by many others since then. Other important IP treaties include the Agreement on Trade-Related Aspects of IP Rights (TRIPS), which was signed by 120 countries in 1994. Although a patent or a copyright grants legal protection only in the country in which it is issued, nations that abide by international IP treaties agree to honor each other's IP laws. For example, a nation that abides by TRIPS does not allow the importation of pirated software or unauthorized generic drugs. However, TRIPS allows for some compulsory licensing to address public safety or public health crises (WTO, 2007). For example, a nation facing a devastating epidemic such as HIV/AIDS could use the compulsory licensing provisions of TRIPS to require a pharmaceutical company to license another company to manufacture HIV/AIDS medications.

As one can see from this brief history, the main rationale that people have offered for IP protection is utilitarian: IP laws promote social welfare by encouraging ingenuity and progress in science, technology, and the arts (Kuflik 1989). They encourage ingenuity and progress because they provide authors and inventors with economic incentives to produce original works and inventions and to share the products of their labor with the public. Without such protections, authors and inventors may decide to not pursue their original works or inventions or to keep them a secret (Foster and Shook 1993). When an inventor is granted a patent, the patent application becomes a public record, which enables other scientists and inventors to learn from the invention. This allows researchers to share information while also granting them IP rights. The IP laws also protect the financial interests of businesses and therefore encourage businesses to invest in research and development (R&D). Businesses view R&D funding as risks that can be justified only if there is some expectation of a reasonable return on investment. IP laws enable businesses to take these risks by allowing them to control the products of their R&D investments (Resnik, 2007; Kuflik 1989).

Another type of justification for IP comes directly from the work of John Locke (1764 [1980]), who was a strong defender of individual rights (i.e., a libertarian). According to Locke, all human beings have some inalienable rights relating to life, liberty, and property. The main function of government is to protect these rights and prevent citizens from violating each other's rights. We can acquire property, according to Locke, through original acquisition or transfer, such as through commercial transactions or gifts. Original acquisition of property occurs when one mixes or adds one's labor to a thing or common resource. For example, if we view the forest as a common resource, if I remove a piece of wood from the forest and carve it into a flute, then the flute becomes my property because I have added my labor to the wood. This libertarian approach implies that laws can be crafted to protect IP rights and that people can acquire IP through original acquisition or transfer. For example, one might acquire a new invention (e.g., a better mousetrap) by adding one's labor to previous ideas and inventions (e.g., the old mousetraps). One could acquire property rights to a song by using or putting together melodies, words, and harmonies from previous songs to make a new one (Kuflik 1989).

Regardless of whether one adopts a utilitarian or a libertarian approach to IP, the most basic theoretical issue with respect to IP rights is finding the proper balance between public and private control of IP (Resnik 2007). Most theorists agree that some form of private ownership is necessary in order to provide rewards and incentives to individuals and corporations, and most theorists agree that a public domain of information is needed to ensure that people have freely available resources to create new inventions and make new discoveries. But finding the proper balance between public and private control is not always easy, and that balance may change as new technologies, such as computers and recombinant DNA, emerge, and social institutions, such as corporations and universities, evolve. This is one reason that it is necessary to reevaluate and revise IP laws as the situation warrants.

TYPES OF INTELLECTUAL PROPERTY

Patents

Under U.S. law, a patent is a type of IP granted by the U.S. Patent and Trademark Office to an inventor. A patent gives inventors exclusive rights to prevent anyone else from using, making, or commercializing their inventions without the permission of the inventors. Inventions may include machines, products of manufacture, methods or techniques, compositions of matter, or improvements on any of these. Individuals as well as corporations or the government can own patents. The length of a patent is 20 years from the filing date of the patent application (Kayton 1995). Patents are not renewable. Inventors can sell their patent rights, or they can grant others a license to use, make, or commercialize their inventions. In exchange for the licenses, the licensee may provide the licensor with royalties in the form of a one-time payment or a percentage of profits. An exclusive license is a license between the licensor and only one licensee. A nonexclusive license allows the licensor to license the invention to more than one licensee. Different companies often reach agreements allowing them to use, make, or commercialize each other's inventions, known as cross-licensing agreements and reach-through licensing agreements. These agreements enable companies to avoid costly and time-consuming patent infringement litigation.

Patent infringement occurs when someone makes, uses, or commercializes a patented invention without permission from the patent holder. If someone infringes a patent, the inventor can file an infringement claim with any U.S. federal court (Foster and Shook 1993). The patent holder can sue the infringing party for damages and obtain an injunction requiring the infringing party to cease infringement. The party accused of infringement may challenge the patent, and the court will determine whether the patent is valid. Because all appeals in patent cases go to the same federal court, the Court of Appeals for the Federal Circuit in Washington, D.C., patent laws are uniform throughout the United States. Appeals of cases heard at this court, such as *Diamond v. Chakrabarty* (1980) (discussed below), are heard by the Supreme Court.

Research (or experimental) use is a narrow provision in patent law that allows a researcher to make or use an invention for research purposes but not for commercial purposes. For many years, academic researchers believed that they were protected from patent infringement under the research use exemption in patent law. However, an important decision made in a legal case, *Madey v. Duke University* (2002), has limited the research use. In this case, the Court of Appeals for the Federal Circuit ruled that Duke University had infringed John Madey's patent on a laser by using the device without his permission. Duke University argued that its researchers could use the laser under the research use exemption, but the court ruled that the university could not claim this exemption because it was using the laser to further its business interests. The court treated the university as similar to a private company. Because most scientists work for either universities or private companies, Madey effectively ended the research exemption in the United States.

To obtain a U.S. patent, the inventor must file an application with the U.S. Patent and Trademark Office. In deciding whether to award a patent, the office considers the following criteria (Foster and Shook 1993; Miller and Davis 2011):

1. Novelty: The invention must be new or innovative. It must not be previously patented or disclosed in the prior art, which includes patents, publications, or public uses. Because publication or public disclosure of an invention can jeopardize the patent, most inventors keep their patentable work secret until they are ready to file an application. In the United States and most other countries, the first person to file a patent application is awarded the patent.
2. Nonobviousness: The invention must not be obvious to a person trained in the relevant discipline or technical field. Whether an invention is or is not "obvious" is subject to a great deal of debate (Duft 1993).
3. Usefulness: The invention must serve some worthwhile practical use. "Trivial" uses, such as filling a landfill or a subject of meditation, do not count as practical uses, nor do uses as research tools. For instance, the U.S. Patent and Trademark Office has recently ruled that basic genome sequence data are not patentable; DNA patents must specify specific uses for DNA in drug development, diagnostics, or bioengineering (Resnik 2004a). If the invention has a military use or implications for national security, the U.S. government has the right to co-opt the invention and compensate the inventor, who may also sign a contract with the government.
4. Enabling description: Inventors must reduce their inventions to practice; that is, they must describe the invention in enough detail so that someone trained in the relevant discipline or field could make and use the invention. This description of the patent becomes a public document and is part of the patenting "bargain."
5. Patentable subject matter: The invention must be the type of thing that can be legally patented. The courts have ruled that natural phenomena, laws of nature, and abstract ideas cannot be patented (Miller and Davis 2011). Deciding whether something is or is not patentable has proven to be very controversial in some cases (see the discussion below).

Although the patent system encourages public disclosure in exchange for IP rights, some corporations use the system not to develop new inventions but to prevent competing companies from developing new inventions (Resnik 2004a). For example, to secure the market for their trademarked drugs, large pharmaceutical companies have purchased patents on competing generic drugs owned by smaller companies. Other companies have developed "blocking" patents designed to prevent competitors from developing new products. For example, if a company is developing a new internal combustion engine, a competing company could block production of this engine by acquiring a patent on a part that is needed to make the engine.

Copyrights

Copyrights are exclusive rights granted by the U.S. legal system that allow the authors of original works to make copies of the work, make other works derived from the original work, perform or display the work, and distribute, sell, or rent copies of the work. People who perform any of these actions without the permission of copyright holders violate copyrights. Original works include written works, such as books, papers, software, databases, and poems; performances, such as plays or dances; audiovisual recordings, such as movies, music, photographs, and television shows; and artistic works, such as paintings and sculpture. A work can be original without being new or novel because the author is the first person to put the work into tangible form. A copyright extends for the lifetime of the author(s) plus 70 years, and it may be renewed. To register copyright, one may file for a copyright with the U.S. Copyright Office at the Library of Congress. However, authors of original works have copyright protections even if they do not take this step. To ensure that others are aware of their claims to a copyright, many copyright holders write "copyright" on their original works, such as "Copyright © 2014 Shamoo and Resnik, all rights reserved." Copyrights protect original works but not the ideas expressed by those works (Chickering and Hartman 1980; Office of Technology Assessment 1990). Although it is illegal to sell copies of the book *Jurassic Park* without permission of the copyright holder, it is perfectly legal to discuss (or profit from) the ideas expressed in the book without the owner's permission.

Many copyright holders sell their rights to publishers or other distributors for a one-time fee or a percentage of profits. A work produced by an employee of a business is considered a "work for hire," so the copyright belongs to the business, unless the business grants the employee some portion of the copyright as part of contract negotiations. For example, most academic institutions allow faculty members to retain copyrights over their works. In some instances, universities or colleges may seek copyrights to special, commissioned works, such as Internet courses or educational software. Works created by U.S. government employees as part of their official duties are considered to be in the public domain, and the employees have no copyrights pertaining to such works.

One important exception to copyright law is the doctrine of fair use. According to this doctrine, it is permissible to copy portions of the author's work or even the whole work, without his or her permission if the copying is for personal, educational, or research purposes and does not jeopardize the commercial value of the work (Miller and Davis 2011). For example, the doctrine of fair use allows a person to use a device to record a television show to watch later, but it does not allow a person to use a device to make or sell copies of the television show for a large audience. During the 1980s, the copying company Kinko's compiled, copied, and sold course packets—selections of readings from journals or books—for professors teaching university or college courses. Publishing companies sued Kinko's for copyright violations, and the courts ruled in their favor in 1991 (*Basic Books, Inc. v. Kinko's Graphics Corp.*). Even though the use was for an educational purpose, it was not a fair use because it defrayed the commercial value of the published works. The dispute over the legality of the Napster website illustrates the continuing evolution of the doctrine of fair use. Many companies from the recording industry sued Napster for copyright violation because the company was distributing copyrighted music over the Internet without permission. Also note that many types of knowledge, such as government documents, public records, weight conversion tables, temperature measures, calendars, known titles, phrases, and lists of ingredients, are considered to be in the public domain and are not copyrighted (Chickering and Hartman 1980).

Trademarks

A trademark is a distinctive symbol or mark, such as a name, phrase, device, stamp, logo, or figure, that businesses use to distinguish themselves. Some examples of trademarks include the name "Coca-Cola," the phrase "have it your way," the McDonald's arches, the Hot Wheels® flame logo, and the Planter's peanut man. Trademarks are useful to businesses for marketing their goods and services, because they provide consumers with a way to easily recognize the business and its products. Trademarks are protected by state and federal laws and are important in commerce, but they play only a minimal role in research. To obtain federal trademark protection, a business may submit an application to the U.S. Patent and Trademark Office. Trademarks are renewable indefinitely for 10-year periods (Miller and Davis 2011).

Trade Secrets

The forms of IP discussed above—patents, copyrights, and trademarks— are rights granted by the government designed to promote the dissemination of information while protecting proprietary interests. The key policy issue in these forms of IP is finding the proper balance of public and private control of information. Trade secrets, on the other hand, are designed to prevent information from becoming publicly available. The law recognizes trade secrets because they promote the interests of commerce and industry and can be more useful than other forms of IP for some businesses (Foster and Shook 1993). For example, consider the formula for Coca-Cola, one of the best-guarded trade secrets. If the company had patented its formula for the product, then the patent would have expired decades ago and the company would have lost its share of the market for this product. As far as the company is concerned, it can make more money by keeping the formula a secret instead of patenting it. The company can do this because the secret is well guarded and difficult to discover. Although many companies have manufactured products that taste similar to Coca-Cola, no company has manufactured a product that tastes just like "the real thing" because it is difficult to master all the subtle variations in ingredients and manufacturing processes that the company employs. Other types of trade secrets may include other formulas, instruments, business plans, customer lists, and company policies. State laws protect trade secrets provided that the company makes an attempt to keep the secret and the secret has commercial value. Someone who discloses a trade secret to a competing business can be prosecuted under civil liability or for theft and can be fined up to and exceeding the monetary value of the secret.

One problem with trade secrets is that they are difficult to protect. First, employees may disclose trade secrets either intentionally or inadvertently. Second, there are legal methods that competitors can use to discover trade secrets, such as reverse engineering. It is perfectly legal for another company to "reverse engineer" Coca-Cola by purchasing some of the product and analyzing it to determine how it is produced. Trade secrets are not protected if they are derived from independent research, open meetings, and a host of other methods. In the biotechnology industry, it is virtually impossible to keep trade secrets due to the open nature of biotechnology R&D. Most of the materials used in biotechnology are available to the public, such as organic compounds, organisms, common tools, and techniques. Thus, in biotechnology and pharmaceuticals, patents are generally a better form of IP protection than are trade secrets (Adler 1993; Office of Technology Assessment 1990; Resnik 2004a).

Data Ownership

Individuals, corporations, universities, and government agencies often assert ownership claims over data. For example, private companies claim to own all the data produced in their laboratories or using their funds. Universities also claim to own data generated by means of university funds or resources. People claim to own research data mainly to protect their financial interests. Suppose a researcher does animal toxicology studies on a drug that a pharmaceutical company is developing. She has a contract with the company and is employed by a university. Suppose a dispute arises over publishing the data: The researcher wants to publish but the company objects to publication. Who owns the data: the researcher, the company, or the university? Or suppose a researcher obtains data at a university through a government grant and then leaves the position for a job at another institution—can he take data with him, or must it remain at the university? If questions such as these are not resolved upfront by means of contracts or agreements, such as Cooperative Research and Development Agreements (CRADAs) or material transfer agreement (MTAs), then costly legal battles may arise concerning the control of data and IP (Shamoo 1989; Shamoo and Teaf 1990).

There is certainly a sense in which one might view data as property, but there are no laws designed specifically to protect data. To treat data as property, one must therefore apply existing copyright, patent, trade secrecy, or property, contract, criminal, or civil laws to research data or enact specific institutional policies. For example, an employee's contract with a university or private company can settle data ownership issues. If the employee discloses or uses data without permission, the university or private company can sue the employee for breach of contract. Similarly, trade secrecy laws can permit companies to prevent employees from disclosing data. Research records, such as lab notebooks or computer disks, are physical objects that can be protected by property laws. Someone who takes a lab notebook from an institution without permission can be charged with theft. Trade secrecy laws can provide companies with some ownership of data, provided that the data are properly protected trade secrets. For example, tobacco companies sought for many years to protect their research on nicotine's addictive properties under the cloak of trade secrecy (Hurt and Robertson 1998; Resnik 1998b).

In the private sector, data are treated as "propriety information." The data submitted by private companies in support of a drug application to the U.S. Food and Drug Administration (FDA) are not all made public, even after the drug has been approved. Although U.S. law protects this type of information, researchers may still face an ethical dilemma in situations where promoting the good of society requires them to break the law. For example, a scientist conducting secret research for a drug company who discovers a problem with the medication, which the company does not want to report to the FDA, must choose between abiding by the company's policies and serving the public good (Resnik 1998b).

Some laws and regulations require researchers receiving government funds to share data. Under the 2002 Freedom of Information Act amendments, data generated by the use of government funds are public property. Interested parties can request research data once a researcher has completed a study by contacting the appropriate agency of the U.S. government. The agency will gather the information and may charge a reasonable fee for its services. However, the public cannot gain access to some types of data, such as confidential information pertaining to human subjects or patients, proprietary business information, classified information, information used in law enforcement, or personnel records (Cohen and Hahn 1999; Fields and Price 1993; Freedom of Information Act 2002). According to the National Institutes of Health (NIH) policy on data sharing, NIH-funded researchers are required to share published research data with qualified scientists. Researchers may charge a reasonable fee for the costs of sharing data with interested parties (National Institutes of Health 2003).

OTHER TYPES OF PROPERTY IN SCIENCE

In addition to IP, many other different types of property are related to scientific research, including the following:

- Research materials, such as pharmaceuticals, reagents, cell lines, antibodies, genetically engineered organisms, fossils, and blood samples
- Research tools, such as microscopes, telescopes, mass spectrometers, satellites, assays, computers, satellites, and test tubes
- Research venues, such as laboratories, greenhouses, archaeological sites, jungles, reefs, and lecture halls

Ethical and legal issues can arise concerning the stewardship of these resources. One might argue that scientists have an ethical obligation to share these resources so that other researchers may benefit from them. However, some reasons that scientists may refuse to share research resources include the following:

- Financial interests: Researchers and research sponsors may have financial interests related to research materials, tools, or venues. Sharing these resources adversely affects those interests.

- Scientific priority: A researcher who shares research materials, tools, or venues may give an edge to his competitors and lose the race for priority.
- Cost and inconvenience: Sharing research materials and tools can be costly and inconvenient. Researchers may not want to maintain stockpiles of materials for others to use or ship them out upon request.
- Scarcity: Some research materials and tools are scarce resources. Researchers may want to limit their sharing to preserve resources for their own work.

The sharing of research resources, therefore, raises many of the same issues that arise in data sharing (see the discussion in chapter 3). Deciding whether, and how, to share resources used in research requires a careful examination of the facts, circumstances, and options pertaining to the decision. Given the importance of sharing information and resources in science, the burden of proof falls on those who refuse to honor legitimate requests to share. Many government agencies require researchers to share not only data but also materials that have been developed or purchased with public funds. Grant applications may include plans for sharing research materials. Researchers may charge a reasonable fee for sharing, or they may license private companies to help them answer requests to share materials. Obligations to share materials need not undermine researchers' plans to publish or patent.

ADDITIONAL ETHICAL CONCERNS

Before concluding this chapter, we return to some more fundamental issues in IP. This first issue is the question of who has an ethically defensible claim to ownership of IP; the second is the question of what ethically can be treated as IP. Here we are not concerned with what the law says about IP, but with what the law should say.

WHO HAS INTELLECTUAL PROPERTY RIGHTS?

Consider an invention or an original work. Many different individuals and institutions may assert ownership claims over an invention, such as a transgenic mouse, or an original work, such as computer software. Who should be granted patent rights on the mouse or copyrights on the software? In many ways, this question parallels questions about authorship discussed in chapter 6, where we argue that authorship and accountability should go hand in hand: An author is someone who makes an important contribution and can be held publicly accountable for the research. If all authors have copyrights, then the question of who should have copyrights is the same as the question of who should be an author. One may argue that the same point applies to patent rights: An inventor, like an author, is someone who makes an important contribution to the invention and can be held accountable for the invention. That is, the inventor could describe the invention, explain how it works and what it does, and show how it is useful and original (Dreyfuss 2000). Interestingly, an invention often has more authors listed in the paper describing it than it has inventors listed on the patent application (Ducor 2000). One might speculate that in these cases people are being listed as authors who do not deserve to be or people are not listed as inventors who deserve to be.

Although relying on some principle of accountability may settle many concerns about IP rights, it does not address the role of "contributors" and any morally legitimate claims they may make to IP. Because contributors do not, by definition, play a significant role in research, most of the IP claims made by contributors relate to concerns about fairness, not about accountability. Consider the following examples:

- A lab technician carries out a great deal of the work in developing a patented mouse and is listed as an author on the paper but not as an inventor on the patent. Should the technician have any patent rights? If she has no patent rights, then should she not be listed as an author on the paper?
- A medicine man in the Amazon jungle teaches a team of botanists and pharmacologists about some of the healing powers of a native plant, and they develop a new drug by isolating and purifying a compound in the plant. Should the medicine man (or perhaps his community) be granted some share of royalties from the patent?
- An oncologist develops a valuable cancer cell line from cancerous tissue extracted from a patient's tumor. Should the cancer patient have IP rights over commercial products from his tissue? (This example is based on the famous *Moore v. Regents of the University of California* [1990]; see Case 1 below.)
- A graphic artist develops images for a textbook and is listed as a contributor but not as an author. Should she be granted a share of copyright on the book?

Questions about "fairness" raise fundamental issues about how to allocate benefits and burdens. According to the libertarian approach exemplified by

Locke, fairness is strictly a matter of contribution or merit: If you contribute something to a project, then your fair share (i.e., your benefits) should be in proportion to your contribution. According to the utilitarian approach, what is fair is what best promotes society's good, and IP principles and laws should promote the social good. Thus, it may follow, on this view, that it is fair not to allocate benefits, such as royalties, on the basis of contribution. The best way to maximize utility may be a system that rewards authors and inventors who are the first to create an original work or invention.

WHAT CAN BE TREATED AS INTELLECTUAL PROPERTY?

The final issue we consider in this chapter concerns the ethical or moral limitations on IP. Are there some things that should not be treated as IP? In recent years, many biological materials have been treated as IP that were previously viewed as belonging in the public domain, such as genetically engineered organisms, cell lines, genes, and proteins, all of which biotechnology or pharmaceutical companies have now patented. Many people find the idea of "owning" products of nature to be morally or even religiously offensive or at least not in the best interests of science, medicine, and technology. For example, James Thomson of the University of Wisconsin and the University of Wisconsin Research Foundation came under attack from many prominent stem cell researchers for patenting human embryonic stem cells (Holden 2007), and researchers and laypeople have objected to patents on human genes since the mid-1990s (Resnik 2004a). Other controversial types of patents include patents on computer software, business plans, and medical diagnostic tests.

In thinking about these controversial cases, the courts, patent offices, and policymakers have wrestled with two distinctions: (1) products of nature (not patentable) vs. products of human ingenuity (patentable); (2) abstract ideas and natural laws (not patentable) vs. methods and techniques (patentable). To delineate the domain of the patentable, patent agencies and the courts have struggled to find the right balance between private control over IP and public access research.

U.S. courts have ruled that natural phenomena and naturally occurring species are products of nature and cannot be patented. In a landmark case for the biotechnology industry, *Diamond v. Chakrabarty* (1980), the Supreme Court ruled that living things could be patented. The Court referred to an earlier patent case, *Funk Brothers Seed Co. v. Kalo Inoculant Co.* (1948), and stated that "anything under the sun made by man" is a human invention. Ananda M. Chakrabarty had filed a patent claim on a genetically modified bacterium useful in cleaning up oil spills. Prior to this case, the only living things that could be patented were hybrid species of plants protected by special plant patenting laws, such as the Plant Variety Protection Act of 1930 (9 USC 2321). A lower court had rejected the patent on the grounds that the genetically modified bacteria were not human inventions, but the Supreme Court negated this decision. This Court decision helped pave the way for patenting many products of biotechnology, including genes, proteins, cell lines, and genetically modified organisms (Eisenberg 1995; Resnik 2004a).

Recently, the U.S. Supreme Court made an important ruling that helped clarify the realm of patentability in biotechnology. The case involved Myriad Genetics' patents on BRCA1 and BRCA2 genes, mutations of which significantly increase the risk of breast and ovarian cancer. The company patented isolated and purified BRCA1/BRCA2 DNA sequences as well as methods for testing for BRCA1/BRCA2 mutations. Some of these methods involved comparing DNA sequences in a patient to mutated forms of the BRCA1/BRCA2. Patient advocacy groups and scientists sued Myriad, claiming that its patents on genes and genetic diagnostic testing methods were invalid. In 2010, a federal court ruled that all of Myriad's patents were invalid. In 2011, an appeals court ruled that Myriad's gene patents were valid but that some of its method patents were not because they were patents on laws of nature. The case went to the U.S. Supreme Court, which upheld the lower court's ruling that some of the methods patents were invalid but reversed its ruling that the gene patents were valid (Kesselheim et al. 2013). In a 9–0 opinion issued on June 2013, the Supreme Court declared that patents on naturally occurring DNA sequences are not valid. The court distinguished between naturally occurring DNA sequences, which are products of nature and not patentable, and modified DNA sequences, which are products of human ingenuity and are patentable. It held that Myriad's gene patents were invalid because they did not involve any significant alteration of the naturally occurring DNA sequences. Patents on complementary DNA (cDNA), which has been synthesized from a messenger RNA template and has had noncoding sequences removed, are valid because cDNA is a product of human ingenuity (*Association for Molecular Pathology et al v. Myriad Genetics* 2013).

Prior to the decision in the Myriad case, the U.S. patent office had granted thousands of patents on isolated and purified DNA sequences because it treated these as similar to patents on isolated and purified chemical compounds found in nature, such as erythropoietin and immune system proteins, which were held to be valid. The thinking that guided agency decisions was that isolated and purified compounds are products of human ingenuity because these chemicals do not occur naturally: They only occur in the context of many other compounds found in nature, such as chemicals in the cytoplasm, cell membrane, cellular organelles, blood, and so on. Myriad's patents described genomic sequence data, not chemical formulas, so they may not be quite the same as patents on chemicals. As a result of the *Myriad* decision, many U.S. patents on genomic sequence data may now be invalid. It remains to be seen whether courts outside of the United States will follow the line of reasoning in *Myriad* and whether the case will have implications for patents on other isolated and purified chemicals found in nature or other isolated and purified biological entities, such as stem cells or antibodies (Kesselheim 2013). If litigants are able to use the Myriad case to mount successful challenges to other isolated and purified chemicals or biological entities, this could have negative impacts on the biotechnology and pharmaceutical industries. Nevertheless, the *Myriad* litigation was a victory for those who hold that patenting naturally occurring DNA sequence information is morally repugnant.

Myriad's methods patents involved the distinction between practical methods and abstract ideas (such as mathematical algorithms) or natural laws ($E = MC^2$). Lower courts had held that one of Myriad's methods patents was invalid because it did little more than restate a natural law, and the Supreme Court allowed these rulings to stand (Kesselheim et al. 2013). The method was to determine breast cancer susceptibility by comparing the patient's DNA to BRCA1/BRCA2 mutations. The court held that this patent was invalid because it was simply restating the statistical association between breast cancer and BRCA1/BRCA2 mutations. This would be like patenting a method treating a disease (such as a heart attack) based on detecting metabolites in the blood (such as cardiac muscle proteins) (Kesselheim and Karlawish 2012). The reason that abstract ideas and natural laws have been regarded as unpatentable is that patents on these things would stifle scientific discovery, engineering, and medical practice. A practical application of an abstract idea or natural law can be patented, however. For example, a computer program that manages the operations of a factory is patentable but the mathematical algorithms used by the program are not (Miller and Davis 2011).

Questions concerning patentability are likely to continue to arise as scientists, engineers, and inventors make new discoveries and innovations. Because these questions involve the interpretation of laws and ethical and policy issues, they are likely to be controversial. Other ethical and social issues raised by patenting include the impact of patenting on access to essential medicines and diagnostic procedures; the role of patenting in the genetic engineering of plants and animals; the impact of patenting human body parts (genes, proteins, cell, etc.) on our respect for human dignity; and the effect of biotechnology patenting on our respect for nature. (For further discussion, see Chapman 1999; Resnik 2004a, 2007; and Nuffield Council 2002.)

QUESTIONS FOR DISCUSSION

1. Do you think that people have a right to IP?
2. Do you think that IP undermines free inquiry, openness, and the academic ethos?
3. How would utilitarians address IP issues? How does the utilitarian approach differ from libertarianism?
4. Is it unethical to copy software without the copyright owner's permission?
5. If you are familiar with the Napster case, do you think the company acted unethically?
6. Should pharmaceutical companies be allowed to charge whatever price the market will bear for patented drugs?
7. Should developing nations violate international IP agreements in order to make drugs affordable to patients with HIV/AIDS, dysentery, or malaria?
8. Do you have any objections to patenting DNA, cell lines, proteins, tissues, genetically modified plants or animals, or other biological materials?
9. Would you have any objections to a patent on a genetically modified human?
10. In some European countries, patents can be rejected because they violate public morals. Do you think this is a useful criterion for awarded patents? What are the possible advantages and disadvantages or applying a morality test to patents?

CASE STUDIES

CASE 1

John Moore went to the University of California, Los Angeles (UCLA), Medical Center in 1976 to receive treatment for a rare type of cancer known as hairy-cell leukemia. Moore's physician, Dr. David Golde, recommended that Moore have his spleen removed. After the surgery, Golde asked Moore to provide samples of blood, skin, bone marrow, and sperm, which required him to travel a considerable distance to make several visits to the UCLA Medical Center. Moore was led to believe that Golde needed the samples to monitor his health, but, in fact, the purpose of gathering the samples was to develop a cell line from Moore's cancerous tissue (Resnik 2004a). Golde was interested in growing this cell line because of its scientific and commercial value. The cell line had a mutation that caused it to overproduce lymphokines, which are proteins that help to regulate the immune system. The estimated market for the lymphokines was $3 billion. Golde signed an agreement with the University of California and several private companies to develop the cell line. Golde and his research assistant Shirley Quan applied for patents on the cell line. When the patents were awarded, they assigned them to the University of California (Resnik 2004a).

Moore eventually discovered the true purpose of his visits to the UCLA Medical Center and became very upset. He sued Golde, Quan, the private companies, and the university for violating informed consent, failing to uphold fiduciary obligations, and conversion (i.e., substantially interfering with another person's personal property). The case went to the California Supreme Court. The court ruled that Moore could not prove his conversion claim because he did not have a property interest in the cell line (*Moore v. Regents of the University of California* 1990). According to the majority opinion of the court, the researchers who isolated and cultured the cell line had property rights on the cell line because they had invested their time and labor in developing it. According to the majority, granting patients or research subjects property rights over their biological samples would interfere with biomedical research and innovation. Only inventors and companies should have property rights over biological materials left over from medical procedures or donated research. In separate dissenting opinions, two judges from the court argued that Moore should have property rights to the cell line because his cells are no different from other materials that are exchanged on the market, such as sperm or hair, and a person should be able to control his own body and its parts (*Moore v. Regents of the University of California* 1990). Although the court did not recognize Moore's property rights pertaining to the cell line, it did rule that Golde had violated his fiduciary obligation to Moore by not disclosing his financial interests in Moore's tissue as part of the informed consent process. One interesting legal (and ethical) question related to the Moore case is whether researchers who are not acting as health care providers have fiduciary obligations to research subjects. Another important question is whether researchers have an obligation to disclose financial interests to research subjects (Morreim 2005; Resnik 2004b). In a more recent case regarding who owns the patient's tissue sample, the federal court in Missouri similarly ruled that the tissue belonged to Washington University in St. Louis and to the patients, because the patients gave up their ownership rights when they donated tissue to the university (Kaiser 2006).

- Do you think that Moore was treated fairly?
- Should Moore have property rights pertaining to the patented cell lines developed from his tissue?
- Do you think patients give up their property rights to tissue when they donate it to research or no longer want it (e.g., it is left over from a surgical procedure)?
- Should Moore's doctors have told him about their financial interests?

CASE 2

A faculty member at a U.S. university met a very bright young postdoctoral fellow at a meeting in Germany. The postdoctoral fellow was working for a company in Germany and had a new chemical entity that could be developed into a product to prevent one type of urinary tract infection. Animal testing had already been conducted, with very promising results. The postdoc then came to the United States to work for the university faculty member, with support from the German company. The German company, through its subsidiary in the United States, submitted an investigational new drug application to the FDA in order to start Phase I clinical trials on humans. Later that year, a French company acquired the German company. In the meantime, the postdoctoral fellow met a colleague at a meeting at a different U.S. university and collaborated to test the new chemical entity. They discovered a new modality to treat another disease with the same chemical entity. At this time, the faculty member's U.S. university was negotiating with the French/German company to have the research conducted at the university's facilities. From the start, the French/German company demanded sole proprietorship of the drug and wanted to control all aspects of its R&D. The university then asked the postdoctoral fellow to sign a visiting fellowship agreement assigning all IP claims to the university. The postdoctoral fellow refused, on the advice of the French/German company. Meanwhile, the French/German company filed for a patent alone without any mention of the part of the work conducted at the university.

- What should the university do? What should the university faculty member do?
- Who owns the patent? Is the patent application valid?
- What should each party have done in the first place?

CASE 3

A university investigator is in hot pursuit of a project that received a medium-sized grant from the NIH. Her grant depends on the use of reagents from an independent company. She has had a long and fruitful relationship with the company—she has given several seminars at the company, and her counterpart in the company has given several seminars at the university. Also, the investigator has earned a few thousand dollars annually from the company through consulting. She has signed a consultancy agreement with the company without clearance from the university. Her agreement relinquishes all her IP rights regarding the subject of the consultancy to the company. The investigator asked the university to sign an MTA so that she could start using the reagents. The university refused because the MTA gave too many rights to IP to the company in exchange for the reagents. The university investigator was anxious to start her project and make progress so that she would be able to renew her grant. One day during her frequent seminars at the company, she was asked to sign the MTA, and she did.

- What should the university do?
- What should the faculty member do?
- What should the company do?

CASE 4

In the early 1990s, a university faculty member was collaborating with a Danish company in a joint venture on a compound with a view toward clinical trials within a year. The company had already submitted a patent application on a portion of the project. In written correspondence between the university faculty member and her counterpart at the Danish company, both pledged full cooperation without mentioning anything about IP. A year later, the Danish company enlisted a U.S. company to conduct certain experiments. The university and the Danish and U.S. companies all entered into negotiation regarding IP. The negotiations failed, and the university ordered the faculty member to stop any further collaboration.

- What should the faculty member do?
- What should the university do?
- What lessons are learned in this scenario?

CASE 5

A member of an NIH study section, while reviewing a grant proposal, realized she could do part of the proposed research faster and better with a method already available in her laboratory. Under normal conditions, she would not be conducting such research. After getting back to her laboratory, she gave the project to her most reliable postdoctoral fellow. One year later, they submitted a paper to a prestigious journal.

One of the reviewers was the investigator who wrote the original grant proposal. The original investigator has not yet published his paper on the subject because he has applied for a patent, which delayed his writing of the paper. The original investigator complained to the U.S. Office of Research Integrity.

- Is this plagiarism?
- What should Office of Research Integrity do?
- What should the reviewer do?
- Who should get the patent?

CASE 6

A National Science Foundation–funded anthropologist and his team from a university have discovered a human skeleton in a national forest in Montana. Carbon dating shows that the skeleton is around 10,000 years old. Further study of the skeleton will prove to be extremely useful in determining human migration to the North American continent. However, a group representing Native Americans is taking legal action to have the skeleton returned to their custody under the Native American Graves Protection and Repatriation Act. The Native Americans say that the skeleton is one of their ancestors and should not be the object of a scientific study.

- Who owns this skeleton?
- How should this dispute be settled?

CASE 7

A tissue collection and storage company has signed a contract with a hospital and medical school to collect human tissue that is left over from surgical procedures and laboratory tests for research purposes. The company plans to collect tissues from patients at the hospital. Patients will sign an informed consent form that gives the company exclusive rights to their tissue. Patients will receive $50 for their tissue. Once the tissue is donated, it will be placed in a tissue bank. All personal identifiers linking the tissue to the donor will be removed. The company expects to profit by charging access to its tissue database. It also plans to patent valuable cell lines and other products. The medical school will help with the tissue collection and receive a portion of the profits.

- Do you see any ethical problems with this proposal?

CASE 8

A private university has decided to treat all of its faculty members' academic writings as "works for hire." Under this arrangement, the private university will own all copyrights for faculty members' writings. Faculty members will receive a 50% percentage of royalties. The university will have the right to decide whether significant writings (such as papers or books) will be published and to negotiate terms with publishers.

- Do you have any concerns with the arrangement?
- Should academic writings be treated as "works for hire"?

CHAPTER 9

Conflicts of Interest and Scientific Objectivity

Researchers and research institutions have various financial, personal, and political interests that sometimes conflict with their professional, ethical, or legal obligations. These situations can create conflicts of interest or the appearance of conflicts of interest. This chapter discusses how conflicts of interest affect research, how they are defined, and how they should be managed. It also describes how government agencies, journals, and research institutions have responded to conflicts of interest in research and discusses some cases from science.

INTRODUCTION: THE JESSE GELSINGER CASE

In 1999, Jesse Gelsinger, an 18-year-old male with a genetic disease known as ornithine transcarbamylase (OT) deficiency, agreed to participate in a Phase I (first in humans) gene therapy study at the University of Pennsylvania. Gelsinger lacked a functional copy of a gene that codes for OT, a liver enzyme involved in protein metabolism. Many patients with this disease die in infancy, but Gelsinger was able to manage his illness by restricting his diet and taking drugs to help him remove protein metabolites from his body. The goal of the study was to transfer functional copies of the OT gene into Gelsinger's liver. Because this was a Phase I study, Gelsinger was not expected to benefit from the research, although there was a chance that he could. The investigators infused an adenovirus vector into Gelsinger's liver that carried copies of the gene. Shortly thereafter, Gelsinger developed a massive immune reaction and died. Subsequently, Gelsinger's family sued the university; the principal investigator of the study, James Wilson; and a private company,

Genovo, which sponsored gene therapy research on campus. The lawsuit was settled out of court for an undisclosed amount of money. The lawsuit alleged that Gelsinger was not properly informed of Wilson's or the university's financial interests in the research. Wilson and the university both owned stock in Genovo, and Wilson had 20 gene therapy methods patents, some of which had been transferred to the university. Wilson held a 30% equity interest in the company, which violated university policies that limited equity interests to 5%. Wilson had started the company several years before the study was initiated. The lawsuit also alleged that Gelsinger was not properly informed about animal studies that showed that the adenovirus could cause an immune reaction (Gelsinger and Shamoo 2008). Investigations by the Food and Drug Administration (FDA) and the Office of Human Research Protections found that informed consent was inadequate and that there were problems with adverse event reporting related to this study. The incident undermined the public's trust in biomedical research, set back the field of gene therapy, and led funding organizations and professional associations to revise their conflict-of-interest policies (Resnik 2007).

CONFLICTS OF INTEREST

The Gelsinger case illustrates, in stark terms, some of the ethical concerns related to conflicts of interest (COIs) in research. Individual scientists and research organizations daily encounter situations where personal, financial, political, and other interests conflict with professional, ethical, or legal obligations or duties. Although conflicts of all types are a normal part of human existence, some, known as COIs, involve conflicts between interests and duties. Most of the concern with COIs in research arises because financial or other interests can undermine duties relating to scientific objectivity and integrity (Resnik 2001b, 2007; Shamoo 1992, 1993). Consider some examples of situations that might be considered COIs in research:

- A clinical investigator with stock in a pharmaceutical company that sponsors his research overestimates the clinical significance of his research on one of the company's drugs, which drives up the price of his stock.
- An academic researcher on a National Institutes of Health (NIH) study section reviews a grant from a competitor in the same field.
- A medical journal runs an advertisement for a new drug.

- A clinical investigator receives $3,000 in patient-care costs from a company for each patient she recruits into a clinical trial even though it only costs on average $2,000 to care for patients in the study.
- A university's institutional review board (IRB) reviews a research proposal sponsored by a company that has recently given $10 million to the university.

In each of these situations, researchers have financial or other interests that may interfere with their ability or tendency to fulfill ethical or legal duties to colleagues, patients, sponsors, or the public. Another way of putting this is to say that these interests compromise the researchers' objectivity, integrity, or trustworthiness. There are two ways that COIs can undermine objectivity and integrity. First, a COI can affect a person's thought processes (i.e., judgment, perception, decision making, or reasoning) (Angell, 2001, 2004; Bradley 2000; Davis 1982; Krimsky 2003; Resnik 1998b, 2007; Shamoo 1993; Thompson 1993). In some of these cases we might say that the person's thought processes are biased; that is, they tend to be skewed in a particular pattern or direction that can be attributed to the particular interest. Second, a COI can affect motivation and behavior (Porter 1993; Resnik 1998b, 2007). A person with a COI may be perfectly capable of sound thinking but may fail to implement it due to temptations that affect his or her motivation and behavior. All people are tempted from time to time by a number of interests and desires, but the problem with COIs, one might argue, is that they place people in situations where only people with extraordinary characters will not succumb to temptation (Resnik 2007). There is a substantial body of literature demonstrating how COIs can undermine the objectivity of research, which we reviewed in chapter 5 (Angell 2004; Krimsky 2003; Resnik 2007).

Because COIs can undermine the objectivity and integrity of research, they can also have a negative impact on the trustworthiness of researchers. Throughout our book, we have emphasized the importance of trust and trustworthiness in research: Research subjects must trust investigators, students must trust mentors or supervisors, principal investigators must trust subordinates, and colleagues must trust each other. Researchers must trust journals, granting agencies, and research institutions. Society must also trust investigators to honor their ethical and legal obligations in conducting research. When investigators have COIs, people may suspect that their research is biased, unreliable, or morally tainted. Because personal, professional, political, or financial interests can threaten trustworthiness, it is incumbent upon the research community to address such concerns.

Putting all of this together, we offer the following definition of a COI for an individual:

> An individual has a conflict of interest when he or she has personal, financial, professional, political, or other interests that are likely to undermine his or her ability to fulfill his or her primary professional, ethical, or legal obligations.

In theory, it is fairly easy to define COIs, but in practice it is often difficult to determine whether people have COIs, because we may not know how their personal, financial, professional, or political interests are likely to affect their thought processes or behaviors. Many people with financial or other interests will acknowledge them but maintain that they have a great deal of integrity and will not allow their interests to undermine their ethical or legal responsibilities. How can we know which conflicts are likely to undermine a person's ability to meet his or her primary obligations? How much money does it take to influence reasoning, judgment, motivation, or behavior—$10,000? $5,000? $500? We cannot address these difficult practical issues adequately here, but we adopt a standard that we call the average person standard: A person has a COI when the average person under similar circumstances would be affected. Although some extraordinary people may be able to maintain their objectivity and integrity when faced with such circumstances, most people will succumb to biases or temptations.

Situations may arise where it is clear that the person does not have a COI, but it might appear to a reasonable outside observer that he or she does. The situation might create an issue related to trustworthiness even if it has little or no impact on integrity. Because trustworthiness is very important in research, situations that affect trustworthiness should be addressed, even when they are not likely to undermine integrity. Thus, it is important to distinguish between real and apparent (or perceived) COIs for individuals:

> An individual has an apparent conflict of interest when he or she has personal, financial, professional, political, or other interests that create the perception of a conflict to a reasonable outside observer.

As discussed elsewhere in this text, scientists frequently have ethical and legal responsibilities to other members of their profession, clients, patients, students, and society. Scientists also have personal, financial, or political interests that could interfere with their ability or tendency to fulfill these responsibilities. Many of these personal interests relate to career ambitions, such as the quest for reputation, fame, power, priority, funding, tenure, and promotion. These interests can affect scientific thinking or behavior. For example, a scientist who has stock options in a pharmaceutical company and is conducting research on that company's drugs has a responsibility to conduct objective research. However, her financial interests may prevent her (or appear to prevent her) from fulfilling that responsibility; she may conduct, or appear to conduct, research that is biased toward the company. Money or ambition can also interfere with a researcher's ability or tendency to promote the rights and welfare of human subjects. A researcher with strong financial or personal interests in recruiting human subjects for a clinical trial may overstate the benefits and understate the risks of the study to his patients, or he may take other steps to compromise the informed consent process (as appeared to occur in the Gelsinger case, described above). When professors are supported by funds from industrial sponsors, conflicts may affect duties to the research profession, patients, and students (Blumenthal 1995).

Because COIs can have such a great impact on scientific objectivity and integrity, they have been linked to fraud and misconduct. For example, due to pressures to obtain funding, a scientist might fabricate or falsify data in a grant application or paper (see discussion of the Poehlman case in chapter 2). Or perhaps a researcher working for a pharmaceutical company manipulates the data to make his results appear to be more statistically or clinically significant than they are. Indeed, money has played an important role in most of the cases of research misconduct (or alleged misconduct) discussed in chapter 2. However, having a COI is not, in itself, research misconduct: A COI is only a risk factor for misconduct (U.S. Congress 1990).

CONFLICTS OF COMMITMENT AND DUTY

It is important to distinguish between COIs and other types of conflicts that occur in research. Consider this example: A molecular biologist who is hired by a public university also consults with several private and public clients, including a biotechnology firm, a hospital, and the local health department. As a result, she often has a difficult time balancing her commitments to the university and to these other organizations. This is a type of situation known as a conflict of commitment (Resnik 1998b). Conflicts of commitment (COCs), unlike COIs, do not normally involve situations that compromise a person's objectivity or integrity. They primarily have to do with the prudent and responsible management of time and effort. People with COCs usually can manage their different commitments. However, if one cannot manage one's many different commitments, the responsible thing to do is to prioritize these commitments and eliminate some of them. Sometimes conflicts of commitments can lead to COIs. For example, a university scientist may become so involved with time-consuming consultations that her objectivity or integrity becomes compromised (Davis 1995a). To deal with COCs, most universities have policies that limit the amount of time and effort that professors may dedicate to outside consulting activities.

A conflict of duties is also not a COI (Davis 1982). For example, a doctor may have to decide between respecting a patient's confidentiality and protecting the public's health when a patient with HIV refuses to tell his spouse that he is infected. A researcher may face a conflict between the duty to share data and the duty to protect intellectual property or confidentiality (see the discussion in chapter 3). Although conflicts of duties can lead to COIs when the person in question also has an interest in meeting a specific duty, COIs are not the same as conflicts of duty. COIs involve the collision between personal interests and duties, not conflicts among duties.

DEALING WITH INDIVIDUAL CONFLICTS OF INTEREST

There are several ways to protect the objectivity, integrity, and trustworthiness research when dealing with COIs. One strategy that has been adopted by many institutions and organizations is known as disclosure (Bradley 2000; McCrary et al. 2000). Researchers should disclose COIs and apparent COIs to the relevant parties. A relevant party would be someone in a supervisory role that does not have a vested interest in the particular conflict situation, such as a department chair, section head, dean, journal editor, or grant review officer. Disclosure embodies the virtue of transparency because it puts conflicts out in the open and allows people to assess them. For example, if a researcher discloses a COI in a paper, scientists may pay more careful attention to the paper's methods, results, and interpretations. The paper may warrant additional scrutiny, though it is not automatically invalidated (Resnik 1998b; Resnik and Elliott 2013). Moreover, disclosure can promote trust because people are likely to be more suspicious and untrusting when they discover previously hidden conflicts that have not been disclosed upfront (Cho 1997).

Funding agencies, universities, scientific journals, and other organizations have adopted financial disclosure policies. For example, the NIH requires that funded investigators disclose financial interests (e.g., stock or consulting fees) in a given year that are greater than $5,000. The NIH also requires institutions that receive funding to adopt policies for disclosing and managing COIs (Department of Health and Human Services 2011). The National Science Foundation (NSF) and other funding agencies have similar rules. The FDA, which regulates medical products, cosmetics, and food additives, has COI rules for individuals who serve on its advisory committees. The rules prohibit committee members from having financial interests that have a direct and predictable effect related to the matters they are reviewing, unless the agency grants a waiver (Food and Drug Administration 2013). Most scientific journals now have rules that require authors to disclose sources of funding and financial relationships (Cooper et al. 2006; Krimsky 1996, 2003; Krimsky et al. 1996, 2003).

Disclosure alone may not always be a sufficient response to a COI, because it does nothing to contain or minimize potential adverse impacts of financial interests, and it may lull people into a false sense of security if they think that there is nothing to worry about since the interests have been revealed (Cech and Leonard 2001; Elliott 2008). A strategy that goes beyond mere disclosure, which has been adopted by many organizations, is known as management of conflicts (McCrary et al. 2000). According to this strategy, people with COIs should disclose them to the relevant parties, who consult with other people to develop strategies for controlling the interests at stake. For example, a university could form an independent committee to review research conducted by an investigator with a COI to make sure that research is being conducted properly.

Most research institutions have policies that require some form of disclosure of COIs, and many have methods for managing COIs (Cho et al. 2000). Fewer institutions make much use of a third strategy, known as avoidance/prohibition. In this strategy, which is frequently used in government, law, and medicine, organizations make rules that prohibit specific situations that create COIs. For example, government ethics rules prohibit employees from overseeing contracts with family members. Medical ethics codes prohibit kickbacks and self-referrals. The NIH has COI rules for its study sections that prohibit scientists from reviewing grant proposals from colleagues at the same institution, collaborators, or former students or supervisors (within five years). As mentioned earlier, the FDA also prohibits COIs among advisory board members. COI avoidance may also occur when a person chooses to remove (or "recuse") himself or herself from the situation that creates the conflict, for example, when a reviewer for a journal declines to review a paper because of a personal or professional relationship with the authors.

Like disclosure and management of conflicts, conflict avoidance can promote objectivity, integrity, and trustworthiness. Elliott (2008) argues in favor of more conflict avoidance in research because he believes that disclosure and conflicts management are insufficient to promote objectivity, integrity, and trustworthiness in research. However, conflict avoidance can sometimes lead to outcomes that are worse (from a utilitarian point of view) than the outcomes that result from nonavoidance. For example, suppose that a scientist submits a paper to a journal on a highly specialized topic and there are a limited number of people who are qualified to review that paper. If most of the potential reviewers have personal or professional relationships with the author (as is sometimes the case), it may be difficult to find unconflicted reviewers.

When dealing with a COI requires more than mere disclosure, how should one decide whether the COI should be avoided/prohibited or managed? Three factors can help guide these decisions:

1. The strength of the COI: How strong are the interests involved? How likely are they to affect thought processes or behavior? If the COI is very strong, perhaps it should be prohibited.
2. The difficulty of managing the COI: How difficult is the COI to manage? Is there an appropriate mechanism or process for managing it? Could one be created? Are there sufficient financial and human resources to manage the COI? Difficulty in managing a COI also favors prohibition.
3. The consequences of prohibiting or not prohibiting the COI: What will happen if the COI is prohibited? Will prohibition have a negative impact on science or society? What will happen if the COI is not prohibited? Will this have a negative impact on science or society? Will this create a public perception problem? A COI might be permitted if the overall good/bad consequences of allowing the COI are likely to be greater than the good/bad consequences of prohibiting it.

INSTITUTIONAL CONFLICTS OF INTEREST

It is important to realize that organizations or institutions can also have COIs. Consider the following situations:

- A television network decides to not broadcast a story that is unfavorable to a company because that company threatens to stop advertising on the network.
- A medical society endorses a medical product made by a company that donates a great deal of money to the society.
- A university's IRB approves a human research proposal over the objections of several members because a failure to approve the proposal could threaten a $10 million grant.
- A university disciplines a faculty member for speaking out on an environmental issue because several state legislators want him punished.
- A university is trying to silence a faculty member because he spoke against research conducted on his campus that in his opinion is unethical.
- A university president owns stock in a company that sponsors research on campus and has made large gifts to the university.
- A wealthy CEO for a media company wants to donate $50 million to the journalism school. In return, he wants the school named after him and to have some input into the school's curriculum.

These examples illustrate how institutions, including research institutions, government agencies, professional associations, and journals, can also have COIs and apparent COIs. These organizations, like individuals, often have collective duties to professionals, clients, students, patients, and the public. Their duties usually stem from their primary missions (or goals), such as research, education, and public service. Institutions, like individuals, may also have financial, political, or other interests that can adversely affect (or appear to affect) their ability to carry out these responsibilities. Although institutions do not "think," they do make collective decisions that result from the judgments, decisions, and actions of their members, and they carry out actions. These decisions and actions occur through the various components of the organization's management structure, such as faculty members, committees, advisory boards, deans, and vice presidents. Institutional COIs, like individual COIs, can also threaten the objectivity, integrity, or trustworthiness of research. Sometimes the financial or other interests of institutional leaders (such as department chairs, deans, vice presidents, or trustees) can create a COI for the institution because these interests may adversely impact institutional decision making (AAUP 2008; Association of Academic Health Centers 1994, 2001, 2002; Bradley 2000; Moses and Martin 2001). We define an institutional COI as follows:

An institution has a conflict of interest when financial, political, or other interests of the institution or its leaders are likely to undermine the institution's ability to fulfill professional, legal, ethical, or social responsibilities.

As with individual COIs, the same three strategies to protect research integrity may apply: disclosure, conflict management, and avoidance. For some organizations, it may be enough to simply disclose the conflict; for others, avoidance may be the best option.

The research community has just begun to think about how to deal with institutional COIs. In some ways, institutional COIs can pose more significant problems for research than individual COIs, because institutional COIs can exert systematic, widespread effects. For example, if a university has a COI resulting from its relationship with a private company, then this COI could affect many different faculty or research projects at the university. Another concern with institutional COIs is that they may be more difficult to manage or control than individual COIs, because often there is no independent body with the authority and willingness to deal with institutional COIs. At a university, a faculty member can disclose her interests to her department chair, who is independent from the faculty member and has the authority to make decisions pertaining to the faculty member. But who can oversee a university's COIs? While there may be some organizations with the oversight authority, such as the board of trustees, these outside authorities may be unwilling or unable to do anything to deal with these COIs. More important, institutional officials who do not take effective action serve as poor moral examples to thousands of members of the organization.

Some authors have suggested some specific strategies for dealing with institutional COIs (AAMC-AUP 2008; Moses and Martin 2001):

1. Build firewalls: An organization builds firewalls to prevent some parts of the organization from having an adverse impact on other parts. For example, a university could try to shield committees that oversee research, such as IRBs and institutional animal care and use committees (IACUCs), from parts of the university that deal with money, such as the contracts and grants office, the technology transfer office, or the development office. While this strategy sounds good in theory, it may not work in practice, because members of a university often know each other and know about the university's business. Subtle or not-so-subtle influences can still occur even when there is no direct line of authority between different parts (Resnik and Shamoo 2002). Moreover, it may not be a good idea to shield these different parts, because they often

need to communicate. For example, an IRB needs to communicate with the contracts and grants office when it is reviewing a research project sponsored by a federal agency or private company.

2. Manage investments and properties: An organization could take steps to manage its investments and properties to prevent inappropriate influences. For example, many universities have established separate, private foundations to hold stock and equity, invest in startup companies, and hold intellectual property. This is another approach that sounds good in theory, but it probably has little effect in practice because there are close connections between universities and their private foundations. The fact that a foundation associated with a university holds stock in a company, instead of the university, probably makes little difference to how decisions are made related to the company, or the public's perception of those decisions (Resnik and Shamoo 2002).

3. Require COI committees to also review institutional COIs: Many institutions have committees to review and deal with COIs disclosed by employees. Some authors have suggested that these committees could also deal with institutional COIs (AAMC-AUP 2008; Moses and Martin 2001). While we think this is also a good idea, there may be some problems with implementing it, because committees that review individual COIs may lack the independence to review institutional COIs. COI committees are usually composed of members of the institution and a few outside members. They are also supported by the institution and report to a leader at the institution (e.g., a vice president or president). We question whether these committees can give an adequate review of institutional COIs, given their composition, funding, and structure (Resnik and Shamoo 2002). A better strategy may be to form a committee at the level of the board of trustees that oversees institutional COIs, but this committee might face some difficulties if the trustees have COIs.

4. Establish policies and rules for institutional officials and other important employees or associates: An institution could establish different policies to prevent some types of COIs or minimize the effect of some COIs. For example, IRB or IACUC members with COIs could be prohibited from voting on or discussing submissions where they have a relationship to the research. Leaders of the institution, such as presidents, deans, or directors, could be prohibited from having some types of stock or equity. While it is a good idea to establish rules and policies to deal with institutional COIs, we wonder whether there will be sufficient interest in developing these, given the lack of independent oversight of institutions and lack of federal policy guidance in this area

(Shamoo 1999). A recent study (Ehringhause et al. 2008) indicates that only 38% of all medical schools have institutional COI policies. This survey indicates that most institutions have little interest in dealing with institutional COIs, while they continue to push for individual COI policies.

CONCLUDING REMARKS

Although we believe that it is important to respond appropriately to individual and institutional COIs, it is not possible (or even desirable) to avoid or prohibit all situations that create COIs or apparent COIs. Individuals and institutions have many different duties and interests. Only a hermit could avoid all COIs and apparent COIs. Because most institutions need private funding to continue to exist, it is also doubtful that they can avoid COIs or apparent COIs. Given the ubiquity of COIs and apparent COIs, the best response is to take appropriate steps to disclose or manage these situations and to sometimes avoid or prohibit them. Many situations in research that create COIs, such as collaborations with industry and intellectual property, also have important benefits (see the discussion in chapters 5 and 8).

COI policies should strike a reasonable balance between objectivity/integrity and freedom in the conduct of research. On the one hand, it is important to have rules that promote objectivity and integrity, because these rules help to ensure that research is scientifically sound, ethical, and trustworthy. On the other hand, excessive and highly strict rules can impede research by interfering with scientific creativity and innovation, undercutting financial rewards, or impeding collaborative work or the private funding of research. Additionally, COI policies should include an educational component. Researchers should help students and colleagues understand what COIs are, how they can occur, why they create serious problems relating to objectivity, integrity, and trustworthiness in research, and how best to respond to them.

QUESTIONS FOR DISCUSSION

1. What is a COI? Do you agree with our definitions?
2. What is the difference between an actual and an apparent COI? Does it matter?

3. How much money (or stock, etc.) has to be at stake before a person has a COI?
4. Do you think that nonfinancial COIs are an important concern in research?
5. Do you think a COI is a risk factor for misconduct?
6. Do you think that disclosing COIs is an effective strategy? What are some limitations of this strategy?
7. Do you think managing COIs can be an effective strategy? What are some limitations of this strategy?
8. Should some COIs be prohibited? Which ones?
9. How important of an ethical issue is the COI in research? Is it a minor problem or a major concern?
10. What is the best way to help young researchers understand the predicaments created by COIs? What about established researchers?
11. Can you give an example of scientific COIs from your own experience or that you have heard about? How was it dealt with? How should it have been dealt with?
12. How do you evaluate the process for managing COIs? Do you view it as primarily preventive or primarily remedial? Is it fair to the individual scientists? To the research institutions? To the public? Do you think that existing policies favor one group over others? Can you think of any changes that would improve the procedures?

CASES FOR DISCUSSION

CASE 1

The Cleveland Clinic Foundation (CCF), with its eight hospitals, is one of the most prominent organizations in health care. It has a prestigious cardiac center and is a national leader in oncology research. It has nearly $4 billion in annual revenue and 30,000 employees. Dr. Delos "Toby" Cosgrove, a world-renowned cardiologist, was the chief executive officer of the CCF until 2005. The clinic created the Foundation Medical Partners (FMP) in 2001 to raise money. Cosgrove was an investor in the FMP (Armstrong 2005). The clinic contributed $25 million of the total limited partnership in FMP and was entitled to 38% of its profits.

FMP invested in several startup companies involved in treating atrial fibrillation, including a $3 million investment in AtriCure. Atrial fibrillation affects 2.2 million Americans; 15% of them will have a stroke due to the illness. The purpose of AtriCure's device was to control heart rhythms by using a radio frequency to scar the tissue near the pulmonary veins that contribute to an irregular heartbeat, which would block the impulses.

Cosgrove and the CCF promoted AtriCure's device in articles, conferences, and brochures. The CCF claimed that Cosgrove mistakenly declared that he had no COIs on forms he was required to fill out by the clinic's board of directors.

AtriCure's device was approved by the FDA for soft-tissue surgery, but it had not been approved to treat atrial fibrillation by the FDA, which has rejected its device application three times. The CCF went ahead with its use for other surgeries on an off-label basis. (An "off label" use of a medical product occurs when the product is used in a purpose or manner other than what it has been approved for.) The device was also used in patients on an off-label basis at other hospitals. Four patients died as a result of using the device, but AtriCure did not notify the FDA. (The FDA requires manufacturers to report adverse events.) The CCF has used the device on 1,247 patients/subjects, which includes 16 subjects who are part of an ongoing clinical trial.

The cardiologist Eric Topol and the blood specialist Alan Lichtin, both at CCF, reported the AtriCure issue to the COI committee at the Cleveland Clinic. In response, Cosgrove announced that Topol would lose his post as a provost of the medical school and thus automatically lose his membership in the COI committee and the board of governors of the CCF. Topol has been an outspoken critic of relationships with industry that create COIs. The COI committee began to investigate the case after it learned about it and after the IRB had informed them of the conflict. The IRB directed the researchers to voluntarily stop their research. The FMP partners receive 2.75% of money raised, plus other fees totaling $1.7 million a year. Cosgrove stepped down from the AtriCure board and promised to resign from the FMP.

The board of trustees, based on a request from Cosgrove, appointed a special committee to oversee the investigation, and the committee hired a law firm to assist them. The board decided that it should tighten the COI policies and that there should be better communications between the COI committee and the IRB. Cosgrove admitted his shortcomings in this case. The chairman of the board of trustees and its members admitted to having continued investments in medical equipment companies (Armstrong 2006).

- Are there any COIs (individual or institutional) in this case?
- Should the clinic have such a relationship with a medical device company?
- Was the IRB doing its job?
- Was the COI committee doing its job?

CASE 2

In 2005, the NIH revised its COI policies for intramural researchers after an investigation by the *Los Angeles Times* found numerous violations of the existing rules.

An internal review by the NIH found that 44 NIH researchers violated the ethics rules on consulting fees with industry. The new rules prohibit all NIH staff from paid consulting with pharmaceutical companies or nonprofit health care organizations. NIH leaders are prohibited from owning any stock in pharmaceutical, biotechnology, or medical device companies, and other researchers cannot own more than $5,000 worth of stock (Kaiser 2005). Researchers are also banned from giving paid lectures to organizations that are affected by the NIH, such as universities, with a few exceptions. These are some of the strictest COI rules for researchers anywhere (Kaiser 2005; Willman 2005).

- Do you agree with these rules?
- Do you think it is fair that the rules governing NIH intramural researchers are stricter than those governing NIH extramural (grant-funded) research?
- Should universities adopt rules as strict as these?

CASE 3

A faculty member of a Midwestern university has a postdoctoral fellow who had been working for three years on one aspect of a new drug that has just been approved by the FDA. The drug company pays the mentor $5,000 per year in consulting fees. This year, the company is sponsoring a three-day conference in San Francisco, all expenses paid. The conference brings together approximately 15 scientists from around the country who are leaders in research on this drug. Their job is to speak to 300 invited guests, physicians who are potential prescribers of the drug. All the physicians' expenses are paid. The speakers will each receive a $3,000 honorarium. The faculty member accepts the invitation, and the postdoctoral fellow hears about it by accident. He informs his mentor that he has new data indicating that the drug may have serious side effects. The mentor points out that the work is not yet published and that she will deal only with the published data for now.

- Under the terms of the COI policies described above, is this a COI?
- If the answer is yes, what is the COI? What type is it?
- Are there COIs in this case that are not covered by the policies?
- Is this a case of misconduct?
- Should the mentor have done anything differently up to the point that the postdoctoral fellow told her about the new data? What should the mentor and postdoctoral fellow do now?

CASE 4

A senior researcher at a major research university has two grants from the NIH and research contracts from two different large pharmaceutical companies. She also serves on the National Heart, Lung, and Blood Institute Advisory Board and on one of the FDA's advisory panels. Her work pertains to drugs that lower cholesterol. The FDA panel that she is on was convened to decide whether to recommend the final approval of a drug for consumer use. The drug is manufactured by one of the two companies with which she has a contract. However, the contract has nothing to do with this particular drug. Prior to the deliberations, she disclosed her research contract as a COI and proceeded to participate in the panel. She was one of those who voted to recommend approval of the drug, but the recommendation would have passed anyway, without her vote.

- Is this really a COI case? Was it necessary for the senior researcher to have disclosed her contract with the company as a COI?
- Should the FDA have allowed her to deliberate on this panel?
- Despite the fact that she was allowed to participate on the panel, do you think she can deliberate without being unduly influenced by the contract she holds?
- Should universities encourage or discourage their researchers from placing themselves in such positions?

CASE 5

A member of an NIH study section was the primary reviewer of a grant proposal submitted by a very close personal friend and colleague. The extent of their relationship was well known among the close-knit research community, and the primary reviewer chose not to recuse himself. He proceeded to review the proposal and gave it his highest ranking. During the deliberation, another member of the study section raised the issue of the perception of COI. The chair of the study section and the reviewer in question rejected the implications of the comments, pointing out that the member's signature on the COI declaration was sufficient indication of his ability to make an objective judgment and that the relationship did not violate any NIH rules. Additionally, the NIH scientific review administrator said that study section members were obligated and expected to put personal relationships aside as part of their commitment to an objective evaluation. The study section proceeded with the overall approval of the grant proposal. However, the administrator informed the chair of the study section that the person who raised the issue concerning the COI has the right to go through the formal appeal process.

- Was the scientific review administrator justified in making the statement about expected objectivity? What should the policy be in such circumstances? Should personal friendships ever be considered as a disqualifier for an objective review?
- Should the member of the study section in question have done anything differently?
- Was the other member of the study section justified in bringing up the subject of COI?

CASE 6

A member of an NIH study section has been asked to review a grant proposal submitted by a direct competitor to her own research. They are both working on practically the same project and are very familiar with each other's strengths and weaknesses. Their mutual animosity is common knowledge; during scientific conferences, their exchanges almost amount to shouting matches. The reviewer prepared a very thoughtful and lengthy evaluation. She highly criticized the proposal and gave it a poor rating. The proposal received an overall average rating, which removed it from consideration for funding.

- Under the terms of existing federal or university COI policies, does this represent a COI?
- Given the general awareness of their competitive positions and their mutual animosity, was the scientific review administrator justified in not intervening? In selecting the reviewer in the first place?
- Should the member of the study section have done anything differently?

CASE 7

A clinical researcher receives $3,200 per patient from a drug company to enroll patients in a clinical trial of a new hypertension medication. The money covers patient-care costs and administrative costs for the duration of the study and includes a $200 finder's fee. After the initial screening and enrollment, patients will make a total of eleven 15-minute office visits during the study. At each visit, nurses will take blood, record vital signs, and ask questions about the patients' hypertension. The clinician will do a physical exam.

- Is this financial arrangement a COI or apparent COI?
- Should it be prohibited?
- During the informed consent process, should patients be told about the clinician's financial interests?

CASE 8

A political science professor is an authority on ancient political theory. His textbook is required reading in his undergraduate class. Some of the students have complained to the department chair that the book is not up-to-date.

- Does the professor have a COI?
- Should the department chair review the professor's decision to use his own textbook in class?

CASE 9

A university has a special IRB to review social science research involving human subjects. The board includes seven institutional members (two sociologists, two psychologists, an ethicist, a statistician, and a behavioral economist) and three community members (a pastor, a homemaker, and a teacher). The board regularly reviews studies submitted by the chair of the department of sociology. Both sociologists on the board are assistant, untenured professors in the department.

- Do the sociologist IRB members have a COI when they review proposals submitted by the department chair?
- How should the IRB deal with this issue?
- Would it make a difference if the professors were tenured?

CASE 10

Two toxicologists published a commentary in an environmental health journal that was critical of a review article published in an earlier issue of the journal on the health risks of bisphenol A (BPA). The review article claimed that BPA can exert toxic effects at very low doses by disrupting the body's endocrine functions. The toxicologists challenged this claim. One week after the toxicologists published their commentary, the journal editors received a letter to the editor claiming that the toxicologists' commentary was biased, because they were receiving support from the chemical industry that they had not disclosed in the commentary.

- Should the journal publish this letter?
- Should it give the toxicologists a chance to respond?
- How should journals enforce their COI policies?

CHAPTER 10

The Use of Animals in Research

This chapter provides a brief history of animal research and examines the ethical arguments for and against animal experimentation. It discusses the animal rights views of Peter Singer and Tom Regan and considers some morally significant differences between animals and humans. The chapter also discusses some principles for the ethical treatment of animals in research, such as the "three Rs"—reduction, replacement, and refinement—as well as animal research regulations.

Experimentation on (nonhuman) animals is one of the most controversial issues in research ethics. Like the abortion debate, the issue has been hotly contested and often violent. Animal rights activists have freed laboratory animals and destroyed research records, materials, equipment, and buildings to protest what they consider to be immoral uses of animals (Koenig 1999). Animal welfare organizations, such as People for the Ethical Treatment of Animals (PETA), have enlisted volunteers to penetrate institutes, spy on researchers, and uncover abuses of animals. In response to threats from individuals and organizations, universities have tightened security measures. Researchers have rallied around the cause of animal research and have formed professional organizations, such as the National Association for Biomedical Research and the Foundation for Biomedical Research, to promote the humane use of animals in research. Given the highly polarized nature of the debate about the use of animals in research, one wonders whether there can be any hope of some consensus (DeGrazia 1991; Garrett 2012).

Estimates of the number of animals used in research vary from 17 to 70 million animals per year (LaFollette and Shanks 1996). Advances in technology have made it possible to eliminate some uses of animals in research and replace animal models with other testing procedures, such as tissue cultures and computer simulations (Barnard and Kaufman 1997). Researchers are also finding ways to obtain valid results using fewer animals. Additionally, universities are using fewer live animals in educating graduate and undergraduate students. The number of animal experimental procedures conducted in the United Kingdom declined from 5.2 million in 1978 to 3 million in 1998. However, this trend may reverse as researchers increase the number of animals used in transgenic research (Stokstad 1999). For example, researchers participating in the National Institutes of Health (NIH) Knockout Mouse Project plan to make approximately 25,000 strains of genetic knockout mice, one for each gene in the mouse genome (Austin et al. 2004). The project will use about 10 million mice (Williams et al. 2003).

The percentages of animals used in different research activities are as follows: 40% in basic or applied research, 26% in drug development, 20% in safety testing, and 14% for other scientific purposes (Pence 1995). Much of what is known about human and animal physiology, anatomy, biochemistry, embryology, development, genetics, cytology, neurology, immunology, cardiology, and endocrinology has been gained through experiments on animals. Animals are commonly used in applied research to test new medical therapies, such as drugs, vaccines, medical procedures, or medical devices. Indeed, the U.S. Food and Drug Administration (FDA) regulations require that new drugs and medical devices be tested in animal populations before they are tested in human populations (Bennett 1994). Animals are used in environmental studies to determine the toxic or carcinogenic effects of compounds that are released into the environment, such as pesticides, herbicides, or pollutants. Animals are also used in agricultural research in the development of hybrid breeds, clones, or transgenic species and in cosmetic research to test the toxicity of mascara, shampoo, hair dye, lipstick, and other products. Transgenic animals are playing an increasingly important role in research: Researchers have developed varieties of transgenic mice that contain genes for specific diseases, such as diabetes, obesity, cancer, and Parkinson's disease. Transgenic animals are playing an increasingly important role in agriculture as well: Researchers have developed sheep that produce human hormones in their milk, and they are attempting to develop pigs that will produce organs suitable for transplantation into human beings (Marshall 2000; Wilmut 1997).

Although people have spoken on behalf of animals for many years, a book by the philosopher Peter Singer, titled *Animal Liberation* (1975

[1990]), spurred and buttressed the modern animal rights movement. But before examining Singer's views on animals, we provide a brief history of the animal rights movement.

HISTORICAL PERSPECTIVE

For many years, scientists who used animals in research were influenced by the views of the 17th-century French philosopher René Descartes (1596–1650), who argued that animals are like machines and that their behavior results from instincts, reflexes, and other internal mechanisms that do not involve consciousness or rationality (Descartes [1970]). Descartes's view probably had a significant influence on early vivisection practices: Seventeenth- and 18th-century vivisectionists nailed dogs to boards and cut them open without anesthesia or analgesia. They interpreted their howls and cries as mere noises produced by machines (LaFollette and Shanks 1996). Pain-relieving measures were not used in animals before the discovery of anesthesia in 1846. In the 20th century, the behaviorists, such as B. F. Skinner and J. B. Watson, wielded considerable influence over researchers' attitudes toward animals. The behaviorists held that science can only study animal and human behavior: It is not possible to have scientific knowledge of the inner workings of the mind, such as thoughts, feelings, and emotions. People who were influenced by this doctrine did not pay much attention to animal pain or suffering, because they believed that it is impossible to know whether animals think or feel (Rollin 1989).

Two intellectual forerunners of the modern animal rights movement were the British philosophers Jeremy Bentham (1748–1832) and John Stuart Mill (1806–1873), who advanced the notion that animals can suffer and thus deserve moral consideration. The views of Mill and Bentham provided a philosophical and moral basis for the 19th century's animal welfare movement. From the mid-1800s until the early 20th century, there was a strong antivivisection movement in England and the United States. Leaders of this movement opposed the use of animals in experiments and opposed all forms of cruelty to animals.

The American Society for the Prevention of Cruelty to Animals (ASPCA) was formed in 1866, and local societies for the prevention of cruelty to animals soon followed. The American Humane Organization, founded in 1874, opposed the use of animals in experiments as well as inhumane experiments on human beings. Many of the leaders of this movement, such as Caroline White and Mary Lovell, were women with strong religious and moral convictions. The antivivisection movement also received support from the Women's Christian Temperance Movement, the Department of Mercy, and *Life* magazine. The antivivisectionists made two main arguments against animal experiments. First, they argued that these experiments cause unnecessary and unjustifiable suffering to animals. Second, they argued that our attitudes toward animals could influence how we treat human beings: Cruelty to animals can lead to cruelty to human beings. In this light, the antivivisection movement also drew connections between exploiting animals in research and exploiting human beings, and they helped draw attention to unethical experiments on children, mentally ill people, poor people, African Americans, and prisoners (Lederer 1995).

In Britain, animal rights activists helped pass the Martin Act in 1822 titled the "Act to Prevent Cruel and Improper Treatment of Cattle." A few years later the Royal Society for the Prevention of Cruelty to Animals (RSPCA) was founded. In 1829, New York State passed a law to protect domestic animals such as horses, oxen, and other cattle. By the end of the 19th century, Britain passed stricter animal protections laws. The feminist and animal activist Frances Power Cobbe became more active in opposing vivisection. Late in the 1800s, all experiments with animals in Britain required a yearly license. During the same period, Darwin's theories on evolution convinced many people that human beings are descended from animals, which heightened sensitivity to subjecting animals to pain. The animal rights movement in England remained dormant until the 1960s. In 1972, Richard Ryder, Ronald Lee, and Clifford Goodman founded the Animal Liberation Front (ALF) in England.

In the United States, the National Academy of Sciences and the American Medical Association formed a coalition to push for legislation in the late 1890s to disarm antivivisectionists and promote medical progress. The animal rights movement was practically nonexistent in the United States until the 1960s and the advent of the civil rights movement. This was followed by Singer's book *Animal Liberation* (1975 [1990]). In the 1980s, two strident activists, Alex Pacheco and Ingrid Newkirk, formed PETA, which has since engaged in numerous high-profile activities to highlight the plight of animals in scientific experiments. Although PETA has not condoned the use of violence, many people have alleged that the organization has used unethical and illegal means to reach its goals (Oliver 1999).

THE ARGUMENT FOR USING ANIMALS IN RESEARCH

Why do scientists use animals in research? The main argument can be understood in utilitarian terms (Botting and Morrison 1997; Cohen

1986): Animal research produces important basic and applied knowledge that promotes human health and well-being. An added benefit of animal research is that it can yield knowledge that improves the health and welfare of animals. The argument is utilitarian because it holds that the ends (e.g., promoting human health and well-being) justify the means (animal research). Those who criticize this argument argue either (1) that the ends do not justify the means or (2) that the means are not effective at achieving the ends. The first type of critique raises moral objections to animal research; the second raises scientific or technical objections. Below we examine both of these critiques as well as replies to them.

MORAL CRITIQUES OF USING ANIMALS IN RESEARCH

Moral objections to using animals in research hold that animals, like human beings, have inherent moral worth and should not be sacrificed for a greater good. There are two very different ways of supporting the idea that animals have moral worth: a utilitarian perspective defended by Singer (1975 [1990]), and a rights-based perspective defended by Tom Regan (1983).

According to Singer, the central question in our treatment of animals is whether they deserve moral consideration. Singer does not believe that all organisms deserve moral consideration; for example, he would not claim that bacteria deserve moral consideration. Merely being a living creature is not a sufficient reason for special moral status. Singer also thinks that the question of whether animals can reason or communicate is not the only relevant issue in deciding whether they deserve moral consideration—what matters is that animals have the ability to suffer. Singer cites Bentham on this point. In discussing the moral status of black slaves, Bentham argued that the color of their skin was irrelevant to determining their moral status. And Bentham extended this argument to animals: The most important question in determining the moral status of a being is not whether the being can think, talk, or reason, but whether it can suffer (Bentham 1789 [1988]). According to Singer, many animals can suffer and therefore pass the key test for determining whether they deserve moral consideration. This view implies that human beings have a moral obligation to refrain from causing animals to suffer.

Most people would likely accept most of this argument: It is certainly wrong to inflict needless suffering on animals, and one should take steps to minimize animal suffering. But most people would say that animal suffering could be justified to promote important causes, such as improving human health and well-being. Animals have some moral worth, but human beings have a higher moral status or worth (Cohen 1986; Frey 1994). Thus, we should consider animal suffering in deciding how to treat animals, but we should give far more weight to human suffering.

However, Singer does not believe that we should give more weight to human suffering. According to Singer, all beings that deserve moral consideration deserve equal moral consideration. Thus, we should give equal weight to human and animal suffering. Our refusal to give equal consideration to animals is a form of bias that Singer calls "speciesism." Singer equates speciesism with racism and sexism because these "isms" discriminate between different classes of beings based on what he believes to be morally irrelevant characteristics. Just as skin color and gender are not relevant to a person's moral standing, species membership is also not relevant. According to Singer, "Speciesism . . . is a prejudice or attitude of bias toward the interests of members of one's own species. It should be obvious that the fundamental objections to racism and sexism made by Thomas Jefferson and Sojourner Truth apply equally to speciesism" (1975 [1990], p. 7).

Singer's view does not prohibit animal experiments on species not considered to merit moral consideration, including plankton, worms, and many other lower species. Nor does it imply that experiments on animals with moral worth can never be morally justified. Because Singer is a utilitarian, he believes that animal experiments could be justified if the experiments promote the greatest good for the greatest number of beings that deserve moral consideration—humans and animals. However, his view implies that most of the animal experiments that are performed today should be stopped and that we should consider performing experiments on human beings that lack the ability to suffer, such as human beings with severe brain damage, instead of performing those experiments on animals.

Many writers have countered Singer's charge of speciesism by arguing that there are morally significant differences between human beings and other animal species (Caplan 1983; Carruthers 1992; Cohen 1986; Frey 1994). The charge of speciesism is unsound because, although there are no significant moral differences among races, there are significant moral differences between humans and other species. Typical, adult humans have the following qualities:

- Rationality: the ability to reason and solve problems, to engage in abstract thinking

- Linguistic communication: the ability to communicate information using a language
- Emotion: the ability to feel and respond to emotions such as empathy, compassion, mercy, guilt, anger, fear, and shame
- Morality: the ability to formulate and follow moral rules, to make moral choices
- Creativity: the ability to come up with new ideas, behaviors, solutions, and expressions
- Spirituality: the ability to form a concept of higher power or being, the need to find meaning in life and a connection to the whole universe
- Self-consciousness: the awareness of one's self in one's environment, of one's own beliefs, emotions, desires, and attitudes
- Self-determination: the ability to make deliberate choices in controlling one's own behavior
- Consciousness: the awareness of sensations, including the capacity to feel pain

Admittedly, not all human beings have all of these characteristics all of the time. Children develop these characteristics as they mature, people with severe brain injuries no longer have all of these characteristics, and people born with mental disabilities may never have some of them. Nevertheless, the typical adult member of the species *Homo sapiens* has all of these characteristics, while the typical, adult animal used in an experiment may have only some of these characteristics. A laboratory rat probably has consciousness, emotion, and perhaps even some degree of self-awareness, but it probably does not have reasoning, linguistic communication, morality, self-determination, spirituality, and other qualities. Some animals have more of these human characteristics than rats. For example, chimpanzees have consciousness, emotion, self-awareness, creativity and rudimentary reasoning, linguistic ability, and self-determination. Accordingly, chimpanzees should be treated differently than rats because they have more human qualities. (We'll return to this point later.)

An additional critique of Singer's view is that his use of the term "suffering" is somewhat naive and simplistic. It would appear that Singer uses the term "suffer" as a substitute for "feel pain," but suffering is not the same thing as feeling pain (Cassell 1991). There are many different types of suffering: unrelieved and uncontrollable pain; discomfort, as well as other unpleasant symptoms, such as nausea, dizziness, and shortness of breath; disability; and emotional distress. However, all of these types of suffering involve much more than the awareness of pain: They also involve self-consciousness, or the awareness that one is aware of something. For a creature to experience suffering, the creature must be at least aware that it is in pain and that the pain is not going away.

If we think of suffering in this fashion, then it may not be at all obvious that animals suffer, because we do not know the extent to which animals are self-conscious. Although one might argue that it is also difficult to prove that animals feel pain, most people find this idea easier to accept (based on behavioral and neurological similarities) than the claim that animals are self-conscious. However, once again, a great deal depends on what species of animal we have in mind. Monkeys, dogs, and cats probably have enough self-consciousness to experience suffering. But what about fish, frogs, and mice? Perhaps Singer has chosen the wrong word to describe animal experiences. If he had said that the key point is that animals can feel pain, rather than suffering, then perhaps his claims would be less contentious (Rollin 1989).

Regan, like Singer, also believes that animals have moral status but, unlike Singer, he argues that animals have rights. This seems like an outrageous claim to those who believe that only moral agents—beings who can formulate and follow moral rules—have rights. Rights and responsibilities go hand in hand: One cannot have a moral right unless one can also accept moral responsibilities. Because animals are incapable of following moral rules and making moral choices, they are not moral agents. Thus, they have no moral rights (Fox and DeMarco 1990).

To make sense of the idea that animals have rights, Regan (1983) draws a distinction between moral agents and moral patients. Regan argues that moral communities include members who have moral rights but not moral responsibilities, such as young children, mentally retarded adults, and permanently comatose adults. We grant moral rights to these people because they still have interests even if they do not have responsibilities. Moral patients do not have all the rights accorded to moral agents. For instance, children do not have the right to vote, the right to enter a contract, or the right to marry, but they do have some basic rights, such as the right to life and the right to health.

Animals, according to Regan (1983), are moral patients because they have inherent value. By this he means that animals are capable of valuing their own experiences and their own lives. They can prefer pleasure to pain, freedom to captivity, and life to death. They have perception, memory, and a sense of their own past and future. Because animals have inherent value, one should treat them just like other beings that have inherent value, because inherent value does not come in degrees. Indeed, it would be a form of speciesism to insist that humans have more inherent value than do animals. Thus, animals should be accorded the same rights that we grant to other moral patients, such as children.

According to Regan, and many other writers, the purpose of rights is to serve as moral "trump cards" to protect and promote individual interests. For example, when we say that a person has a right to vote, we imply that this right should not be taken away in order to promote a greater good. Animal rights also function as moral trump cards that forbid us from sacrificing animals for some "greater good." In particular, we should not use animals in experiments that are not designed to promote their interests. Because more than 99% of animal experiments yield no benefits for the experimental subject, almost all animal experiments are immoral (Regan 1983). The only kind of animal experiment that could be justified would be an experiment that is designed to benefit the animal or promote its interests.

Many different writers have criticized Regan's view. Some of the critiques address the theoretical underpinnings of his position and argue that he has not adequately explained how animals can have rights (Carruthers 1992). First, one might ask whether the claim that animals really value their own experiences and their own lives has any plausibility. The word "value" connotes more than having a preference, want, or desire: To value something, one must make a judgment about the worth of that thing. Wanting a drink of water is not the same thing as valuing a drink of water: A person who values a drink of water also makes a judgment that the water is good in some respect, for example, good for quenching thirst. It is not at all clear that animals have the cognitive capacity to make judgments about value even if they have desires or preferences.

Second, according to most accounts of rights, rights promote or protect interests (Feinberg 1973). An interest, in this view, is something that one needs in order to promote one's overall well-being. For example, people need food, shelter, freedom, companionship, freedom from pain, and many other things that promote well-being. Regan's view implies that animals also have various interests, such as interests in living, in freedom of movement, in food and water, and in freedom from pain. But how can we make sense of the interests of animals? If we are not careful, we may find ourselves accepting the idea that plants have interests, if we maintain that animals have interests. Plants need water, sunlight, and soil to grow and flourish. But do plants have interests? This view seems patently absurd. So there must be some difference between an interest and a biological need. One might argue that interests are different from biological needs in several ways. First, beings with interests are aware of those interests. Second, beings with interests can communicate those interests. Although a plant may need water, it is not aware of this need, nor can it communicate it (as far as we know). Although laboratory mice may be aware of their biological needs in some sense, they cannot communicate those needs.

Finally, other writers have objected to the practical problems with making sense of animal rights (LaFollette and Shanks 1996). One problem would be how we should resolve conflicts of rights among animals. For example, if a lion and a zebra both have a right to life, should we stop the lion from killing the zebra in order to protect the zebra's rights? How do we weigh the rights of a beaver to make a dam against the rights of those animals who will have their homes flooded if it does so? If we accept the idea that animals have rights, and that these rights are held equally, then there are no satisfactory solutions to these types of problems. To solve these issues, we would need to have some way of assigning value to various rights claims, for example, that the lion's right to food is more important than the zebra's right to life. But this opens the door to assigning greater value to the rights of human beings, which is a move that Regan wishes to avoid. If we say that animals and human beings both have rights but that human rights are more important, then we can also justify animal experimentation on the grounds that human rights to health and welfare outweigh animal rights to life, freedom from pain, and so on.

Although we think that Singer's and Regan's critiques of animal research have some serious flaws, they offer society and the research community some important lessons about our treatment of animals. In particular, these critiques clarify the importance of developing an account of the moral status of animals that is sensitive to both the similarities and differences between humans and animals (LaFollette and Shanks 1996). Singer and Regan, incidentally, do recognize that there are moral differences between humans and animals (Regan and Singer 1989). Singer (1975 [1990], 1985) holds that it is worse to kill a normal human adult than to kill a mouse, and Regan (1983) admits that if one must choose between saving the life of a human and saving the life of an animal, greater harm will occur if one does not save the human. But these concessions offer little comfort to those who place much greater value on human life than on animal life.

However, it is also important to remember that for many years many researchers held very little respect or consideration for animal pain or suffering. Some, such as the Cartesians and the behaviorists described above, adopted this stance based on their judgment that animals are unthinking and unfeeling beings, much like robots (Rollin 1992). We believe that the most sensible view lies somewhere between the extreme positions staked out by Singer and Regan on the one hand, and the Cartesians and behaviorists on the other. Most people, including most researchers, believe that we have moral duties toward animals and that we should respect and promote the welfare of animals (Bulger 1987). For example, most researchers favor extending the Animal Welfare Act (1966, 1996) to laboratory animals, including rats and mice (Plous and Herzog 2000). However, many people, including researchers, also recognize the importance of using animals in research (Botting and Morrision 1997). The only way to make sense of the competing claims is to adopt the view that animals have moral status (or moral value) but that human beings have a greater value (Frey 1980). There are degrees of moral value, and not all species have the same moral worth. We believe that the value of a species depends on its degree of similarity to the human species: Species that closely resemble humans, such as chimpanzees, have greater moral worth than species with little in common with humans, such as rats or cockroaches. (We do not explain why we consider human life to be valuable—we consider this to be a basic assumption of ethics and morality).

If animals have some moral value but less value than human life, how should we treat animals? To answer this question, it will be useful to distinguish between intrinsic and extrinsic value. Something has intrinsic value if people value it for its own sake; something has extrinsic value if it is valuable for the sake of something else. Some things can have both intrinsic and extrinsic value. For example, most people would agree that happiness has intrinsic value. The value of money, however, is extrinsic: Money is valued not for itself but for what you can buy with it. Education may be valuable for its own sake and also because it can help one to obtain employment.

Most people will agree that animals at least have extrinsic value because they are valuable as sources of food, clothing, labor, amusement, companionship, and so on. But saying that animals have extrinsic value provides very little in the way of any moral restriction of our conduct toward animals. One might appeal to the extrinsic value of animals in many different ways to justify restrictions on our conduct toward animals. For example, one might argue the following:

- It is wrong to torture a cat because people find this to be degrading or offensive.
- It is wrong to kill dolphins because people like dolphins.
- It is wrong to kill lions because people think lions are beautiful.
- It is wrong to exterminate prairie dogs because they play a vital role in the ecosystem of the Great Plains of North America.
- It is wrong to cause an animal species to become extinct because the species is an important source of biodiversity.

- It is wrong to harm an animal because a person who harms an animal is more likely to harm a human being.

These arguments, while important, are contingent and relativistic because they depend on human wants, beliefs, and desires or features of the ecology. For instance, if no one liked dolphins, then it might be acceptable to kill dolphins; if prairie dogs did not play a vital role in the ecology, then it might be acceptable to exterminate them; if people were not offended by someone who tortures a cat, then it might be acceptable to torture a cat. For these reasons as well as others, it is important to show that animals have intrinsic value, not just extrinsic value (Taylor 1986). Thus, it is wrong to torture a cat because this act harms a valuable life, not just because people find it offensive.

So how might one prove that animals have intrinsic value? How does one prove that anything has intrinsic value, for that matter? We suggest that the process of assigning intrinsic value to something is not entirely rational, in that one does not arrive at judgments of intrinsic value based solely on empirical evidence or logical argument. In ethics and morality, judgments of intrinsic value are basic premises (i.e., assumptions or axioms). More than 2,300 years ago, Aristotle argued that one cannot "prove" basic premises; one accepts basic premises and then makes arguments on the basis of those premises (McKeon 1947). (As noted above, we consider the premise "human life has intrinsic value" to be a basic axiom of ethics and morality.)

So how does one come to accept basic premises, assumptions, or axioms? Arguments can be helpful, but experience is also important. For example, consider how one develops an appreciation for a piece of classical music, such as Mozart's *Eine Kleine Nachtmusik*. You might start to like this piece after someone convinces you by means of an argument that this is good music. Someone might argue that the music is well ordered, creative, intelligent, expressive, lively, and so on. But you will probably only come to appreciate this piece after listening to it. You experience the value or worth of the music after becoming familiar with the music. Some might even describe this psychological phenomenon as a "conversion" experience or a gestalt shift: You simply come to "see" the value of the music much as you come to "see" that a picture of a witch is also a picture of a young woman (a classic gestalt figure). We suggest that the same psychological mechanisms apply to coming to appreciate the intrinsic value of animals (and humans): Arguments can play a role in helping us to accept the value of animals, but we also must have some experience with those animals in order to fully appreciate their value. For instance, if you have never had a pet pig, then an argument may convince you of the worth of the pig, but you will not truly appreciate the worth of the pig until you have come to know the pig, much in the same way that one would come to know the worth of Mozart's music.

Although we admit that it is not possible to conclusively prove that animals have intrinsic value, we do believe that arguments by analogy can play a role in helping people come to appreciate the value of animals. As noted above, we assume that people already accept the claim that human beings have intrinsic value. To show that animals also have intrinsic value, one may construct an argument by analogy with human beings: Animals have value insofar as they are like human beings. As the analogy increases in strength, the value of animals should also increase (LaFollette and Shanks 1996). An argument by analogy does not conclusively establish basic premises about moral worth, but it can help people become more willing to accept those premises. To develop the analogy between humans and animals, one must consider the above list of characteristics of human life and ask whether animals are like us in relevant ways.

Many of these questions are very difficult to answer and require a great deal of scientific investigation and research. After many years of treating questions about animal cognition and emotion as "unscientific," we are just now beginning to understand in greater detail important aspects of animal consciousness, experience, emotion, self-consciousness, and communication (Bonner 1980; De Waal 1996; Griffin 1992; Rollin 1989). Evidence that can help us answer these questions can come from the study of animal behavior, evolution, genetics, physiology, neurology, or endocrinology. Because different animal species have different behavioral, physiological, neurological, genetic, and biochemical traits, as well as different evolutionary histories, it is likely that some species will be more like humans than others. As mentioned above, given what we know about chimpanzees and mice, we have reasons to believe that chimpanzees are more like humans than are mice. Thus, chimpanzees have greater moral worth than mice have. One can make similar comparisons for other species, such as dogs, cats, elephants, dolphins, monkeys, and birds. The more the species is humanlike, the greater its moral value.

ETHICAL ANIMAL EXPERIMENTATION AND SCIENTIFIC VALIDITY

We now consider arguments dealing with objections to the scientific validity of animal experiments. Before deciding whether to conduct an experiment on animals, we must decide whether it is morally acceptable to use the animal in the experiment, given the purpose of the study, the experimental design, the methods used, and the species of the animal. If we decide that the animal has some moral value and that the experiment would harm the animal in some way (e.g., by causing pain, suffering, disability, or death), then we must argue that the experiment can be ethically justified, given the expected benefits. Researchers can conduct experiments on animals, provided that they provide a sufficient moral justification for the experiments (LaFollette and Shanks 1996). Because many different animal species may have some degree of moral value, the moral burden of proof rests with researchers who plan to conduct experiments on animals; researchers do not simply have a moral "free ticket" or "blank check" regarding animal experimentation. Moreover, because animal species may differ with respect to their moral worth, an experiment can be morally acceptable for one species but not be morally acceptable for a different species. For example, it may be morally acceptable to create a transgenic mouse that is prone to various forms of cancer (i.e., an oncomouse), but it may not be morally acceptable to create an "oncochimp" or an "oncomonkey," because chimpanzees and monkeys have greater moral value than mice by virtue of their higher degree of similarity to human beings.

Because animal species have some degree of intrinsic value, our view implies a commonly accepted policy known as the "three Rs" of animal experimentation (Russell and Birch 1959):

- Replacement: When it is possible to answer a research question without using an animal, replace the animal with a methodology that does not use animals, such as cell studies or computer modeling. When it is possible to answer a scientific question using a morally "lower" species of animal, replace the "higher" species with a lower one.
- Reduction: When it is possible to answer a research question using a smaller number of animals, reduce the number of animals used.
- Refinement: Wherever possible, refine research methods, techniques, concepts, and tools to reduce the need for animals in research and to reduce harms to animals.

The three Rs can be justified on the grounds that they minimize harm to animals and promote animal welfare within the context of animal experimentation. Of course, these three Rs make sense only if one believes that the research protocols are likely to yield results with scientific, medical, or social value. Thus, a fourth R should also apply to animal research:

- Relevance: Research protocols that use animals should address questions that have some scientific, medical, or social relevance; all risks to animals need to be balanced against benefits to humans and animals.

Finally, a fifth R is also important (and plays a key role in U.S. animal research regulations):

- Redundancy avoidance: Avoid redundancy in animal research whenever possible—make sure to do a thorough literature search to ensure that the experiment has not already been done. If it has already been done, provide a good justification for repeating the work.

Avoiding redundancy is important so that one does not use animals unnecessarily and waste research resources.

This approach to the ethics of animal experimentation suggests that researchers also need to address the five Rs relating to the scientific validity of every research protocol they propose, because these issues can affect the ethical soundness of the research. Some of the scientific issues that researchers need to address are as follows:

1. The scientific necessity of the experiment: If the experiment has already been done, it may or may not be worth repeating. Although it is often important to repeat new experimental findings, unnecessary repetition should be avoided.
2. The appropriateness of the animal model: Animal research protocols specify the species used to answer a research question. These protocols should therefore provide a rationale for the particular species chosen; they should describe how the experiment would provide evidence that is relevant to the research question. For example, if one is interested in learning about the conduction of nerve signals along axons, then a species of squid may be a good animal model because it has long axons that are easy to study. Moreover, knowledge about squid axons may be generalized to other species. If one wants to know whether a specific chemical is likely to be toxic or carcinogenic in humans, then it is important to use an animal species that is metabolically similar to the human species. For many years, researchers have more or less assumed that toxicity studies in mice can be generalized to humans, but this assumption is now being questioned (Anonymous 1993; LaFollette and Shanks 1996). For example, researchers at one time thought that saccharin can cause bladder cancer in humans based on studies in which mice were fed huge doses of the saccharin and then formed tumors in their

bladders. However, we know that laboratory mice have a mechanism of waste elimination that is different from the human mechanism. When mice eliminate saccharin, they build up uric acid crystals in their bladders. Human beings, on the other hand, do not form these crystals. Thus, conclusions about the carcinogenic effects of saccharin in laboratory mice probably do not apply to human beings (Cohen 1995).

3. The number of animals used: The principle of reduction implies that researchers should reduce the number of animals used, whenever this does not affect their ability to obtain useful data, but researchers must also make sure that they use enough animals to obtain statistically significant data and results. Otherwise, the experiment causes unjustifiable harm to the animal subjects. Here, good statistical design and ethical practice go hand in hand (see the discussion of statistics in chapter 3).

4. Efforts to promote animal welfare and reduce animal harm: Because animal research should promote animal welfare and minimize animal harm wherever possible, researchers need to take measures to minimize pain, suffering, disability, and death. Researchers must consider the appropriate use of analgesia and anesthesia; humane forms of euthanasia, when this is required for pathological findings; appropriate and sterile surgical procedures; disease control; and living conditions, such as nutrition, living space, and exercise. The United States and many other countries have many regulations addressing these issues (discussed below). However, although regulations govern this important aspect of research, we want to stress that these regulations have a sound moral justification; they are not needless rules or "red tape" (LaFollette and Shanks 1996).

5. Alternatives to the animal model: As mentioned above, the principle of replacement implies that researchers should find alternatives to animal models, wherever possible. In the last few decades, scientists have made greater strides in developing alternatives to animal models, such as cell and tissue cultures and computer simulations (LaFollette and Shanks 1996; Office of Technology Assessment 1986; Stokstad 1999). We encourage further developments in this direction. However, it is unlikely that researchers will be able to completely eliminate the need for animal subjects, because many complex physiological, behavioral, and developmental phenomena can be understood only within the context of a whole organism. For example, to understand how a vaccine protects an organism against infection, one must eventually use the vaccine in whole organisms. Inferences about the vaccine from tissue cultures or computer models simply will not provide relevant knowledge about

whole organisms. Most research questions related to animal behavior, such as research on Parkinson's disease, obesity, aggression, and addiction, will probably require whole organisms.

TRANSGENIC ANIMALS

As noted above, transgenic or genetically modified (GM) animals play an important role in biomedical research. Researchers have made GM animals that model various human diseases, such as cancer, hypertension, diabetes, Parkinson's disease, and so on. Researchers can also study the function of different genes by developing knockout animals that lack those genes. GM animals also are playing an increasingly important role in agriculture and agricultural biotechnology. Scientists have created GM salmon that grow faster than those found in the wild; GM cows that have more lean muscle than normal ones; and GM sheep that secrete human hormones in their milk.

Although the production of GM animals offers important benefits for science and society, it also raises some ethical issues. Chief among these is the potential suffering experience by a GM animal. Some diseases may cause GM animals considerable suffering: animals with cancer may develop tumors that press on nerves, crowd out organs, or break through the skin; animals with Parkinson's disease may experience muscle tremors, rigidity, and difficulties with movement. Animals may also experience suffering as a result of inadvertent genetic engineering mistakes that produce dysfunction and pain. Another issue concerns the sheer number of animals needed to produce transgenic varieties, as it can take hundreds of animals to produce a GM strain. Scientists should keep the 5 Rs in mind when developing transgenic animals and strive to minimize pain and suffering and the unnecessary use of animals in research (Resnik 2012b).

CHIMERAS

One of the important techniques that researchers have developed in the last decade is using human–animal chimeras to study human diseases. The word "chimera" comes from Greek mythology. A chimera was a monster composed of parts from a lion, human, snake, and goat. In modern biology, a chimera is simply an organism composed of parts from different species or different parts from the same species. Biomedical science and technology have helped to create many different types of chimeras, such as mice with human genes, cells, or tissue or containing cells with different genomes. Some humans have pig heart valves to replace their defective valves. Chimeras are playing an increasingly important role in biomedical research, because they can help scientists to study basic biological processes, such as embryonic development and cell differentiation, and to model human diseases, such as cancer, obesity, heart disease, and Parkinson's disease (Robert 2006).

Chimeras raise some interesting and important ethical issues (Robert and Baylis 2003). Animals with human parts could be like human beings in many important ways. It is possible, in theory at least, that an animal–human chimera might be created that is subhuman. For example, suppose that researchers transfer human genes or stem cells into chimpanzees, which cause the chimpanzee to develop linguistic and reasoning skills. How should we treat this animal: like a chimpanzee or like a human being? Would it have moral or legal rights? What kind of impact would the creation of a subhuman have on the idea that human beings have inherent worth and value? Would the creation of subhumans degrade the value we place on human life? Although H. G. Wells anticipated some of these issues in *The Island of Doctor Moreau*, the possibilities involved in human–animal chimeras are so novel and fantastic that most people have not had time to think clearly about the ethical issues. For this reason, research proposals that aim to create human–animal chimeras with significant human characteristics need careful review and oversight (Moreno and Hynes 2005).

REGULATIONS

Here we briefly review some of the regulations that govern research on animals in the United States. Many of these rules embody the ethical and scientific considerations mentioned earlier in this chapter. The two main federal laws that govern animal research in the United States are the 1966 Animal Welfare Act (AWA), since revised several times (in 1970, 1976, 1985, 1996), and the U.S. Public Health Service (PHS) Policy on the Humane Care and Use of Laboratory Animals (Rollin 1992; U.S. Public Health Service 2000). The PHS policy applies only to animal research conducted using PHS funds, but the AWA applies to all animal research. Many research institutions and professional societies have their own guidelines for the humane care and use of animals in research (Bennett 1994). There are also private organizations, such as the Association for the Assessment and Accreditation of Laboratory Animal Care (AAALAC), which accredit research institutions. Institutions can legally conduct animal research without AAALAC accreditation, but accreditation still plays an important role in shaping research practices, because many research sponsors require AAALAC accreditation (Association for the Assessment and Accreditation of Laboratory Animal Care 2007). States also have their own laws pertaining to animal welfare, but we do not review them here because these laws all allow animal research that conforms to the federal laws.

The PHS policy applies to all vertebrate animals used in research supported by PHS funds. The NIH is one of the units of the PHS and the largest one supporting research with animals. The PHS policy requires compliance with the AWA and the National Research Council (NRC) *Guide for the Care and Use of Laboratory Animals* (1996). The NIH Office for Laboratory Animal Welfare (OLAW) is responsible for monitoring recipients of PHS funds for compliance with the regulations, which takes the form of a written assurance of compliance by the research institution. OLAW can inspect animal care facilities "for cause."

The AWA, originally titled the "Laboratory Animal Welfare Act," promulgates rules that apply to the commercialization and use of animals, including the use of animals in research. Animals originally covered by the AWA included (nonhuman) primates, dogs, cats, guinea pigs, hamsters, and rabbits (Bennett 1994). In 1970 the AWA was expanded to cover all warm-blooded animals, but in 1976 the Secretary of Agriculture excluded rats, mice, birds, farm animals, and horses from being covered under the AWA. The U.S. Department of Agriculture (USDA) oversees compliance with the AWA. In 2000 the USDA announced a plan, later suspended, to once again include rats, mice, and birds under the AWA (Malakoff 2000). Although some researchers have objected to including rats, mice, and birds under the AWA, polls suggest that many researchers would welcome this change (Plous and Herzog 2000).

Both the AWA and the PHS policies stipulate rules and guidelines for the humane care and use of animals in research. These regulations address a variety of issues, including living conditions, such as cage sizes, temperature, environmental stimulation, food, and exercise; efforts to reduce pain and discomfort, including analgesia and anesthesia; surgical procedures, including antisepsis and euthanasia; veterinary care and disease prevention and control; procurement and transportation; and the qualifications, health, and safety of personnel. The NRC's *Guide for the Care and Use of Laboratory Animals* (1996) spells out many of the standards for animal experimentation contained in the AWA and PHS regulations. The NRC established the Institute for Laboratory Animal Research to study, prepare, and distribute documents on the care and use of animals in the research community. The AAALAC also considers the NRC guide when deciding whether to accredit an institution. All researchers and students are advised to consult the NRC guide when preparing animal experimentation protocols and proposals (Bennett 1994).

The AWA and PHS regulations also address institutional responsibilities for ensuring and promoting the humane care and use of animals in research. These rules require institutions that conduct animal research to establish an institutional animal care and use committee (IACUC) to review and approve animal research protocols and to monitor animal research. IACUCs are also charged with educating researchers about scientific and ethical aspects of animal research and relevant regulations. IACUC members should include a veterinarian, a scientist, and a community representative. Many IACUCs also include an ethicist or a lawyer. IACUCs have the authority to stop any animal research protocol that does not meet the standards set forth in relevant policies. IACUCs also conduct inspections of laboratories on a biannual basis. IACUCs function much like institutional review boards (IRBs) in that both of these research committees are charged with ensuring institutional compliance with relevant regulations and with protecting research subjects.

QUESTIONS FOR DISCUSSION

1. How can we know whether an animal can feel pain or suffer?
2. What is the difference between the ability to feel pain and the ability to suffer? Do you agree with this distinction? Why or why not?
3. Do you agree with Singer that speciesism is like racism? Do you think speciesism can be justified? Why or why not?
4. What is the moral status of nonhuman animals? Do they have rights? Should we promote their welfare?
5. What criteria should we use to decide whether a being has moral status?
6. Are there some types of animal experiments that you regard as unethical? Why?
7. Would you add any ethical principles for the 5 Rs described in this chapter?
8. Do you think that animal research always has important benefits for human beings? Are there some types of research that are not very beneficial?
9. Do you think animal research is overregulated, underregulated, or is regulated just about the right amount? Why?
10. Do you have any ethical concerns about creating human–animal chimeras?

CASE STUDIES

CASE 1

In the spring of 1984, head-injury experiments on baboons conducted by investigators at the University of Pennsylvania drew protests from animal rights groups, intense media coverage, and a review by Congress and the NIH, the federal agency sponsoring the research. The primary aim of the experiments was to develop and test a model for brain injuries that occur in automobile accidents and some sports, such as football or boxing. The secondary aims were to measure the effects of the experimentally induced trauma on brain tissue. In the experiments, baboons were outfitted with helmets, which were fastened to their heads with cement. The baboons were sedated with a tranquilizer. A hydraulic piston hit would hit the helmet with a force 2,000 times the force of gravity. The piston was not designed to cause a penetrating wound to the animal's head, but to produce trauma to the soft tissue of the brain. The experiments resulted in brain injuries, paralysis, and coma. The baboons were kept alive for two months following the experiments and then euthanized for pathological analysis. Although the animals were sedated prior to the experiments, some animals were awake when the piston hit their helmets. Some animals received more than one blow to the head (Orlans et al. 1998).

On May 18, 1984, five members of ALF, an animal rights organization, entered the Head Trauma Research Center at the University of Pennsylvania and stole 30 videotapes the researchers had made of the experiments. They also vandalized equipment in the laboratory and wrote "ALF" on the walls. ALF gave the videos to PETA, which released excerpts to the media. The video excerpts showed the piston hitting the heads of the baboons, with some of them apparently writhing in great pain and distress. These grotesque images shocked researchers, convinced many people to support the animal rights movement, and instigated public debate about animal research. Researchers and leaders at the University of Pennsylvania defended the experiments as important studies with potential benefits for human health. They also maintained that the experiments were in full compliance with federal regulations. A congressional committee held hearings on the experiments, which included testimony from officials from the NIH, the FDA, and PETA. The NIH, the FDA, and the University of Pennsylvania continued to maintain that the experiments were ethical and in compliance with the law. The NIH even renewed the $300,000 grant it had awarded to Thomas Gennarelli, a professor of neurosurgery at the University of Pennsylvania who was the principal investigator for the baboon experiments (Orlans et al. 1998).

PETA and other animal rights groups continued to protest against the experiments. They held peaceful demonstrations at the University of Pennsylvania and the NIH. PETA put together a 20-minute video from 60 hours of stolen videotape titled

Unnecessary Fuss, after a remark Gennarelli had made about the experiments. In the summer of 1985, animal activists petitioned members of Congress to stop the experiments. Sixty members of Congress signed a letter to the director of the Department of Health and Human Services, Margaret Heckler, asking her to stop funding the experiments. When Heckler refused to stop the experiments, animal activists staged a sit-in at the NIH and occupied several offices. Four days later, Heckler suspended the funding for the study. The NIH then conducted a full investigation of the experiments and found that the University of Pennsylvania had failed to comply with the NIH's animal welfare policies. The investigation determined that the researchers had failed to provide adequate anesthesia, analgesia, nursing care, training, and supervision. The University of Pennsylvania reprimanded Gennarelli and Thomas Langfitt, the chair of the department of neurosurgery, who was associated with the study. The USDA fined the university $4,000 for violating the Animal Welfare Act. The NIH eventually removed its funding restrictions, but by that time the university had abandoned its primate head trauma program (Orlans et al. 1998).

- Was this experiment ethical?
- Would it be possible to do an experiment like this one with a design that causes less pain and harm?
- How does the fact that the experiment was conducted on baboons affect your ethical assessment of it?
- Would the experiment be ethical if it were conducted on rhesus monkeys, dogs, or mice?
- Did the NIH and the FDA act ethically the first time? The second time?

CASE 2

You are a graduate student conducting an experiment for Dr. Beeson on repairing spinal chord injuries in rats. During the experiments, you sever the spinal chord, allow the rat to heal, determine the degree of paralysis, and then inject neural stem cells into the site. You will use 25 rats in your protocol. In one of the experiments, one of the rats died after surgery, and Dr. Beeson replaced the rat. You asked him what he planned to do in response to this death, and he said nothing. You prod him a bit further, and he says that he knows why the rat died—he gave the rat too much anesthetic—and he doesn't think the death will have any effect on the experiment's results. He also does not want the IACUC to know about the death.

- How should you respond?
- What should the IACUC do if it finds out about this incident?

CASE 3

A researcher is planning to test a new analgesic medication in dogs. The medication may prove useful in relieving pain associated with severe burns. To conduct the experiment, she will use two groups of 12 dogs each, an experimental group and a control group. Both groups will receive a burn on the back. Both will receive treatment for the burn, but only one group will receive the medication under study. She will also attempt to measure their degree of pain and discomfort by touching the burn to evoke a response, such as behavioral cues, heart rate, and blood pressure.

- Would you approve of this experiment? Why or why not?

CASE 4

Surgeons are developing a robotic device for performing heart surgery. The device, if successful, would be a safer and more reliable way to perform heart surgery than current human techniques. One of the main benefits of the robotic system is that it minimizes unstable movements. It is also expected to reduce the risk of infection. In developing the device, the surgeons are planning to test it on dogs, cats, and pigs. They also plan to use animals to teach surgeons how to use the device. For each animal, the protocol will include a surgical procedure followed by a postoperative recovery period, followed by euthanasia and pathological analysis. One of the research protocols also involves using the device for emergency surgery to respond to heart trauma, such as gunshot or knife wounds. For this protocol, animals will be shot or stabbed and prepared for surgery. All animals will be given appropriate analgesia and anesthesia.

- Would you approve of this protocol? Why or why not?

CASE 5

Researchers are developing an animal model for a rare genetic disorder known as osteogenesis imperfecta. Children born with this disorder have a genetic mutation that prevents them from forming strong bones. Neonates usually have many broken bones at birth and usually die within six months or a year at most. They usually also have severe brain damage, organ damage, and a variety of infections. Researchers plan to develop a transgenic mouse with a genetic defect that results in a condition similar to osteogenesis imperfecta. They will study the etiology of the disease in mice as well as a variety of treatment modalities.

- Do you have an ethical problem with this experiment? Why or why not?

CASE 6

A researcher is conducting experiments on tumor suppression with transgenic on-comice. In his experiments, he allows the mice to develop cancerous tumors, and he then treats them with different gene therapy vectors designed to inhibit cell cancer growth. Two graduate students and two lab technicians work with him on his project. Last week, one of his graduate students informed the IACUC chair that several mice had developed tumors that impeded their free movement in the cages. The tumors were growing around their front legs and on their chests. This was a violation of the researcher's animal protocol. A graduate student also reported that the researcher has been out of town consulting with biotech companies and has not been paying close attention to work being conducted in his lab.

- Was the graduate student justified in reporting this protocol violation?
- How should the IACUC handle this problem?

CASE 7

Dr. Murphy is studying aggression in rats. She is experimenting with a variety of environmental and hormonal influences on aggression in order to study the relationship between aggression and overcrowding, stress, food deprivation, and levels of sex hormones. In some of her experiments, rats will be placed in crowded cages; in others they will be deprived of food; in others they will receive high doses of testosterone. She will also include control groups for the various conditions. She will attempt to minimize pain and discomfort to the rats, but they are likely to fight and injure each other.

- Would you allow Dr. Murphy to do this experiment?
- Would you require Dr. Murphy to modify the protocol in any way?

CHAPTER 11

The Protection of Human Subjects in Research

This chapter discusses the history of human experimentation, giving special attention to cases that have helped to shape ethical guidelines and policies. It discusses important ethics codes and provides an overview of U.S. federal regulations. The chapter also addresses some key concepts and principles in human research, such as informed consent, risks versus benefits, privacy and confidentiality, protection of vulnerable subjects, and research versus therapy.

The use of human subjects in research came into sharp focus during the Nuremberg war crimes trials, when the world discovered the atrocities committed by Nazi doctors and scientists on tens of thousands of prisoners held in concentration camps. While these tribunals were unfolding, the American Medical Association (AMA) was developing a set of principles to be followed in experiments using human subjects (Advisory Committee on Human Radiation Experiments 1995). After the tribunals concluded in 1947, the research community adopted the world's first international code for research on human subjects, the Nuremberg Code (Advisory Committee on Human Radiation Experiments 1995). The code emphasized the importance of informed consent of research subjects, minimization of harms and risks to subjects, scientific validity of the research design, and the social value of the research. Since then, many documented cases of unethical or questionable research have also been conducted in the United States and other countries (Advisory Committee on Human Radiation Experiments 1995; Beauchamp and Childress 2001; Capron 1989; Washington 2006). There have also been many ethical controversies in human subjects research (Egilman et al. 1998a, 1998b; Shamoo and Irving 1993; Washington 2006). As a result, federal agencies and scientific and professional associations have developed regulations and codes governing human subjects research, and there have been a great deal of discussion and debate about ethical standards that should govern the use of humans in research (Levine 1988; Pence 1996). This chapter reviews these regulations after providing a historical perspective on these issues.

HUMAN EXPERIMENTATION BEFORE WORLD WAR II

Alexander Morgan Capron (1989, p. 127) has observed that "the darkest moments in medical annals have involved abuses of human research subjects." A brief survey of the history of human subjects research supports this view. Before the Scientific Revolution (ca. 1500–1700 A.D.), medicine was an observational rather than experimental science. Medical research was based on the teaching of Hippocrates (460–377 B.C.), the father of scientific medicine. Hippocrates developed theories and principles that explained diseases in terms of natural rather than supernatural causes. According to his teachings, health was a state of balance among the four humors of the body: blood, phlegm, yellow bile, and black bile. Disease occurs when the body becomes out of balance as the result of too much or too little of one or more humors. The goal of medicine is to use various treatments and therapies to restore the body's proper balance. For example, Hippocratic physicians believed that bloodletting could restore health by eliminating excess blood.

Hippocrates' method was observational rather than experimental because he did not use controlled interventions (or experiments) to obtain medical knowledge. Instead, Hippocrates gathered knowledge through careful observation of disease conditions, signs, symptoms, and cures. He also developed detailed case histories. Hippocratic physicians believed in the body's ability to heal itself, and they tended to prescribe nonaggressive and noninterventional therapies, such as special diets, herbal medications, exercise, massage, baths, and prayer. The Hippocratic School developed a code of medical ethics that emphasized the importance of promoting the welfare of the individual patient. Two of the Hippocratic Oath's key tenets, which evolved hundreds of years after Hippocrates' death, are to keep patients from harm and injustice ("do no harm") and to benefit the sick. Although Hippocratic physicians sought to improve medical knowledge, their code of ethics and their philosophy of medicine implied that medical advances would occur slowly and would not sacrifice the welfare of the individual patient for scientific progress (Porter 1997).

This conservative approach to medical research began to change during the Scientific Revolution, as physicians such as Paracelsus (1493–1542), Andreas Vesalius (1514–1614), and William Harvey (1578–1657) challenged medical dogmas and sought to apply the new experimental method to medicine. However, these physicians still did not conduct many controlled experiments on human beings. Although Paracelsus, Vesalius, and Harvey dissected human bodies, they did not gain their knowledge of anatomy from experiments on living people. While Harvey conducted some experiments on human beings, his experiments were relatively benign and noninvasive. For example, he used a tourniquet to demonstrate the direction of the flow of blood in human veins, and he measured pulse and blood pressure. He conducted his more invasive procedures, such as vivisections, on animals (Porter 1997).

As physicians began to apply the experimental method to medicine, experiments on human beings became more common and more risky. One famous 18th-century experiment conducted by the English physician Edward Jenner (1749–1823) illustrates some recurring ethical concerns. Jenner observed that dairymaids who developed cowpox did not develop smallpox. He hypothesized that exposure to cowpox provided protection against smallpox. To test his hypothesis, he inoculated James Phipps, an eight-year-old boy, with some material from a cowpox pustule. The boy developed a slight fever but suffered no other ill effects. Six weeks after this inoculation, Jenner exposed Phipps to the smallpox virus and he did not develop the disease (Porter 1997).

During the 19th century, experiments on human beings became even more common. For example, William Beaumont (1785–1853) treated Alexis St. Martin for a bullet wound in the stomach. The wound healed but left a hole in the stomach. Beaumont hired Martin as a servant and used him as an experimental subject, because he could observe the process of digestion through the hole in Martin's stomach (Pence 1995). During the 20th century, physicians began to accept the germ theory of disease developed by Louis Pasteur (1822–1896) and Robert Koch (1843–1910). Despite Pasteur's unquestioned place in science, there are now historical studies indicating that his behavior was not above ethical reproach. For example, Pasteur treated a patient for rabies without first ensuring the safety of the treatment in animal experiments (Geison 1978). The surgeon Joseph Lister (1827–1912) performed a variety of experiments to develop and test antiseptic methods in medicine. For instance, Lister observed that carbolic acid was effective at reducing infections among cattle, and he hypothesized that this compound has antiseptic properties. To test his idea, he applied lint soaked in carbolic acid and linseed oil to a boy's wound. He also took measures to prevent germs from entering the wound. The boy, James Greenlees, did not develop an infection. Lister applied his method to dozens of other cases of compound fractures and amputations and published his results in *The Lancet* in 1867 (Porter 1997).

One of the most disturbing experiments in the United States before World War II took place in 1874 in Cincinnati, when Robert Bartholomew inserted electrodes into the brain of Mary Rafferty, a 30-year-old "feeble-minded" patient who was dying of terminal cancer, which had spread to her scalp. Bartholomew saw a research opportunity and for several hours electrically stimulated Rafferty's brain and recorded her responses, which were often cries of pain (Lederer 1995).

Many of the human experiments were inspired by the work of Pasteur and Koch, who developed vaccines for bacterial infections. To implement this methodology, researchers needed to establish a link between a pathogen and a disease, isolate a disease pathogen, develop a vaccine, and then test the vaccine. In 1895, Henry Heiman, a New York pediatrician, infected two mentally retarded boys, 4 and 16 years old, with gonorrhea. In 1897, the Italian researcher Giuseppe Sanerilli injected yellow fever bacteria into five subjects without their consent in order to test its virulence. All five subjects became severely ill, although none died (Lederer 1995). Many physicians, including William Osler (1849–1919), condemned this experiment. In his textbook *The Principles and Practice of Medicine* (1898), Osler discussed Sanerilli's experiments as well as some other studies of yellow fever.

U.S. Army physician Walter Reed and his colleagues in Cuba conducted their well-known yellow fever experiments around 1900. Yellow fever had become a major health problem for military operations in Cuba, the Caribbean, and Central America. At the time, researchers hypothesized that yellow fever was transmitted to humans by the *Aedes aegypti* mosquito. Because there were no animal models for the disease, human subjects were required to study its transmission. The risks to human subjects were great, because medicine had no cure for the disease, which often resulted in death. Two investigators working with Walter Reed, James Carroll and Jesse Lazear, allowed themselves to be bitten by mosquitoes in order to test the hypothesis. Reed had also agreed to participate in these experiments, but he was in Washington, DC, when his colleagues exposed themselves to the disease. Both colleagues contracted yellow fever, and Lazear died from the disease. After Lazear died, Reed decided not to use himself as an experimental subject, but he continued experimenting on human beings. A total of 33 subjects participated in the experiments, including 18 Americans and 15 Spanish immigrants. Six subjects died from yellow fever (Lederer 1995).

Because the risks of participating in these experiments were so great, Reed and his colleagues had volunteers sign written documents stating that they understood the risks of the experiment and that they agreed to participate. Informed consent documents were translated into Spanish. Volunteers were also given $100 in gold and free medical care for their participation. Although other researchers obtained undocumented informed consent from subjects, this is believed to be the first case of the documentation of informed consent in research. Research subjects who participated in these yellow fever experiments came to be regarded as heroes and martyrs. Surviving military volunteers received gold medals and government pensions (Lederer 1995). Although some scholars claimed that the ethical/legal doctrine of informed consent evolved in the 1950s and 1960s (Advisory Committee on Human Radiation Experiments 1995), Reed's work shows that he followed this paradigm before it became more broadly accepted.

There have been numerous unethical experiments on vulnerable African Americans, such as the Tuskegee study (discussed below). Harriet Washington's 2006 book *Medical Apartheid* cites many examples of such experiments. For instance, in the early 1800s, 250 out of 251 subjects in an experiment testing inoculations of smallpox vaccine were African Americans. In 1846, Dr. Walter F. Jones of Virginia poured boiling water on patients with typhoid pneumonia. Washington describes many dangerous and humiliating experiments on African-American slaves. The author recognizes that progress has been made in research with black populations.

Before World War II, physicians and surgeons had ambivalent attitudes toward human experimentation. On the one hand, most physicians accepted the Hippocratic idea that they should not harm their patients. Claude Bernard (1813–1878) restated the principle in his *Introduction to the Study of Experimental Medicine* (1865 [1957]). According to Bernard, physicians should never perform on humans an "experiment, which might be harmful to him to any extent, even though the result might be wholly advantageous to science" (p. 101). On the other hand, physicians regarded many risky and untested interventions as therapeutic and believed that it was sometimes necessary to try these treatments in order to benefit the patient. While physicians condemned many of the unethical experiments that were brought to their attention, they also had a strong commitment to medical experimentation and did not want to place any burdensome restrictions on research. Most physicians thought that self-experimentation was noble and virtuous, but they did not think that informed consent was always necessary. Indeed, most physicians at the time thought that it was more important to avoid harming the research subject than to obtain the subject's consent. For several decades, the AMA considered adopting a code of ethics for research on human subjects, but it did do so until 1946 (Lederer 1995).

In 1900, Prussia was the first nation in the world to formalize the prohibition of medical interventions other than for therapeutic purposes (Capron 1989). The Prussian directive required that consent be given and that prospective subjects be informed of adverse consequences. It also excluded minors from research. These directives were not given in a vacuum or without a cause: They came as a reaction to numerous and repeated abuses of patients in medical research. For example, Amauer Hansen (1841–1912), who discovered the bacillus strain that causes leprosy, carried out an appalling experiment on an unwitting 33-year-old woman when he twice pricked her eye with a needle contaminated by nodules of a leprous patient (Bean 1977). Hansen was later merely reprimanded.

In the early 1900s, the eugenics movement flourished in Europe and in the United States. In the 1930s, one Canadian province and 28 U.S. states passed laws requiring the sterilization of the criminally insane, presumed "feeble-minded," psychopathic personalities, and the mentally ill (Ollove 2001; Proctor 1988). By the late 1930s, California alone had sterilized 13,000 persons, and the U.S. total is estimated at between 30,000 and 100,000 persons (Ollove 2001; Proctor 1988). The State of Virginia in the early 20th century was a leader in sterilization efforts. A *Baltimore Sun* reporter, Michael Ollove, chronicled the ordeal of a Virginian who was sterilized for being "feeble-minded." Later, this Virginian became a soldier, winning the Purple Heart, the Bronze Star, and Prisoner of War honors during World War II (Ollove 2001). The eugenics movement helped provide impetus for the Nazi atrocities committed in World War II. Hitler was a strong advocate of eugenics, and he believed it was necessary to control human breeding in order to prevent the Aryan race from being corrupted by "inferior" races, such as the Jews and Gypsies (Proctor 1999).

Human Experimentation during World War II

The Nazi experiments conducted during World War II have been regarded by many as the worst experiments ever performed on human subjects. None of the subjects gave informed consent, and thousands were maimed or killed. Many of the experiments were not scientifically well designed or conducted by personnel with appropriate scientific or medical qualifications. Moreover, these experiments were planned, organized, and conducted by government officials. Subjects included Jews, homosexuals, convicted criminals, Russian officers, and Polish dissidents. Some of the experiments included the following (Müller-Hill 1992; Pence 1995; Proctor 1988):

- Hypothermia studies where naked subjects were placed in freezing cold water
- Decompression studies where subjects were exposed to air pressures equivalent to the pressures found at an altitude of 70,000 feet
- Wound-healing studies, where subjects were shot, stabbed, injected with glass or shrapnel, or otherwise harmed to study how their wounds healed
- Vaccination and infection studies, where subjects were intentionally infected with diseases, such as typhus, staphylococcus, malaria, and tetanus, in order to test the effectiveness of vaccines and treatments
- Josef Mengele's (1911–1979) experiments designed to change eye color, which resulted in blindness
- Mengele's human endurance experiments, where subjects were exposed to high levels of electricity and radiation
- Mengele's twin studies: exchanging blood between identical twins, forcing fraternal twins to have sex to produce children, creating conjoined twins by sewing twins together at the back, placing children in virtual isolation from birth to test the role of nature and nurture in human development

Although historians and ethicists have focused on Germany's horrific experiments with human subjects during World War II, less attention has been given to Japan's atrocities during this era. From 1932 to 1945, Japanese medical researchers killed thousands of human subjects in medical experiments. Most of the experiments took place in China while the country was under Japanese occupation. The experiments included intentionally wounding and operating on human beings for surgical training, vivisection of live humans, infecting humans with pathogens, exposing subjects to extremes of temperature, and biological and chemical warfare research. Most of the human subjects were people of Chinese ancestry, but victims also included Allied prisoners of war. At the end of the war, the U.S. government made a deal with Japan to gain access to the data from chemical and biological warfare experiments. In exchange for the data, the U.S. government agreed not to prosecute Japanese physicians and scientists for war crimes. As a result of this coverup, the Japanese atrocities were not widely known until the 1990s, and Japanese political leaders have been reluctant to acknowledge that these crimes against humanity occurred (Tsuchiya 2008).

Human Experimentation after World War II

By the mid-20th century, human experiments, ethical and otherwise, were becoming more common, but the research community had not put a great deal of thought into the ethics of research on human subjects. Although some physicians, most notably Bernard and Osler, had written about the ethics of human experimentation, and the AMA had drafted some documents on human experimentation, there were no well-established ethical codes for experimentation on human subjects before 1947. This is one reason that the Nuremberg Code has such an important place in history: It was the first internationally recognized code of ethics for human research.

Although the Nuremberg Code did help to define and clarify some standards for the ethical conduct of human experiments, many abuses took place after the code was adopted. Some of these ethical problems in research were discussed by Henry Beecher (1904–1976) in an exposé he published in the *New England Journal of Medicine* in 1966. Beecher described 22 studies with ethical problems, including the now well-known Tuskegee syphilis study, the Willowbrook hepatitis experiments on mentally disabled children, and the Jewish chronic disease case study (Beecher, 1966).

The Tuskegee study took place from 1932 to 1972 in a public health clinic in Tuskegee, Alabama. The purpose of the study was to follow the natural etiology of later-stage syphilis in African-American men. Six hundred subjects were enrolled in the study, which was funded by the U.S. Department of Health, Education, and Welfare (DHEW), the precursor to the Department of Health and Human Services (DHHS). The subjects were divided between an "experimental" group of 399 subjects with untreated syphilis and a "control" group of subjects without syphilis. The initial plan was to conduct the study for one year, but it lasted nearly 40 years. The subjects who participated in the study were not told that they had syphilis or that they were participating in an experiment. Subjects with syphilis only knew that they had "bad blood" and could receive medical treatment for their condition, which consisted of nothing more than medical examinations. Subjects also received free hot lunches and free burials. An effective treatment for syphilis, penicillin, became available in the 1940s, but the subjects were not given this medication or told about it. In fact, study investigators took steps to prevent subjects from receiving treatment for syphilis outside of study. The study also had scientific flaws: Key personnel changed from year to year, there were no written protocols, and records were kept poorly. Even though Beecher brought the study to the attention of the public, it was not stopped until Peter Buxton, who worked for the U.S. Public Health Service (PHS), reported the story to the Associated Press. The story soon became front-page news, and a congressional investigation followed. In 1973, the U.S. government agreed to an out-of-court settlement with families of the research subjects, who had filed a class-action lawsuit (Jones 1981; Pence 1995). In 1997, the Clinton administration issued an official apology on behalf of the U.S. government.

From 1956 to 1980, a team of researchers, led by Saul Krugman and Joan Giles, began a long-range study of viral hepatitis at the Willowbrook State School for mentally retarded children. Viral hepatitis was endemic at Willowbrook: Most children who entered the institution became infected within 6 to 12 months of admission. Although the disease is usually not life-threatening, it can cause permanent liver damage. Victims of the disease usually have flulike symptoms, such as fever, fatigue, and nausea. The disease is transmitted orally through contact with feces or body secretions. In their research, Krugman and Giles infected healthy subjects with viral hepatitis. This allowed them to study the natural progression of the disease, including its incubation period, and to test the effectiveness of gamma globulin in preventing or treating the disease. They collected over more than 25,000 serum samples from more than 700 subjects. The two researchers justified their study on the grounds that it offered therapeutic benefits to the subjects: The children in the study would receive excellent medical care, they would avoid exposure to other diseases, and they would acquire immunity against more potent forms of hepatitis. Krugman and Giles obtained written informed consent from parents, although some critics have charged that the parents did not understand the nature of the study. Krugman and Giles also obtained appropriate approvals for their study: The study was approved by the New York State Department of Mental Hygiene, the New York State Department of Mental Health, and the human experimentation committees at the New York University School of Medicine and the Willowbrook School (Munson 1992).

The Jewish chronic disease case study took place in Brooklyn, New York, in 1964. In this case, researchers introduced live cancer cells into 22 unsuspecting patients (Faden and Beauchamp 1986). The purpose of the study was to learn more about the transplant rejection process. Previous studies had indicated that healthy subjects and subjects with cancer have different immune responses to cancer cells: Healthy subjects reject those cells immediately, whereas cancer patients have a delayed rejection response. Researchers claimed that they obtained informed consent, but they did not document the consent. They claimed that there was no need for documentation because the procedures they were performing were no more dangerous than other procedures performed in treating cancer patients. Investigators also did not tell the subjects that they would receive cancer cells, in order to avoid frightening them unnecessarily (Levine 1988).

Human radiation experiments took place in the United States from 1944 to 1974, during the cold war era (Advisory Committee on Human Radiation Experiments 1995). These experiments were funded and conducted by U.S. government officials or people associated with government institutions on more than 4,000 unsuspecting citizens and military personnel. Many of these experiments violated standards of informed consent and imposed significant risks on the subjects. Most of these experiments were conducted in order to aid U.S. cold war efforts by providing information about how radiation affects human health. Most of these studies used radioactive tracers and did not result in serious harm to the subjects. However, several of the studies that involved children exposed them to an increased lifetime cancer risk, and several studies caused death shortly after the administration of radiation.

In 1994, the Clinton administration began declassifying documents related to these experiments and appointed a commission to develop a report on this research. Although the commission openly discussed some ethical problems with the research, it also found that most studies contributed to advances in medicine and public health (Advisory Committee on Human Radiation Experiments 1995; Beauchamp 1996; Guttman 1998; Moreno 2000). It also judged the experiments by the standards that existed at the time that they were conducted: According to the commission, most of these experiments did not violate existing ethical or scientific standards. Nevertheless, as Welsome (1999) observed: "Almost without exception, the subjects were the poor, the powerless, and the sick—the very people who count most on the government to protect them" (p. 7). Some of the more noteworthy studies that came to light that may have violated the existing ethical standards included the following:

- Researchers at Vanderbilt University in the late 1940s gave pregnant women radioactive iron to study the effects of radiation on fetal development; a follow-up study found that children from these women had a higher-than-normal cancer rate.

- In Oregon State Prison from 1963 to 1971, researchers X-rayed the testicles of 67 male prisoners, who were mostly African Americans, to study the effects of radiation on sperm function.
- During the late 1950s, researchers at Columbia University gave 12 terminally ill cancer patients radioactive calcium and strontium to study how human tissues absorb radioactive material.
- Researchers released a cloud of radioactive iodine over eastern Washington State to observe the effects of radioactive fallout.
- From the 1940s to the 1960s, researchers injected encapsulated radium into the nostrils of more than 1,500 military personnel; many developed nosebleeds and severe headaches after exposure.

Perhaps the most troubling aspect of these studies is that most of them took place after the international community had adopted the Nuremberg Code. It is ironic that the U.S. government, which had been so outspoken in its criticism of Nazi research, would also sponsor human experiments that many would consider unethical (Egilman et al. 1998a, 1998b).

Besides these important cases from the history of biomedical research, there have also been some noteworthy cases in social science research. One of the methodological problems with social science experiments, known as the Hawthorne effect, is that research subjects may change their behavior as a result of knowing that they are participating in an experiment. As a result, the experiment may be biased. To minimize this bias, many social science researchers believe that it is sometimes necessary to deceive human subjects about the experiments in which they are participating, which is what Stanley Milgram did in his 1960s experiments relating to obedience of authority. These experiments involved three participants: an authority figure (such as a scientist), a learner, and a teacher. The teacher was led to believe that the purpose of the experiment was to test the effects of punishment on learning. The teacher provided the learner with information that the learner was supposed to recall. If the learner failed to learn the information, the authority figure instructed the teacher to give the learner an electric shock. The severity of the shock could be increased to "dangerous" levels. Learners would cry out in pain when they received a shock. Most teachers continued to give shocks even when they reached "dangerous" levels and when the learners asked to stop the experiment. In reality, the learners never received an electric shock; they faked agony and discomfort. Milgram was attempting to learn about whether the teachers would obey the authority figures (Milgram 1974). At the end of each session, Milgram debriefed the teachers and told them the real purpose of the experiment. Many of the teachers said that they suffered psychological harm as a result of these experiments because they realized that they were willing to do something that they considered immoral (Sobel 1978).

Another noteworthy case of deception in social science research took place in Wichita, Kansas, in 1954. During these experiments, investigators secretly recorded the deliberations of six different juries in order to gain a better understanding of how juries make their decisions. The judges of the Tenth Judicial Circuit and the attorneys in the cases approved of the study, although the litigants were not told about it. When this study came to light, the integrity of the jury system was cast into doubt. In 1955, a subcommittee of the Senate Judiciary Committee held hearings to assess the impact of this research on the jury system. As a result of these hearings, Congress adopted a law forbidding the recording of jury deliberations (Katz 1972).

During the 1990s, the research community learned about a variety of ethically questionable studies on mentally ill patients. The national media also covered many of these stories. As a result, the National Bioethics Advisory Commission (NBAC) issued a report recommending changes in federal regulations on research on people with mental disorders (National Bioethics Advisory Commission 1998; Shamoo 1997a). Many of these problems originally came to light through a series of papers delivered at a conference held in 1995 (Shamoo 1997b, 1997c) and a series of articles published in journals (Shamoo and Irving 1993; Shamoo and Keay 1996; Shamoo 1997a, 1997c). This was followed by a major series of articles in the *Boston Globe* (see Kong and Whitaker 1998). Many of these research projects were washout studies in which subjects stop taking medications for a period of time (usually 30 days) before exposure to an experimental drug. The purpose of the washout period is to conduct a controlled clinical trial that reduces biases and complications due to interactions between drugs subjects have been taking and experimental drugs. After the washout period, the protocol randomly assigns patients to groups that receive either an existing treatment or a new drug. The protocols may also include a placebo control group. In some washout studies, the harms to subjects are fairly minimal, especially if the washout period is short and subjects are carefully monitored under inpatient settings, but in others the harms may be substantial, due to the absence of necessary treatment during the washout period.

In the studies that many people regarded as unethical, the subjects were taking medications for depression, schizophrenia, and other serious mental disorders. Some studies on schizophrenia patients found that many subjects suffered the effects of withdrawal from medications and experienced relapses, which included increased psychosis or rehospital-ization (Baldessarini and Viguera 1995; Crow et al. 1986; Gilbert et al. 1995; Wyatt 1986; Wyatt et al. 1999). As a result, more than 10% of sub-jects dropped out of these studies (Shamoo and Keay 1996; Shamoo et al. 1997c) for a variety of reasons. Because 10% of schizophrenics commit suicide, a relapse of this disease can be very dangerous. In 1991, Craig Aller, a patient with schizophrenia at the University of California at Los Angeles, and his family argued that he suffered permanent brain damage due to a relapse caused by a medication washout as part of his participa-tion in the research protocol (Aller and Aller 1997). Another patient in this study allegedly committed suicide (Aller and Aller 1997). In some of these studies, researchers asked the subjects to consent, but critics ques-tioned whether the patients were capable of giving informed consent, due to their mental illness (Koocher 2005; Shamoo and Keay 1996). Many of these experiments did not even give the subjects the opportunity to con-sent. Other experiments that were criticized included studies in which mentally ill subjects were given ketamine to induce psychosis and delu-sions, to study the mechanism of the disease, and healthy children 6–12 years old who were given fenfluramine (an obesity drug) to test whether they were prone to violence (Sharav and Shamoo 2000). Children were se-lected for these studies because their siblings were incarcerated.

During the 1990s ethical problems and concerns related to research in developing countries also came to light. In 1996, Pfizer conducted a clinical trial in Kano, Nigeria, to test whether its new antibiotic, trova-floxacin (Trovan) was effective at treating meningococcal meningitis, which was endemic in the region. In the trial, 100 children received the experimental drug and a control group received a standard therapy (ceftriaxone). A lawsuit against the company alleged that investigators gave children a reduced dose of ceftriaxone to bias the results in favor of trovafloxacin and that the children and their families were not told that they were in a study. The company disputed these allegations but later admitted that it reduced the dose of ceftriaxone to minimize pain resulting from the injections. Five children in the study who were given trovafloxacin died, and six who received ceftriaxone died. The Nige-rian government determined that the lead investigator of the trial, Dr. Abdulhamid Isa Dutse, had provided a letter of ethics committee ap-proval that was falsified. The Nigerian government claimed that the trial was an illegal study involving an unregistered drug. In 2011, Pfizer reached a settlement with families whose children died in the study. In 1999, the FDA restricted the use of trovafloxacin. The drug is banned in Europe (Lenzer 2011).

A controversy concerning the use of placebos in clinical trials emerged in 1997, when two members of Public Citizen's Health Research Group, Peter Lurie and Sidney Wolfe (1997), published an article in the *New England Journal of Medicine* (NEJM) in which they argued that fifteen clinical trials taking place in sub-Saharan Africa and other developing nations were unethical. The editor of the NEJM, Marcia Angell (1997a), also argued that the clinical trials were unethical. She compared the trials to the infamous Tuskegee syphilis study, and she also accused the researchers of accepting a double standard: one for the developed world and one for the developing world. The National Institutes of Health (NIH) director Harold Varmus and the Centers for Disease Control (CDC) director David Satcher (1997) published a response to the allegations by Lurie and Wolfe in the next issue of NEJM, and an international debate ensued.

The controversial studies attempted to determine whether perinatal (mother-to-child) transmission of HIV could be effectively prevented by using a method that was much less expensive than the method currently being used to prevent perinatal HIV transmission in developed nations. The standard of care for preventing perinatal transmission of HIV in developed nations, known as the 076 protocol, involved the administration of $800 worth of azidothymidine (zidovudine; AZT) to the mother during pregnancy and labor and to the child following birth. Breast-feeding mothers also received AZT. This method was shown to reduce the rate of perinatal HIV transmission from 25% to 8%. The controversial studies attempted to determine whether perinatal HIV transmission could be reduced by using about $80 worth of AZT and fewer health care services. The drug was administered less frequently than it was under the 076 protocol. None of the nations where the studies took place could afford the medications needed to administer the 076 protocol on a large scale. The countries also did not have sufficient health care infrastructure to execute the 076 protocol. The trials were approved by the local leaders and authorities, by the World Health Organization (WHO) and the U.N. Joint Programme on HIV/AIDS (UNAIDS), and by the CDC and NIH, which helped to sponsor the trials (Resnik 1998c). Local researchers helped to design and implement the trials and recruit subjects. Less than a year after the controversy began, the investigators showed that a 10% dose of AZT given at the end of pregnancy can reduce the rate of transmission of HIV by 50% (De Cock et al. 2000).

Most of the ethical controversy concerning these trials focused on the research design, because the trials included control groups of subjects who received placebos. The reason for including placebo groups was to prove that the lower dose of AZT was more effective than a placebo. It was already known that the higher dose was effective, but it was not known whether the lower dose would be. The reason for attempting to determine whether the lower dose would be effective is that few people in developing nations can afford the higher dose and they were receiving nothing. The researchers wanted to test a cheaper method of preventing perinatal HIV transmission.

Lurie, Wolfe, and others objected to this research design on the grounds that it denied subjects in the control group a proven, effective therapy. They argued that since AZT has already been shown to prevent perinatal HIV transmission, all of the subjects should receive the drug. Giving placebos instead of an effective therapy was unethical and exploitative, they argued. The investigators were sacrificing the health of research subjects for scientific or public health goals. Lurie and Wolfe argued that the studies should have used active controls rather than placebo controls. An active control group is a control group where subjects receive an effective treatment. They argued that the protocol should have examined the effectiveness of different doses of AZT.

Varmus, Satcher, and other defenders of the trials argued that an active control design would lack the scientific rigor of a placebo control design. An active control design would also require a much larger sample size to ensure that the studies had sufficient statistical power. The sample would need to be much larger because a study that used active controls would be attempting to detect a very small difference between treatment groups. It would probably also take a much longer time to complete active control trials. Placebo control trials would take less time, cost less money, and would yield clearer, more rigorous results. Defenders of the controversial studies also argued that the subjects who were receiving placebos were not being exploited or mistreated, because they did not have access to AZT in any case. Participation in the study did not make the subjects who received placebos any worse off, and it could have benefited them by giving them access to medical care (other than AZT therapy). Critics of the studies argued that it did not matter whether subjects lacked access to the treatments needed to prevent the perinatal transmission of HIV, since the treatment had been proven effective and was available in developed countries. The medical standard of care should be universal, not local. The studies were exploitative because they were taking advantage of the fact that subjects did not have access to AZT (London 2001; Resnik 1998c).

In 2008, Susan Reverby, a professor of history and women's and gender studies at Wellesley College, was conducting research on the Tuskegee study when she discovered some disturbing materials pertaining to previously unpublished experiments conducted by the U.S. Public Health

Service from 1946 to 1948, in which investigators exposed hundreds of Guatemalans to syphilis. The goal of the study was to determine whether penicillin taken prophylactically can prevent syphilis. One of the study's main procedures involved asking prisoners to have sex with prostitutes known to have the disease. When this mode of transmission was not very effective, the investigators inoculated subjects' cheeks, forearms, and penises with syphilis. Out of 696 subjects, 427 developed syphilis. After Reverby published her findings in 2010, the U.S. government launched an investigation of the episode and issued an official apology to the Guatemalan government (Semeniuk and Reverby 2010).

Human Research Guidelines and Regulations

In response to various ethical problems involving research with human subjects, countries and organizations have adopted regulations and guidelines. In addition to the Nuremberg Code, other prominent ethical guidelines include the World Medical Association's Helsinki Declaration, first adopted in 1964 and revised many times since then, mostly recently in 2013 (World Medical Association 2013); the Council for Organizations of Medical Sciences (2002) guidelines; and the International Conference on Harmonization (1996) guidelines. Many professional associations, such as the AMA and the American Psychological Association, have also developed ethical guidelines for human subjects research.

Although ethical guidelines are very useful, they lack the force of laws or regulations, because they usually have no enforcement mechanism. We recognize that many different countries have laws and regulations dealing with research on human subjects, but we focus on the U.S. laws and regulations in this text. The laws and regulations adopted by other countries are similar to those adopted by the United States. We also address only the U.S. federal laws, although we recognize that some states, such as California, have their own research ethics laws. For a compilation of laws from various countries, we refer the reader to the Office of Human Research Protections (2013) website.

The first steps toward developing human research regulations in the United States took place in 1953, when the NIH opened the Clinical Center, which oversaw human experiments conducted at the NIH's intramural campus in Bethesda, Maryland, and reviewed protocols in order to avoid unusual hazards to subjects before proceeding with experiments (Advisory Committee on Human Radiation Experiments 1995; Capron 1989; Hoppe 1996). In 1965, the National Advisory Health Council, at the prodding of then NIH director James Shannon, issued the first prior review requirement for the use of human subjects in proposed research (Capron 1989). In 1966, this action prompted the U.S. Surgeon General to generalize the prior peer-review requirement to all NIH-funded research on human subjects. In 1971, the Food and Drug Administration (FDA) issued its own similar regulations for testing new drugs and medical devices.

In response to research scandals, most notably the Tuskegee syphilis study, the United States enacted the National Research Act in 1974, which required that the DHEW (a precursor to the DHHS) to unify all of its policies into a single regulation, which is codified in the Code of Federal Regulations at Title 45, Part 46, abbreviated as 45 CFR 46. These regulations required each research institution that conducts intramural or extramural research funded by the DHEW to establish or use an institutional review board (IRB) to review and pass judgment on the acceptability of the proposed research according to the detailed requirements listed in the regulations. The regulations set forth rules for IRB composition, decision making, oversight, and documentation. IRBs should be composed of people from different backgrounds, including scientific and nonscientific members, male and female members, as well as members from within the institution and members from the local community. Other countries use similar boards, sometimes called research ethics committees (RECs) or research ethic boards (REBs). Institutions are responsible for reporting serious or continuing noncompliance or unanticipated problems to agencies that oversee research. In 1976, the NIH also developed the Office for Protection from Research Risks to provide oversight for research with human subjects. This office was later renamed the Office for Human Research Protection (OHRP) and relocated to report directly to the DHHS, in order to provide it with a stronger, more independent, and broader governing authority.

In 1979, the first presidentially appointed commission on human experimentation, the National Commission for the Protection of Human Subjects of Biomedical and Behavioral Research, known simply as the National Commission, issued the Belmont Report. The 1974 National Research Act mandated the formation of the National Commission. The Belmont Report provided a conceptual foundation for major revisions of the federal research regulations (National Commission 1979). In 1978, the DHEW revised its regulations to add additional protection for pregnant women, fetuses and embryos, children, and prisoners. From 1981 to 1986, changes in U.S. regulations included revisions to DHEW's regulations for IRB responsibilities and procedures, changes in the FDA regulations to bring them in line with DHHS regulations, further protections for children, and a proposed federal common policy for the protection of human research subjects (Advisory Committee on Human Radiation Experiments 1995, p. 676). Institutions that receive DHHS funding for human subjects research must agree to abide by the ethical principles of the Belmont Report as well as DHHS regulations. These agreements are known as Federalwide Assurances (FWAs).

The Belmont Report describes three ethical principles for research with human subjects: respect for persons, beneficence, and justice. Respect for persons requires researchers to protect the autonomy and privacy of competent research subjects and to provide protections for subjects who cannot make their own decisions. Beneficence requires researchers to minimize the risks and maximize the benefits of research to subject and society. Justice requires researchers to ensure that the benefits and burdens of research are distributed fairly and to ensure that vulnerable subjects are not taken advantage of in research. According to the Belmont Report, one should carefully weigh and balance these different principles when making an ethical decision (National Commission 1979). This is similar to the approach to ethical decision making defended in chapter 1.

In 1991, DHHS issued its final federal policy—the Common Rule, 45 CFR 46—which was adopted by 16 agencies and departments (Federal Policy for the Protection of Human Subjects). However, three federal departments, including the U.S. Environmental Protection Agency (EPA) and FDA, never adopted the Common Rule. The EPA adopted the Common Rule for EPA-sponsored research and has developed a different set of rules for privately funded research submitted to the EPA (Resnik 2007, 2009a). The FDA adopted rules similar to the Common Rule that apply to privately funded research conducted to support applications for new products submitted to the FDA. The Common Rule requires that IRBs can approve research only if they find that (1) risks to subjects are minimized; (2) risks are reasonable in relation to the benefits to the subjects or society (through the knowledge expected to be gained; (3) informed consent is sought and documented; (4) selection of subjects is equitable; (5) privacy and confidentiality are protected; (6) there are additional protections for vulnerable subjects; and (7) there are appropriate provisions for data and safety monitoring (45 CFR 46.111). The Common Rule also describes requirements for consent and its documentation, but it allows these requirements to be waived under certain conditions.

The Common Rule does not require all research to undergo review by the full IRB board. First, if a research activity does not involve a human subject, then the Common Rule does not apply. A human subject is a "living individual about whom an investigator (whether professional or student) conducting research obtains (1) Data through intervention or interaction with the individual, or (2) Identifiable private information (45 CFR 46.102f)." If investigators obtain de-identified samples or data, then this would not qualify as human subjects research. Also, it would not be human subjects research if the samples or data come from someone who is now dead. Second, the Common Rule treats some research involving human subjects as "exempt," meaning that the regulations do not apply to it. Some categories of exempt research include some types of educational research; research relating to existing, publicly available data if subjects cannot be identified directly or through links to the data; research that evaluates public benefit programs; and food quality research (45 CFR 46.101b). If research is exempt, then it does not require IRB review. However, the IRB, not the investigator, should make the determination of whether research qualifies as exempt. Third, if human subjects research is classified as minimal risk, then it can be reviewed on an expedited basis by the IRB chair or a designee (45 CFR 46.110). Minor changes to IRB-approved studies can also be reviewed on an expedited basis. "Minimal risk" is defined as follows: "The probability and magnitude of the harm or discomfort anticipated in the research are no greater in and of themselves than those ordinarily encountered in daily life or in routine physical or psychological examinations or tests (45 CFR 46.102i)."

Although the federal regulations cover a great deal of human subjects research, they have potential loopholes or gaps. For example, privately funded medical research that is not conducted in support of an application for a new drug or medical device is not covered by any existing federal regulations. This is in contrast to the Animal Welfare Act (1966, 1996), which covers use of all animals in research. In order to close this regulatory gap and provide uniform protection for human subjects, Jay Katz was the first to suggest in 1973 that the United States adopt a law to govern the use of all human subjects in research (Katz 1993, 1996; Shamoo 2000; Shamoo and O'Sullivan 1998; U.S. Department of Health, Education, and Welfare 1973). Various bills have come before Congress to close the loopholes in the federal research regulations, but none have passed so far.

In recent years, researchers from the social and behavioral sciences, journalism, and oral history have argued that the U.S. research regulations are excessively burdensome and are better suited to biomedical research (American Association of University Professors 2006; Hambruger 2005). In 2011, the OHRP and the FDA put out an Advanced Notice of Proposed Rulemaking (ANPRM) that would reduce regulatory burdens for low-risk research by expanding the scope of exempt research, enhance the informed consent process and confidentiality protections, and provide better oversight for research involving biological samples and data collections (Office of Human Research Protections 2011). Although the agency has held public hearings on the ANPRM and received hundreds of written comments, it has not implemented these proposed changes as of the writing of this book.

Ethical Dilemmas in Research with Human Subjects

As indicated by our historical review, human subjects research has been controversial for quite some time. Although various regulations and guidelines provide substantial guidance for investigators, controversies remain, because the regulations and guidelines are subject to interpretation and they do not cover every topic. In the remainder of this chapter, we will highlight some of the major ethical issues, most of which involve the perennial conflict between the good of the individual and the good of society (see the discussion in chapter 1). Because we cannot hope to cover every topic in our brief review, we refer the reader to other sources of information (see Emanuel et al. 2003, 2011; Levine 1988).

Research vs. Therapy

As we noted in our historical review, physicians often did not make a distinction between research and therapy and often experimented on their patients. The authors of the Belmont Report recognized that it was important to distinguish between research and therapy, because health care professionals often perform interventions on patients that are innovative or unproven (National Commission 1979). For example, a surgeon may try a new technique when performing a splenectomy, or a general internist may use nonstandard drug combinations and doses when treating an HIV patient. If these interventions are conducted in order to benefit the patient, then, according to the Belmont Report, they are not research, but innovative therapy. As such, they do not need to conform to standards of research ethics, but they should be based on standards of acceptable medical practice. If, on the other hand, interventions are conducted to develop scientific knowledge, then they should be regarded as research (National Commission 1979; President's Commission 1983a, 1983b). The Common Rule defines research as "a systematic investigation, including research development, testing and evaluation, designed to develop or contribute to generalizable knowledge (45 CFR 46.102d)."

Although distinctions between research and therapy make sense in the abstract, they become blurry in concrete cases. For example, consider the case of Baby Fae, an infant born with a defective heart who received a baboon heart when no human hearts were available (Pence 1995). The cross-species transplant (or xenograft) was conducted despite very low odds of success. She lived with a baboon heart from October 26 to November 15, 1984. Clearly, this was a highly innovative procedure that probably benefited transplant science much more than it benefited the patient. Health care quality improvement studies and public health intervention also test the limits of the definition of research. For example, suppose a dozen hospitals collaborate on a project to study procedures for reducing medication errors. The study will compare different procedures for reducing errors used at different hospitals. The hospitals plan to collect and analyze the data and publish it in a journal. Although the goal of this study is to determine the best way to reduce medication errors, one might consider it to be a form of research (MacQueen and Buehler 2004).

Cases that challenge the definition of research pose a difficult problem for human research ethics and regulation. On the one hand, it is important to ensure that with activities inherent risks have adequate oversight to protect people from harm. On the other hand, if an activity is classified as research, it may need to undergo an IRB review, which could pose an undue burden on health care professionals or institutions and interfere with medical or public health practice, or quality improvement activities. While it is important for an IRB to oversee research involving human subjects, there need to be limits on the IRB's jurisdiction, so that institutions and investigators can carry out activities that are designed to benefit patients, institutions, or society without unnecessary burdens that offer little additional protection (Kass et al. 2013; King 1995; MacQueen and Buehler 2004).

The distinction between research and therapy can pose a challenge for investigators who are conducting clinical trials, because there may be a conflict between their ethical duties to their patients (who are also human subjects) and their obligations as researchers (Resnik 2009b). Physicians have an ethical obligation to act in the best interests of their patients by providing them with the best available medical care (treatment, diagnosis, etc.). In some research contexts, this duty may be compromised. For example, many clinical studies require subjects to undergo additional tests or procedures (such as blood draws, x-rays, etc.) that pose risks or discomforts that they would not receive if they were not in a research study. More controversially, in some clinical trials subjects may receive a placebo instead of an accepted therapy. In randomized controlled trials

(RCTs), subjects are randomly assigned to two or more treatment groups (an active control or a placebo control). Many RCTs involve some form of blinding: Neither the subjects nor the investigators know who is receiving a particular treatment. Blinding and the use of placebos help to reduce biases related to the placebo effect, and random assignment helps to reduce biases that may result if subjects or investigators decide who receives a particular treatment. Most RCTs have a data and safety monitoring board (DSMB) that reviews data and safety reports to protect subjects from harm. The DSMB may recommend that the trial be stopped if an experimental treatment is too risky, or if it is so effective that it should not be withheld from subjects receiving placebos or a standard treatment.

The ethical issue in placebo-controlled RCTs is that physicians appear to be violating their duties to patients because they are withholding effective therapy. Some have argued that it is ethical to use placebos in an RCT only when there is no effective treatment (so subjects are not denied treatment), or withholding treatment poses no serious or permanent risks to subjects. This is the position adopted by the Helsinki Declaration (World Medical Association 2013). For example, one could argue that it is ethical to use placebos in an RCT comparing an experimental medicine to a placebo in the treatment of moderate arthritis pain, because withholding pain medications is not likely to result in serious or permanent harm. Using a placebo group in an RCT to test the effectiveness of a blood pressure medication for managing severe hypertension would be unethical, in this view, because a patient with severe hypertension who does not receive effective treatment can suffer serious and permanent harms, such as stroke or heart attack. Some commentators argue that using placebos in RCTs (such as studies comparing surgical interventions to a sham procedure) can be ethical even when subjects face serious or permanent risks, as long as the benefits of the research outweigh the benefits and the subjects' consent. The rationale for this view is that competent adults should be allowed to choose to take some risks for their own potential benefit or to contribute to the advancement of human knowledge (Emanuel and Miller 2001; Miller and Brody 2002).

Another issue related to the research/therapy distinction concerns returning individualized results to research subjects. As noted earlier, the purpose of research is to collect information used to develop scientific knowledge. However, information collected in research is often useful to subjects in making medical decisions pertaining to disease prevention or treatment. When research results have clinical relevance, research becomes similar to medical diagnosis (Resnik 2009b). For example, a clinical study might collect information concerning vital signs, blood composition,

DNA, etc. One could argue that researchers have an ethical obligation, based on the principle of beneficence, to provide research subjects with results about dangerous conditions, such as high blood pressures, elevated blood sugar, and so on, because proper use of this information can protect subjects from harm. A subject who learns that he has moderately high blood pressure can be advised to see his doctor. If a subject's blood pressure is dangerously high, he may need to go to the hospital for emergency treatment. Sometimes the research results are incidental findings, that is, results that researchers were not looking for but happened to discover (Wolf et al. 2008). For example, suppose that a woman undergoes a sonogram for a study of uterine fibroids. The sonogram might indicate that she has abnormal growths that could be uterine cancer. Most people would agree that the investigator should report these incidental findings to the participant so she can follow them up.

While there is little question that investigators should inform subjects about high blood pressure or abnormal growths that could be cancer, controversies can arise concerning the return of other results, such as genomic/genetic data, information concerning paternity, and data from unvalidated biomarker studies, because sharing this information with subjects might do more harm than good. For example, suppose that researchers conducting a study of genetics of heart disease discover that several mutations are associated with a 5% increased risk of heart disease. Should they share these results with participants? On the one hand, one could argue that the investigators should share these findings with subjects, because the results may be useful to them and the subjects would want to know about them. On the other hand, one might argue that the investigators should not return these results to participants because the clinical value of knowing that one has a genetic mutation associated with a 5% increased risk of heart disease is unclear, and the laboratory tests used to detect this mutation may be unreliable or inaccurate. In the United States, medical tests used to diagnose and treat diseases must be conducted by laboratories that have been certified as meeting standards for reliability and accuracy. Research laboratories that conduct genetic/genomic tests for investigators do not need to meet these standards. Returning results with uncertain clinical value produced by uncertified laboratories could cause subjects needless worry and lead to poor decisions (Beskow and Burke 2010; Ravitsky and Wilfond 2006; Wolf et al. 2008).

A final research vs. therapy issue concerns providing subjects in clinical research with medical care beyond what they receive as part of the study. This could include medical care provided during the study (known as ancillary care) or medical care following completion of the study, such as continued access to medications (Resnik 2009b). This issue is especially important in a research setting in which most subjects lack access to care, such as clinical trials conducted in developing nations. For example, suppose investigators are conducting a clinical trial comparing the effectiveness of two different HIV treatment regimens in a Ugandan population. During the course of the study, they might discover that some participants are infected with parasites. They would need to decide whether to offer treatment for these parasites in addition to the other care that is provided (Richardson and Belsky 2004). Once the trial is completed, most subjects would probably no longer have access to HIV medications, and researchers would need to decide whether to help subjects obtain post-trial access to these medications (Millum 2011). The ethical rationales for providing medical care beyond what is needed to conduct a clinical study are to benefit subjects and avoid exploitation. However, providing this additional medical care can add to the costs of research and may constitute an undue burden on investigators. Some investigators and sponsors may decide to forego conducting research if they are required to provide medical care beyond what is called for in the study protocol. Additionally, providing additional medical care may obscure the distinction between research and therapy in the subjects' minds and thereby undermine the consent process (see the discussion below) (Resnik 2009b).

Risk vs. Benefit

Many issues in human subjects' research pertain to risks and benefits, such as developing and implementing procedures and study designs to minimize risks, assessing risks and benefits, and deciding when risks to subjects are justified in relation to the benefits to subjects and society. Although scientific studies pertaining to likely risks and benefits can provide useful information for the evaluation of risks and benefits, risk/benefit decisions always involve an ethical dimension, because one must compare risks and benefits (Kopelman 2000a, 2000b). To determine the overall risks of a study, one must summarize the risks of the different procedures, interventions, and tests used in the study. In a clinical study, interventions, procedures, or tests that patients would have received if they were not in the study should not be included in this risk analysis (Wendler and Miller 2011b). For example, if a study is collecting and analyzing tissue samples from patients who receive lung transplants, the risks of the study would not include the risk of the lung transplant.

Some studies involve significant risks to human subjects. For example, subjects in a clinical trial testing the safety and efficacy of a cancer treatment may face serious risks, such as liver toxicity, kidney failure, dangerous immune reactions, hospitalization, or even death. These risks are usually regarded as acceptable as long as the subjects may potentially benefit from their participation. For example, patients could benefit from having their cancer effectively treated or cured, or from increased longevity or reduction in symptoms (Wendler and Miller 2011b).

Imposing significant risks on subjects is more controversial when the participants are healthy, adult volunteers who are not likely to derive any medical benefits from the study. For example, the subjects in Walter Reed's yellow fever experiments were healthy adult volunteers. Phase I trials of new drugs, biologics, or medical devices are usually conducted on healthy volunteers who are not expected to derive any significant benefits from participation. Phase I studies attempt to generate data concerning safety, dosing, pharmacokinetics, and so on. If the FDA decides that a new product is considered safe for human use after completing Phase I testing, then the agency may allow a sponsor to conduct Phase II studies on subjects with a disease or medical condition, to determine whether the product is effective. If the product completes Phase II testing successfully, then sponsors may begin larger, Phase III studies. If the product completes these studies successfully, the FDA may decide to allow it to be marketed. Thus, the ethical rationale for Phase I studies is that they offer important benefits to society because they are a necessary part of the process of developing new medical treatments (Shamoo and Resnik 2006b). Not all studies on healthy volunteers involve the testing of new medical products, however. Many healthy volunteer studies investigate human physiology, metabolism, immunology, psychology, or behavior (Resnik 2012c).

Although there are no systematic data on the risks that healthy volunteers typically face, anecdotal evidence suggests these can be significant. For example, in 1996 Hoiyan Wan died after receiving a fatal dose of lidocaine during a bronchoscopy performed at the University of Rochester as part of an air pollution study on healthy volunteers. In 2001, Ellen Roche died after developing respiratory distress due to inhaling hexamethonium as part of an asthma study conducted at Johns Hopkins University in 2001. In 2006, six healthy volunteers in a Phase I trial, conducted at Parexel's clinical pharmacology research unit at Northwick Park Hospital in London, developed a dangerous immune reaction and multiple organ dysfunction after receiving a monoclonal antibody known as TGN1412 (Resnik 2012c). Three of these subjects nearly died. There were serious lapses in the design and safety considerations in this trial. For example, the investigators did not wait long enough before administering doses to new volunteers. When testing a drug on a human being for the first time, the usual procedure is to wait and see how the first volunteer reacts to the drug before administering it to other volunteers. The researchers in this study did not observe this and other safety rules (Shamoo and Woeckner 2007).

Exposing healthy adult volunteers to significant risks raises the issue of whether there should be any limits on the risks the healthy subjects face in research. The federal research regulations require that risks be reasonable in relation to the benefits of the knowledge gained, but they do not place any limits on the risks to subjects. One might argue that there should not be any limits on risks that adult subjects face, as long as they provide their informed consent and the research offers important benefits to society. To place limits on research risks would be paternalistic interference in the autonomy of competent adults (Miller and Wertheimer 2007). Some have argued that paternalistic limits on risks can be justified to protect subjects from hazards they may not understand fully and to protect investigators, institutions, and the research enterprise from the impacts of negative publicity when healthy adults are significantly harmed in research (Resnik 2012c).

In medicine, there is also a long and honorable history of self-experimentation, such as Walter Reed's experiments. Self-experimentation is usually a highly altruistic act and morally praiseworthy. However, one might ask whether there should be limits on the risks that a researcher may take in the name of science. A few years ago, a group of researchers said they would test an HIV/AIDS vaccine on themselves (Associated Press 1997). Although this is certainly a worthy cause, one might argue that these researchers should not be allowed to take the risk of contracting HIV/AIDS. There can also be methodological problems with self-experiments, such as a small sample size and bias, that could affect the balance of risks and benefits (Davis 2003).

Some risk/benefit issues involve questions about the benefits of research. One of the many problems with some of the Nazi experiments (discussed above) is that they had questionable benefits. Some commentators have argued that pesticide experiments on human subjects conducted by private companies have dubious benefits (Krimsky and Simocelli 2007). In these experiments, private companies have exposed healthy adult human subjects to pesticides to generate safety data to submit to the EPA. The EPA has had to decide whether to accept these types of data for regulatory purposes. The agency has formulated new regulations pertaining to "third-party" research, or research sponsored by private companies, to submit to the EPA. One of the key issues in pesticide experiments is whether the benefits to society of the research outweighed the risks to human subjects (Robertson and Gorovitz 2000). Some environmental groups have argued that all pesticide testing on human subjects is unethical because the benefits of the research accrue mostly to the private companies and not to society. Others have argued, however, that society can benefit from pesticide experiments that lead to better knowledge of pesticides, which can be used for regulatory and public health purposes (Resnik and Portier 2005). A report by the Institute of Medicine (2004) determined that some types of low-risk pesticide experiments are acceptable, if they meet stringent ethical and scientific standards.

A final risk/benefit issue pertains to dealing with risks and benefits to third parties impacted by research, such as the subjects' community or family. For example, consider a hypothetical study on alcoholism, drug abuse, venereal disease, and sexual behavior in a Native American population. It is conceivable that the study might generate results that could be embarrassing to community members or could lead to discrimination or stigma. Researchers conducting this study would need to consider how best to protect the community's interests while advancing scientific knowledge. Consider a hypothetical study on the efficacy of allergy management education. As part of the study, investigators will hire private contractors to treat the home with insecticides to kill cockroaches. Although the homeowners provide consent for the study, other people who enter the home (such as children) may be affected by the insecticides. Investigators would need to decide how best to protect the third parties from risks. Finally, consider a hypothetical study of a drug to treat depression. If women in the study are lactating, their infants could be exposed to the drug through breast milk. Investigators would need to decide whether to exclude women from the study who are lactating.

The U.S. research regulations have nothing to say about protecting third parties, with the exception of regulations pertaining to enrolling pregnant women in research. U.S. research regulations focus on risks to the subject, not on risks to other people affected by the research. Although the regulations have little to say about third-party risks, the principle of beneficence, from the Belmont Report, implies that investigators should address risks to third parties, because the principle requires researchers to maximize the overall balance of benefits/risks and does not limit benefit/risk maximization to research participants. While most people would agree that investigators have an ethical obligation to address third-party risks, difficult questions can arise concerning how best to meet this obligation. In some cases, informing subjects about third-party risks and urging them to take steps to minimize harm will provide sufficient protection for third parties. In other cases, it may be necessary to obtain the consent of third parties before conducting a study. When a study is likely to have a significant impact on a community, investigators may need to consult a community advisory board concerning research design and implementation (Resnik and Sharp 2006; Weijer and Emanuel 2000).

Informed Consent

Informed consent promotes respect for the subject's autonomous decision making. Though informed consent has been widely recognized as a fundamental principle of ethical research since the adoption of the Nuremberg Code, it raises many different ethical issues. The most basic issue is whether informed consent of the subject (or the subject's representative) is ethically required. Some studies involve research conducted under emergency conditions in which it may not be possible to obtain the consent of the subject or the subject's representative. For example, if an unconscious victim of a car accident with a rare blood type is bleeding to death, it might be reasonable to provide the victim with an experimental, artificial blood product if no matching human blood is available and the subject's representatives (such as close relatives) are not available to provide consent. The ethical rationale for foregoing informed consent under these circumstances is that consent can be implied, because most people would consent to participation in a life-saving emergency research study. In 1996, the FDA developed special regulations for emergency research. Even though federal regulations allow emergency research under some circumstances, controversies may still arise concerning risks and benefits of the study. Fairness may also be an important issue if the majority of participants will be enrolled from low-income groups (Karlawish 2011).

Another fundamental issue is whether the informed consent process can be modified under some circumstances so that subjects are not fully informed. In Milgram's obedience to authority experiments, the subjects were told they were in a study, but they were not told about the exact nature of the research to avoid biasing the results. The subjects were deceived about their role in the study. The Common Rule allows IRBs to alter or waive informed consent when the research is regarded as minimal risk, it could not be conducted without an alteration or waiver, and the subjects will be debriefed after the study is complete (45 CFR 46.116d). Deception is a controversial topic in social science research, because people may disagree about the risks of research and the ability to obtain research objectives without deception. Some have argued that useful knowledge can often be gained in social science research without deception, and that deception can pose more than minimal risks, because people may experience emotional distress after learning that they have been intentionally deceived (Wendler and Miller 2011a).

Many issues in informed consent pertain to the disclosure and understanding of information (Capron 2011). Although the federal regulations specify types of information that must be disclosed (such as risks, benefits, alternatives, procedures, etc.), they do not cover everything that might need to be disclosed and they do not provide specific guidance concerning disclosure (45 CFR 46.116). For example, the regulations do not say that conflicts of interest must be disclosed. The regulations say that reasonably foreseeable risks must be disclosed, but they do not say what makes a risk reasonably foreseeable or the types of risks that must be disclosed (Resnik 2013).

Studies of the informed consent process indicate that subjects often do not understand key concepts related to research, such as randomization, research risks and procedures, and the difference between research and therapy (Flory et al. 2011). Research has shown that subjects in clinical studies often mistakenly think the study is designed to benefit them when its main purpose is to develop scientific knowledge. This mistaken belief, known as the therapeutic misconception, can pose a significant challenge for the consent process (Appelbaum et al. 1987). Researchers have an obligation to help subjects understand information they receive as part of the consent process. They should provide subjects with an ample opportunity to ask questions. Because many potential research subjects are not skilled readers, consent documents should be written at an eighth-grade reading level or lower (Capron 2011).

Some consent issues concern conditions that affect the voluntariness of the subject's choice. Federal research regulations require that investigators minimize the potential for coercion or undue influence (45 CFR 46.116). Prisoners, military personnel, employees participating in company-sponsored studies, and students in studies conducted by their professors may face different types of pressure to participate in research (Bonham and Moreno 2011). Ethical issues can arise concerning enrolling these subjects in research and ensuring that they can make a free choice. Ethical issues can also arise concerning compensating subjects for their participation, because payment for participation may be considered undue inducement if the amount of money subjects can receive is so high that it is likely to compromise their decision making (Dickert and Grady 2011). Not paying subjects enough for participation can also be unethical if it constitutes exploitation of subjects by private sponsors or investigators (Shamoo and Resnik 2006b).

Cultural factors often are relevant to the consent process. As noted in chapter 1, in some cultures women do not make their own medical decisions; medical decisions are made by a woman's husband or older male relative. In other cultures tribal leaders must be consulted in medical decision making (Hyder and Wali 2006). In Western cultures, competent adults make their own decisions. Investigators who conduct studies in cultural settings where individual consent is not the norm must decide how to enroll subjects in research. One possible way of dealing with this dilemma is to allow individuals to make their own choices while consulting other culturally appropriate decision makers (Council for the Organizations of Medical Sciences 2002).

Consent for the use of samples and data is an emerging consent issue. Consent documents often inform subjects that their samples or data may be shared with other researchers and used for various studies other than the one they are participating in. Some commentators have argued that subjects should have to provide consent for specific uses of their samples or data, while others have argued that consent to a broad use of samples or data is permissible (Wendler 2006). The advantage of specific consent is that it maximizes subjects' autonomy. The disadvantage of specific consent is that it can be difficult to implement and may constitute an unnecessary burden for subjects and investigators, because subjects would have to give their permission each time that an investigator wants to share samples or data with other researchers. The advantage of broad consent is that it reduces the burden on subjects and investigators and promotes sharing of samples and data; the disadvantage of this approach is that it may not completely respect subjects' autonomy, as subjects might not want their samples or data used in some types of studies (such as research involving cloning or the production of human–animal chimeras). A compromise position (known as the tiered approach) is to present subjects with a menu of options for use of their samples or data. Subjects can give permission for broad sharing of their samples or data or sharing only for specific studies or uses (Salvaterra et al. 2008). For example, subjects might allow their samples or data to be used only in research related to their disease or condition, or they might allow their samples or data to be used for only noncommercial research.

Privacy and Confidentiality

Privacy and confidentiality are different, but related, concepts. Privacy refers to a domain of personal space, dominion, or information that one has a right to keep from the public. Some threats to privacy have little to do with confidentiality. For example, a stranger who sees a person naked without their permission would be violating that person's privacy. Confidentiality refers to measures used to protect private information, such as medical or research records. Some confidentiality protections used in research include limiting access to research records and specimens, using computer security measures (such as encryption) to protect data, keeping paper records and specimens in locked rooms, and using a code to identify data or specimens. U.S. research regulations require that investigators take appropriate steps to protect privacy and confidentiality (45 CFR 46.111a7) but they say nothing specifically about how to do this. The Health Insurance Portability and Accountability Act (HIPAA) includes rules designed to protect medical privacy that apply to research conducted in hospitals or other clinical settings (Department of Health and Human Services 2013). The rules prohibit unauthorized disclosure of personal health information, with some exceptions, such as disclosure for public health reporting purposes.

Ethical dilemmas can arise in research when investigators share data or specimens from human subjects. The principle of openness (see chapter 1) instructs investigators to share data and samples as widely as possible to promote the progress of science. However, sharing data and samples may threaten confidentiality if not done properly. Researchers have used three different methods for sharing data and samples. Under the first method, recipients sign data use agreements (to receive data) or material transfer agreements (to receive samples). These agreements state conditions for the use of samples and data and require recipients to protect confidentiality. Recipients are not allowed to share samples or data with others without permission. The advantage of these agreements is that they provide strong confidentiality protections. The disadvantage is that they take time and effort to execute and can therefore inhibit sharing. Under the second method, researchers remove personal identifiers (such as name, phone number, address, etc.) from samples or data and share them with recipients. Recipients do not need to sign a data use agreement to receive data though they may still need to sign a material transfer agreement to receive samples. The advantage of this method is that it is less burdensome than signing a data use agreement and therefore promotes sharing. Under the third method, researchers may make de-identified data available to the public on a website. Investigators can download data without signing any agreement. The advantage of this approach is that it maximizes data sharing. A disadvantage of this approach is that it may not adequately protect confidentiality because it may be possible to re-identify individuals in de-identified databases. Statisticians have developed methods to identify individuals in genomic databases from a sample of the individual's DNA, as well as methods for identifying individuals from demographic information (e.g., gender, age, race, etc.) and a postal code. The upshot of these developments is that it may not be wise to place de-identified human subjects data on publicly accessible websites, because this may not adequately protect confidentiality (Homer et al. 2008; Lin et al. 2004; Lowrance and Collins 2007; McGuire and Gibbs 2006; Resnik 2010). Some investigators are promoting "recruitment by genotype" from so-called de-identified data (Beskow et al. 2012) for tissue samples stored in biobanks. There are serious ethical challenges to the use of tissue samples. Rial-Sebbag and Cambon-Thomsen (2012) have suggested a new governance model for the use of such samples, acknowledging the potential for breach of confidentiality.

Similar sorts of concerns can also arise when researchers publish data. Researchers who report data on individuals usually use case numbers, pseudonyms, codes, or other labels that do not identify individuals. However, sometimes it will be possible to identify individuals based on their demographic information, especially in studies on small communities. Sometimes it may be necessary to protect the confidentiality of an entire community to prevent stigma or discrimination. To protect confidentiality, it may be necessary to redact demographic data that could identify individuals or communities. However, redaction may reduce the value of the data for other researchers, because they may need this demographic information. Researchers need to be aware of these issues when they publish data and take appropriate steps to protect confidentiality (Kaiser 2009).

Protecting the confidentiality of subjects' family members also raises ethical issues. Researchers sometimes ask participants questions about their family history. In some cases family members can be readily identified based on an answer to a question; in other cases they may not be. For example, if the question is "was your father an alcoholic?" the answer readily identifies the subject's father. If the question is "did any of your siblings have problems with alcohol?" and the subject has more than one sibling, the answer does not readily identify a sibling. If family members can be readily identified from the answer to a question dealing with a highly sensitive topic (such as medical or psychiatric history, substance abuse, or criminal history) then researchers should obtain consent from those family members (Botkin 2001). A study known as the Personal Genome Project (PGP) raises some interesting issues concerning the confidentiality of family members. Human subjects in the PGP agree to forego traditional confidentiality protections and allow their identified genomic and medical information to be made available on a public website. The subjects understand the threat that this poses to their own privacy and confidentiality, but they have made this choice to help advance scientific research (Ball et al. 2012). While foregoing traditional confidentiality is an admirable gesture, it may threaten the privacy and confidentiality of the subjects' family members, since it may be possible to identify family members based on genomic or other information about the subjects. Some commentators have argued that a project like this should not be conducted unless the subjects' family members also consent to making this information publicly available (Resnik 2010).

Protecting privacy can become a significant issue when conducting research in homes or workplaces. Some research studies include interviews and sample collections that take place in the home or workplace. When researchers enter these areas, they may observe unethical or illegal activities that they feel they have an obligation to report, such as child abuse/neglect, illicit drug use, violations of occupational health or environmental laws, and so on. When this happens, researchers may face a conflict between protecting privacy and preventing harm to individuals or promoting public health and safety. Most states have laws requiring health professionals, educators, and social workers to report suspected child abuse and neglect. Researchers should inform research subjects about their obligations under these laws and report their suspicions. In other situations, researchers must use good judgment when deciding whether to report something they observe. For example, if a workplace safety violation poses a risk of serious harm to employees, researchers should inform management and possibly the relevant authorities. They may decide to only report a minor safety violation to management and not the authorities (Resnik 2011).

Vulnerable Subjects

Vulnerable research subjects are individuals who have difficulty providing informed consent or protecting their own interests, due to age, mental disability or illness, poverty, lack of education, language barriers, or other cultural or social factors (Macklin 2003). The Common Rule and FDA regulations require investigators to provide additional protections for vulnerable subjects (45 CFR 46.111b), and the Common Rule includes special protections for pregnant women, fetuses, and neonates (45 CFR 45, Subpart B); prisoners (45 CFR 46, Subpart C); and children (45 CFR, Subpart D). The FDA has also adopted the Common Rule's protections for children. International ethical guidelines, such as the Helsinki Declaration (World

Medical Association 2013) and the Council for Organizations of Medical Sciences guidelines (2002), also include additional protections for vulnerable subjects. The Belmont Report articulates the ethical rationale for providing additional protections for vulnerable subjects. According to the authors of the report, additional protections are needed to protect vulnerable subjects from exploitation. As described in our historical review (above), investigators have used prisoners, mentally disabled people, and children in studies that placed them at serious risk of harm but offered them no benefits. Such practices were unfair, harmful, and exploitative (National Commission 1979).

Some of the additional protections for vulnerable subjects found in research regulations and ethical guidelines include the following:

- Using a legally authorized representative (LAR), such as a parent, guardian, or family member, to provide consent for subjects who lack the ability to provide informed consent;
- Using procedures (such as a mental status assessment) for determining whether adults have the ability to provide informed consent for research participation;
- Ensuring that subjects who cannot provide informed consent nevertheless provide their assent (i.e., acknowledgment, cooperation), if assent would be meaningful to them;
- Including members on the IRB who have the knowledge and expertise to evaluate research involving vulnerable populations;
- Ensuring that there is a legitimate scientific reason for including vulnerable subjects in a study; vulnerable subjects should not be used if knowledge can be gained by using subjects who are not vulnerable; and
- Placing limits on the risks that vulnerable subjects are permitted to encounter in research.

Concerning the last point, the Common Rule places limits on the risks that may be imposed on pregnant women, fetuses, neonates, children, and prisoners. Pregnant women may not participate in research that poses more than minimal risks to the fetus if the research does not offer direct benefits to the fetus or the woman (45 CFR 46.204). Neonates of uncertain viability may not participate in research unless the research is likely to enhance the viability of the neonate or the research is a minimal risk (45 CFR 46.205). Prisoners may participate in more than minimal risk research only if it offers them direct medical benefits or affects prisoners as a class; other types of minimal risk prisoner research should focus on the causes or conditions of incarceration or criminal behavior (45 CFR 46.306).

The Common Rule allows four categories of research involving children: (1) minimal risk research (45 CFR 46.404); (2) more than minimal risk research that offers medical benefits to subjects (45 CFR 46.405); (3) minor increase over minimal risk research likely to yield knowledge about the subject's disorder or condition (45 CFR 46.406); and (4) research that is not otherwise approvable that represents an opportunity to address a serious problem affecting the health or welfare of children (45 CFR 46.407). An IRB cannot approve research that falls into this last category; the research can be approved only upon recommendation from a special DHHS panel. There is a concern that this category of research on children (45 CFR 46.407) has no explicit limits on the risks allowed for clinical trials on children (Wendler 2013).

The net effect of protective regulations and guidelines pertaining to vulnerable subjects is that some vulnerable groups, such as children and pregnant women, have been routinely excluded from research, which adversely affects the welfare of these groups (Mastroianni and Kahn 2001). For example, 90% of drugs prescribed to children have not been tested on pediatric populations. Physicians prescribe these drugs to children on an "off-label" basis by extrapolating from their effects on adult populations. For example, physicians may use body weight to guide drug dosing. This practice assumes that children are physiologically similar to adults, which is often a faulty assumption. Since the 1990s, pediatricians and advocacy groups have urged investigators and sponsors to include more children in research (Friedman Ross 2006; Tauer 1999). The U.S. government has taken some steps to encourage drug testing on children. In 1998, the FDA mandated that the pharmaceutical industry test drugs and biological products on children if they are to be used on children (Tauer 1999). In 2002, Congress passed the Best Pharmaceuticals for Children Act, which gives pharmaceutical companies an additional six months of market exclusivity for new drugs tested on children (Food and Drug Administration 2002).

The concept of minimal risk plays an important role in the pediatric research regulations, because IRBs can approve nonbeneficial research that is a minimal risk or a minor increase over minimal risk. A minimal risk is defined in the federal regulations as "the probability and magnitude of harm or discomfort anticipated in the research are not greater in and of themselves than those ordinarily encountered in daily life or during the performance of routine physical or psychological examinations or tests (45 CFR 46.102(i))." The definition consists of two ways of defining minimal risk. Minimal risk is either a risk not greater than risks ordinarily encountered in daily life or a risk not greater than routine physical or psychological tests. Because the federal regulations do not define risks "ordinarily encountered in daily life," there has been considerable disagreement about the meaning of this phrase, and there is evidence that different investigators and IRBs interpret it differently. In one study, 23% of IRB chairpersons classified allergy skin testing as minimal risk, 43% classified it as a minor increase over minimal risk, 27% classified it as a more than a minor increase over minimal risk, and 7% answered "don't know" (Shah et al. 2004).

There are two ways of interpreting risks "ordinarily encountered in daily life": a relativistic interpretation and an absolute one. According to the relativistic interpretation, daily life risks can vary according to the population and circumstances. For example, a child living in a ghetto probably encounters more risks than a child living in the suburbs. A child with a serious, chronic disease encounters more risk than a healthy child. Kopelman (2000a) argues against the relativistic interpretation on the grounds that it would lead to unequal protections of children and injustices. The relativistic interpretation leads to unequal protections because different IRBs could classify different studies as minimal risk, depending on the population and circumstances. A study approved as minimal risk by one IRB might not be approved by another. The relativistic interpretation leads to injustices because some populations might be required to bear a greater burden of research risks than other populations, because they already encounter higher risks in their daily lives. To avoid these ethical problems, an absolute interpretation should be used. The daily life standard of minimal risk should be the risk that a typical, healthy child ordinarily encounters (Wendler et al. 2005).

Involving pregnant women in research presents investigators and institutions with difficult ethical and legal questions. On the one hand, pregnant women have a right to decide whether to participate in research, and they can also benefit from research that provides them with medical or psychological therapy. Additionally, it is important to learn about prescribing drugs during pregnancy and how to treat medical problems during pregnancy. On the other hand, including pregnant women in research may expose the fetus to risks. Even if one does not consider the fetus to be a human being with full moral or legal rights, one must still be concerned about the harms that may occur to the future child while in the uterus. The thalidomide tragedy of the 1950s and 1960s provides a stark reminder of the dangers of fetal drug exposures. Thousands of children (mostly in Europe) were born with severe birth defects (such as missing or deformed limbs) as a direct result of in utero exposure to thalidomide, prescribed as a treatment for morning sickness (Stephens and Brynner 2001).

Investigators and research sponsors have been wary of including pregnant women (or even women who could become pregnant) in research out of fear of the legal liability resulting from birth defects related to research. A concern about how research procedures and interventions might affect the fetus is a reason why women were routinely excluded from research for many years (Dresser 2001). In the mid-1980s, feminist activists and politicians pressured the NIH to include more women in research studies. As a result, the NIH now has policies for the inclusion of women and minorities in research (Dresser 2001).

Prior to the National Commission's report in 1979, the use of prisoners in research was common. Current federal regulations reflect the National Commission's recommendation for special restrictions on the recruitment and use of this population as human subjects in research. Prisoners are compensated only for discomfort and time spent in research. The normal compensation package for adults outside the prison could be regarded as exploitative in the prison environment because most prisoners would prefer research participation to the daily boredom of prison life. One might argue that most prisoners would not participate in research if they were not in prison. There are also problems with maintaining confidentiality in the prison environment. In his book *Acres of Skin*, Hornblum (1998) chronicles how in the 1960s and 1970s researchers used the skin on the backs of prisoners to test numerous drugs and perfumes for toxicity and carcinogenicity. Several ethical issues came to light: Subjects received payment, housing for the experiment was better than that provided for other prisoners, the human interactions during the experiments were coercive, and informed consent was barely informative. Even though there are good reasons for excluding prisoners from research, some have argued that exclusionary regulations and policies unfairly restrict prisoners' autonomy. Some prisoners may want to participate in research in order to make a contribution to society and make amends for the harms they have caused (Bonham and Moreno 2011).

Although both the National Commission recommended extra protections for adults who may have difficulty providing informed consent due to mental disability or illness, the federal government did not issue special protections for these subjects as a separate subpart of 45 CFR 46 when it revised this document in 1991, due to insufficient advocacy for the mentally ill or disabled at that time (Shamoo and Irving 1993). To understand issues pertaining to adults who may have a compromised ability to provide consent, it is useful to distinguish between competence and decision-making capacity (DMC). Competence is a legal concept that refers to the right to make decisions. Adults have the legal right to consent to research participation unless a court declares them to be legally incompetent for that task and appoints a guardian. DMC is a psychological concept that refers to the ability to make reasonable choices. Adults who are legally competent may lack DMC because they have not been adjudicated incompetent (Berg et al. 2001). For example, a demented nursing home patient who has not been declared incompetent would lack DMC but be legally competent.

If an adult lacks sufficient DMC to consent to research participation, then it is necessary to obtain consent from an LAR. The preferred order for selecting an LAR in most jurisdictions is a guardian, health care power of attorney, spouse, or close family member (such as an adult offspring or sibling). An LAR may also assist in the consent process when an adult has the ability to give consent if there are some questions concerning the adult's DMC. If the adult's DMC declines, the LAR may be available to make decisions (National Bioethics Advisory Commission 1998). In some cases, an adult may use a legal document, such as a living will or health care power of attorney form, to express a desire to participate in research if he or she loses DMC. Researchers should honor wishes expressed in these documents (Berg et al. 2001).

One of the controversial issues relating to conducting research on adult subjects who may lack the ability to provide informed consent is whether there should be an independent assessment of their DMC (National Bioethics Advisory Commission 1998; Shamoo 1994b). The argument in favor of an independent assessment is that researchers have a conflict of interest when it comes to assessing DMC, because it would be in the researcher's interests to find that a person has sufficient DMC to participate in research to meet enrollment goals. The argument against independent assessment is that this can be very burdensome, expensive, and time-consuming, and is not necessary in low low-risk research. A compromise position, which we recommend, is that the need for an independent assessment of prospective subjects' DMC should vary with the benefit/risk ratio of the research. When the risks of research are more than minimal and the subjects will receive no direct benefits, an independent assessment of prospective subjects' DMC should be required. For example, a Phase I clinical trial of a new drug on healthy subjects should have independent assessment of prospective subjects' DMC. When the risks of research are more than minimal but the subjects are likely to benefit from participation, an independent assessment of DMC is advisable but not required. For example, an independent assessment of prospective subjects' DMC would be advisable in a Phase II clinical trial for a new chemotherapy agent. When the risks of research are minimal, an independent assessment of DMC is not required.

For example, there would be no need for an independent assessment of prospective subjects' DMC for a study that only requires subjects to fill out a health information questionnaire and have five milliliters of blood drawn every five years.

Another important issue concerning adults who cannot provide consent is whether they should be excluded from nonbeneficial, more than minimal risk research. The argument for exclusion is that people who cannot make their own decisions should be protected from harm. The argument against exclusion is that it is important to conduct some types of more than minimal risk studies on adults who lack DMC to learn more about their diseases or conditions. If these adults are excluded, this will adversely affect the welfare of individuals with the disease or condition and stigmatize the group (Miller and Fins 1999). For example, consider a hypothetical long-term study of Parkinson's disease (PD). Adults are recruited into the study when they have DMC, but they may lose DMC as their disease progresses and they develop dementia. The study includes yearly muscle biopsies, which are more than minimal risk procedures that provide important information about how PD affects the muscles. Excluding subjects from this study when they develop dementia may compromise the usefulness of the research, since it is important to understand muscle function as PD progresses. One way of handling this situation would be to ask adults with DMC to fill out an advance directive that allows them to undergo more than minimal risk study procedures if they lose DMC.

One of the most controversial episodes of military research with human subjects occurred during the first Gulf War (1990–1991), when the U.S. Department of Defense obtained an informed consent waiver from the FDA to administer the anthrax vaccine to thousands of soldiers in the war without their consent. The military wanted to vaccinate soldiers against anthrax because it was thought that Iraq had developed and stockpiled biological and chemical weapons, including weapons-grade anthrax dust. The vaccine was an investigational new drug (IND). There were no published studies of the safety or efficacy of the vaccine in humans prior to the war. The military's main rationale for giving the vaccine without informed consent is that if soldiers refused the vaccine, they could endanger other soldiers and military operations if they contracted anthrax. Some soldiers did refuse the vaccine, and they were court-martialed and punished. Many soldiers suffering from Gulf War illness claim that their mysterious disease was caused by exposure to the anthrax vaccine. An FDA review of the military's procedures found that they deviated from the FDA's approved plan for testing the vaccine. For example, the military convened a second IRB to approve the experiment after the first one determined that it was unethical (Cummings 2002; Moreno 2000).

Employees are sometimes asked to participate in research studies conducted by their employers. Like prisoners and soldiers, employees may face coercion or intimidation during the consent process. As mentioned earlier, pesticide companies used employees as test subjects in ethically questionable pesticide experiments (Resnik and Portier 2005). As mentioned in chapter 2, Woo Suk Hwang asked technicians working in his laboratory to donate eggs for his therapeutic cloning research. For employer-sponsored experiments involving employees to be ethical, great care must be taken to safeguard the employees' ability to freely consent as well as their privacy and confidentiality. One way to do this is for the employer to hire an independent contractor to conduct the study. The contractor, not the employer, would have access to the names of people who volunteer for the study. Since the employer would not know who participates (or does not participate) in the research, the employer will not be able to reward employees for participating or penalize employees for not participating. Employees who volunteer for this type of research should be assured that their participation will in no way affect their employment status, salary, and so forth.

Students often participate in research conducted by their professors. These studies range from filling out self-administered surveys distributed in psychology or sociology classes, to providing biological samples for chemical or genetic analysis, to participating in controlled behavioral experiments (Moreno et al. 1998). Students, like employees, may face coercion, undue inducement, or intimidation during the consent process. They may also not want to disclose private information to their professors. For students to participate in research, professors must take steps to ensure that consent is valid and to protect privacy. Participation in research should not be a part of the course grade, unless the professor gives the student an alternative to research participation that takes the same amount of time and effort, such as writing a short essay. Professors should not have access to private information that students disclose in research. Professors may only review private information if personal identifiers have been removed.

Research participants from developing nations represent a unique class of vulnerable subjects. Participants from developing nations may be vulnerable due to poverty, lack of education, language barriers, or cultural or political factors. Individuals that lack access to medical care may be highly motivated to participate in research that offers (or appears to offer) them the prospect of some medical benefit. They may be willing to take extraordinary risks to receive medical care and may have difficulty understanding the information that is conveyed to them during the consent process. Vulnerable subjects or their communities may be the victims of exploitation if the research exposes them to significant risks and is not likely to offer any significant benefits to the participants or the population. For example, if a pharmaceutical company tests a new drug (such as a treatment for sexual dysfunction) in a developing nation and it is not planning to market the drug in that nation, this could be considered exploitative. To avoid exploitation when conducting research in developing nations, it is important for researchers and sponsors to address diseases or conditions that are relevant to people living in those nations and to offer to share benefits with the population, such as new treatments that are developed as a result of research, education, or improvements to health care infrastructure. They should also take steps to ensure that consent is valid and culturally appropriate and that there is adequate local oversight, such as an IRB or REB review of research (Ballantyne 2005; Participants in the 2001 Conference on Ethical Aspects of Research in Developing Countries 2002; Resnik 2003a; Shamoo 2005; White 2007).

Though racial and ethnic minorities are not considered vulnerable subjects per se, studying members of these groups can pose ethical challenges for investigators, due to the legacy of the Tuskegee study and others forms of exploitation of racial and ethnic minorities in research (Lo and Garan 2011). Studies indicate that African Americans have a distrust of medicine and biomedical research that can affect their willingness to participate in research (Corbie-Smith et al. 1999, 2002; Rajakumar et al. 2009). Other minorities, such as Native Americans and Latinos, have experienced discrimination and exploitation that may also affect their willingness to participate in research. Difficulties with recruiting racial and ethnic minorities can adversely impact the generalizability of research findings. For example, if a medication for treating heart failure is tested on a population that is 98% Caucasian, the applicability of this study to other racial and ethnic groups may be limited, due to possible racial or ethnic differences in drug metabolism or cardiovascular physiology (Alessandrini et al. 2013; Saul 2005). To address problems with enrollment of racial or ethnic minorities, researchers may need to focus recruitment efforts on these populations in some cases. Additionally, it may be appropriate to conduct studies that focus exclusively on minority populations in order to learn more about those groups and fill in gaps in the literature (Lo and Garan 2011). However, researchers must use great care when focusing on racial or ethnic identities to avoid conveying the impression that these groups are being targeted unfairly. Research that focuses on racial or ethnic minorities should be conducted in order to learn more about these populations and offer them potential benefits, not to take advantage of them (Lo and Garan 2011).

To summarize this section, there is an ethical tension between including and excluding vulnerable subjects in research (Mastroianni and Kahn 2001). The Belmont Report's principle of justice requires that the benefits and burdens of research be distributed fairly (National Commission 1979). While most would agree that it is unfair to include vulnerable subjects in research unnecessarily, it may also be unfair to exclude them from research without a good scientific or ethical reason, because exclusion prevents investigators from obtaining knowledge that may benefit members of vulnerable groups (Mastroianni and Kahn 2001; National Bioethics Advisory Commission 1999). The key is to strike a reasonable balance between protecting vulnerable groups from harm and exploitation and enhancing their welfare.

QUESTIONS FOR DISCUSSION

Is the media paying too much, just enough, or too little attention to questionable research with human subjects? Why do you think that is so?

In your opinion, should there be a difference between informed consent for volunteering as a human subject and informed consent for medical treatment? What would those differences be, if any? Why?

Do you think children should be able to participate in more than minimal risk research that offers them no direct benefits?

Do you think informed consent documents are too long? Too complicated? What can be done to make them shorter and simpler?

What additional safeguards would you suggest to protect subjects with serious mental illness who enroll in clinical trials?

Do you think IRBs are doing a good job of protecting human subjects? How would you improve the system, if you believe improvement is needed?

Which ethical theory described in chapter 1—utilitarians, Kantianism, or virtue ethics—provides the best approach to research with human subjects? How might these theories disagree about some of the controversial cases discussed in this chapter?

Would you participate in a Phase I study of a new drug that offers you generous compensation but no medical benefits?

Do you think investigators should share individualized research results with participants?

Do you think it is ethical to use placebos in clinical trials?

Do you think deception in research, such as occurred in Milgram's experiments, is ethical?

CASES FOR DISCUSSION

CASE 1

Oscar Cabanerio is a 41-year-old immigrant living in the United States without any legal documentation. He is poor and needs cash to send to his family in Venezuela. SFBC International, Inc., is a large contract research organization (CRO) testing drugs in human subjects for drug companies in Miami, Florida. Cabanerio agreed to be in a trial to test Oros Hydromorphone, made by the Alza Corporation. The study paid each research subject $1,800. The subjects are instructed to swallow the tablets and not chew them, because chewing can cause overdosing. Adverse reactions include heart attacks, allergic reactions, and even death. Informed consent for this study is usually very quick. The subjects are eager to earn money, so they just look over the document and sign. Many of them have limited English-speaking abilities.

- What are some ethical problems with this study?
- Are there any problems with the selection of subjects, the consent process, or safety?
- Is there a fair subject selection in these studies and why?
- How would you run such a facility ethically?

CASE 2

An announcement in the newspaper and radio encourages people to enroll in research protocols to test a new antiflu medication. The announcement emphasizes that each subject will receive a free physical exam, free health care for 60 days, and $400 compensation. The new drug is very promising in either stopping the full-blown symptoms of the flu or preventing it altogether. The protocol has already been approved by an IRB.

- What questions would you ask if you were a potential subject?
- Should the IRB have approved the protocol? Why?

CASE 3

A hospital associated with a research university has a policy that every new employee must provide a blood sample. The employees are told that the blood samples will be frozen for a long time. The hospital's purpose in collecting the blood samples is to reduce their liability in case anyone contracts HIV. From the frozen samples, the hospital can determine whether the employee had the HIV virus prior to employment. A few years later, a researcher at the hospital is developing an HIV diagnostic instrument directly from the blood. The instrument, if it works, would advance HIV screening. The researcher wants to use the samples without any names attached to them (the samples are de-identified). The researcher wants to test different samples from different people.

- What concerns would you have if your blood sample was included in this research?
- Is this study ethical?
- Does this study need to be reviewed by an IRB?

CASE 4

A psychology professor teaching a seminar on human sexuality invites her students to complete a survey on their sexual experiences for course credit. The survey asks questions about sexual activity, sexual orientation, sexual fetishes, and sexual abuse. Students provide detailed, written answers to the questions, but they do not sign their names. There are ten students in the seminar. As an alternative to participating in the survey, students can write a short paper for equivalent credit.

- Do you have any ethical concerns with this study?
- Would you participate in it?
- Do you have any suggestions to improve this study?

CASE 5

Subjects for a research study will be recruited from private pain treatment clinics and the medical school's pain service. Preliminary studies have shown that the drug thalidomide may provide some relief for migraine headaches, arthritis, and neuropathy conditions. Because thalidomide's harmful effects on fetuses are well known, women of childbearing age will be excluded from this study.

- Are there benefits from this study?
- If you are a member of the IRB, what questions would you ask?
- What risks should be addressed?

CASE 6

A company is developing a pesticide for use on various crops, including tomatoes, corn, apples, green beans, and grapes. Previous animal studies indicate that it may be safer than other commonly used pesticides. The company plans to use healthy subjects (its employees) to test the pesticide for toxic effects. Each subject will be paid $500 and will be monitored carefully for three days. Investigators will collect data pertaining to toxicity and pharmacokinetics. Subjects will report adverse effects they experience, such as dizziness, nausea, headache, fatigue, shortness of breath, and anxiety.

- What are the risks to subjects?
- What are the benefits to subjects?
- Would you put any conditions on the protocol before going forward? What would they be?
- Are there any conflicts of interest? Can they influence the outcome of the study?

CASE 7

An untenured assistant professor at a medium-sized university is a member of her university's IRB. One of the human subject protocols the IRB is reviewing is from a world-renowned professor in another department at her university. This world-renowned professor is a member of the promotion and tenure committee. The assistant professor's package for promotion to tenured associate professor will go to the committee in six months. The assistant professor has a great deal of concern about the proposed protocol. She feels that the risks are watered down and the benefits or potential benefits are exaggerated.

- What should the assistant professor do? What would you do?
- How should the IRB handle the problem?

CASE 8

A research proposal and its informed consent forms were submitted to an IRB of an independent nonprofit research facility in San Francisco. The protocol will enroll 30 heroin addicts, of whom 20% are likely to have HIV. The protocol is a study of social habits of these addicts. The surveyor will follow the addicts around in their daily routine for one week to register their food intake, drugs used, sexual habits, and so forth. The researcher considered the study to be minimal risk research and said so on the proposal submitted to the IRB.

- Do you have any ethical concerns about this study?
- Is it minimal risk?
- Does the study raise any issues concerning privacy and confidentiality or the research subjects or other affected individuals?
- What information should the informed consent form contain?
- Should the IRB approve this study? Should it require any modifications for approval?

CASE 9

A researcher has submitted a proposal to an IRB for a clinical trial of a new drug to treat depression in adolescents (ages 12–17). The drug has been tested in adults and approved for use in adults but not in adolescents. The manufacturer of the drug is seeking approval for its use in adolescents. The study will enroll 75 adolescents with a history of depression. Subjects will be randomly assigned to one of three groups: Group A will receive the new drug; Group B will receive a standard treatment; and Group C will receive a placebo. Subjects and investigators will be blinded so that they will not know who is receiving the drugs or the placebo. All subjects will receive psychological counseling for depression and will be carefully monitored during the study. The study includes a 30-day washout period in which subjects stop taking medications for depression. Subjects will be closely monitored during the washout period. The study will follow subjects for 90 days while they are receiving the drugs. Each subject will receive free medication and psychological counseling and $1,200 once the study is completed.

- Do you have any ethical concerns with this proposed study?
- Should the study include a placebo group? A washout period?
- Do you have any suggestions for improving the study?
- Should the IRB approve this study?

CASE 10

An anthropologist is planning to study the culture of an experimental physics laboratory at Whitmore University. The anthropologist will observe the daily activities of people in the laboratory for three months and keep a detailed record of her field notes. She will also conduct semistructured interviews with members of the laboratory. There are 38 people in the laboratory, including senior scientists, junior scientists, postdoctoral fellows, graduate students, and technicians. She plans to summarize her findings in a series of articles that she submits for publication. She has submitted the study to her institution's IRB as minimal risk research. She has obtained the permission of the director of the laboratory to conduct this study and is planning to submit it to the Whitmore IRB as well.

- Do you have any ethical concerns with this study?
- What are the risks of this study? Is it minimal risk?
- Do you have any concerns about confidentiality or privacy in this study?
- Should consent for this study be obtained from all of the members of the laboratory?
- What should the anthropologist do if she observes or learns about unethical or illegal activity in the laboratory, such as data fabrication or falsification?

CHAPTER 12

Science and Social Responsibility

Scientists have ethical obligations to benefit society and avoid causing harm. Scientists can benefit society by conducting research that advances human knowledge or produces useful results (or both); educating the public about their research through lectures, media interviews, websites, and popular books; developing nutritional or health guidelines; providing expert testimony in legal proceedings or on government committees; or contributing informed opinions to public policy debates. Though social responsibility is an important principle for scientific research, it can lead to some ethical dilemmas, because it may conflict with other principles, such as openness and freedom. Conflicts may also arise within the principle itself when scientists consider how best to balance benefits and risks to society.

INTRODUCTION

Scientists have ethical responsibilities not only to each other but also to other members of society. Scientists who work with human subjects, for example, have an obligation to respect their rights and dignity and protect them from harm and exploitation. Social responsibilities may also arise even when scientists do not work with human subjects. All scientists have ethical obligations to benefit society and avoid causing harm. Scientists can benefit society by conducting research that advances human knowledge or produces useful results (or both); educating the public about their research through lectures, media interviews, websites, and popular books; developing nutritional or health guidelines; providing expert testimony in legal proceedings or on government committees; or contributing informed opinions to public policy debates. Scientists can avoid causing harm by refraining from publishing or conducting research that may be used to harm the environment, the economy, species, or society (Committee on Science 2009; Forge 2008; Kitcher 2001; Pielke 2007; Resnik 1998a, 2009a; Shrader-Frechette 1994; Weed and McKeown 2003).

The basis for social responsibilities in science is twofold.

First, like other members of society, scientists have a moral obligation to avoid causing harm and to benefit the others. Most moral theories support a general duty to avoid causing harm (nonmaleficence), which manifests itself in prohibitions against murder, manslaughter, rape, assault, theft, fraud, and so on. Most moral theories also support an obligation to do good when one can be reasonably expected to do so. For example, most people would agree that if you see a person drowning in a pool you should take some action to save that person, such as throwing that person a life preserver or calling a lifeguard. Scientists should benefit society by conducting research that contributes to human health, happiness, liberty, and reducing disease, injustice, and psychosocial distress. Scientists should treat all human beings as having equal worth, regardless of gender, sexual orientation, nationality, religion, and economic status (Shamoo 2012). Scientists' obligations related to benefits and harms extend beyond human society and include other species, habitats, and ecosystems. Scientists have obligations to avoid causing environmental damage (Resnik 2012b).

Second, scientists receive various forms of support from society. Even those scientists who are not directly funded by government agencies usually take advantage of publicly owned or supported laboratories, offices, universities, computers, research sites, and so on. Scientists who work for private companies have usually benefited from public support during their education. Scientists have an obligation to provide public benefits in return for the support they receive (Resnik 1998a; Shrader-Frechette 1994). If scientists cause harm to society, mismanage funds or resources, or fail to produce social benefits, they may endanger their public support.

In 1945, Vannevar Bush, who was a science advisor for Presidents Roosevelt and Truman, wrote an influential report, *Science: The Endless Frontier*, which laid the foundation for U.S. science policy since then. At that time, there was a dispute about how the government should invest money in scientific research and development (R&D). Some argued that government R&D funding should focus on projects with clear and definite practical applications that could be expected to provide immediate benefits to society. Bush argued that focusing on applied R&D was short-sighted and that the government should also fund basic research because basic research has significant long-term impacts on science, technology, private industry, and society. For example, basic research in subatomic physics during the late 19th and early 20th centuries laid the foundations for nuclear power, radar, x-ray imaging, radio, television, and many other technologies. Moreover, private industry is not likely to fund basic research, even though it benefits from it. Basic research can be considered a public good similar to infrastructure (e.g., roads, bridges), the police, firefighters, and the military.

For many years scientists have recognized that they have social responsibilities. The imminent English scientist and philosopher Francis Bacon (1561–1626), who inspired the first scientific association, the Royal Society of London, argued that the goal of science was to produce knowledge that would have practical value and would benefit humankind (Bacon 2000). Though Bacon believed that scientific knowledge should be sought for its own sake, he was confident that knowledge would benefit society by giving people control over nature. The father of microbiology, the French scientist Louis Pasteur (1822–1895), made many important discoveries that helped prevent disease and saved thousands of human lives. Pasteur helped found the germ theory of disease and developed vaccinations against rabies and anthrax (Robbins 2001). The physicist and philosopher Albert Einstein (1879–1955) believed that he had a responsibility to help the Allied forces stop the threat posed by Germany, Japan, and Italy in World War II. Einstein, whose special theory of relativity ($E = MC^2$) provided evidence of the tremendous power represented by nuclear fission, wrote several letters to President Roosevelt urging the United States to take steps to develop an atomic bomb before the Germans did. Roosevelt heeded Einstein's advice and initiated the top-secret Manhattan Project, which led to the development of atomic bombs that were dropped on Japan in 1945 (Isaacson 2007). The marine biologist Rachel Carson (1907–1964) published an influential book, *Silent Spring* (1962), which warned the public about the dangers of DDT (dichlorodiphenyltrichloroethane) and other pesticides for wildlife and human beings. Carson's work helped launch the modern environmental movement and led to increased government regulation of pesticides (Resnik 2012b).

Though social responsibility is an important principle for scientific research, it can lead to some ethical dilemmas, because it may conflict with other principles, such as openness and freedom. Conflicts may also arise within the principle itself when scientists consider how best to balance the inherent benefits and risks to society of their research. The remainder of this chapter will discuss some common ethical dilemmas related to social responsibility.

Communicating with the public and the media about one's research raises ethical issues because the public and media may misunderstand and misinterpret scientific information. Laypeople and reporters may misunderstand or misinterpret scientific evidence, concepts, theories, and recommendations. For example, if a study shows that a gene increases the chances of homosexuality in males by 10%, a reporter may write a headline saying "Scientists Discover Gay Gene." If a small but vocal minority of the scientific community does not accept the hypothesis that human activities that produce greenhouse gases are causing the Earth to warm, the public may interpret this as showing that there is no evidence for human-caused global warming. If a study shows that having a glass of red wine a day can reduce the risk of heart disease, some people may conclude that having three or more glasses of wine a day would be even better at preventing heart disease (Resnik 2001c).

Some scientists are so concerned about being misunderstood, misinterpreted, or misquoted that they decide not to communicate with the public or the media about their research. Others decide to oversimplify or "dumb down" their research to avoid misunderstandings or misinterpretations. While these reactions are understandable, one could argue that they are not socially responsible. Scientists who refuse to communicate with the public or the media about their research ignore their obligation to benefit society. People can benefit in many ways from learning about science. Scientific knowledge can help people learn how to take care of their health and the environment, as well as understand the world and their place in it.

Oversimplification of scientific information can be problematic when it undermines the public's understanding of research and interferes with informed decision making (Elliott 2006; Resnik 2001a). For example, since the 1980s, there has been an ongoing controversy concerning the recommended daily intake of sodium (Kolata 2013; Taubes 1998). Evidence shows that reducing sodium intake can lower blood pressure. High blood pressure is a risk factor for stroke and heart disease (Aburto et al. 2013). A severely restricted sodium diet (less than 500 mg per day) can lead to a dangerous condition known as hyponatremia (Goh 2004). Public health officials recommend that healthy individuals should not consume more than 2,300 mg of sodium per day and that individuals with risk factors, such as hypertension or kidney disease, should not exceed 1,500 daily (Centers for Disease Control and Prevention 2013; Institute of Medicine 2009). However, most people consume much more than 2,300 mg of sodium per day in the form of sodium chloride (salt). Salt is used widely to enhance the flavor of food and as a preservative. Thus, it is difficult for most people to avoid exceeding the recommended daily sodium allowance. Moreover, the evidence has not shown that reducing sodium intake has a significant impact on mortality or morbidity in healthy adults (Aburto et al. 2013; Graudal et al. 1998). Adults without risk factors may derive no significant health benefits from a restricted sodium diet, other than lowering their blood pressure marginally. If your blood pressure is normal and you have no risk factors, then reducing sodium intake to 2,300 mg daily or less may offer you no benefits (Graudal et al. 1998).

Even though the evidence does not show, conclusively, that all healthy adults should consume no more than 2,300 mg of sodium daily, most public health researchers and officials have stuck by the 2,300-mg recommendation, because they want to promote public health and they don't want to confuse people by giving them conflicting evidence (Kolata 2013; Resnik 2001c; Taubes 1998). It is better to give the public a simple recommendation that is not completely accurate, according to this line of reasoning, than to disclose the whole truth, which may be complex and difficult to understand. Enacting policies that help to lower blood pressure in the population will have a beneficial impact on public health by lowering the incidence of stroke and heart disease even if these policies oversimplify the scientific debate somewhat (Taubes 1998). One might argue, however, that withholding or distorting information in order to ensure that people make the "correct" decisions is paternalistic interference in the public's right to make informed choices (Resnik 2001c). The appropriate response to concerns that the public will misunderstand or misinterpret scientific information is to enhance the public's understanding by explaining scientific ideas in lay language and discussing the implications of conflicting evidence.

EXPERT TESTIMONY

Scientists are often asked to provide expert testimony in court cases, including criminal prosecutions and medical malpractice and products liability litigation. Scientists are also asked to provide expert opinions for government committees dealing with such issues as chemical regulation, pollution, food and drug safety, water quality, electric power generation, and highway and airline safety (Elliott 2006; Resnik 2004c). When scientists serve as experts they are usually asked to provide testimony concerning knowledge within their area of expertise, including their own research and scientific evidence, theories, concepts, methods, or principles. Expert witnesses in legal cases can answer questions concerning facts (e.g., "is asbestos listed as a known human carcinogen?") and opinions (e.g., "in your judgment, did exposure to asbestos cause cancer in these workers?"). Attorneys on opposing sides of legal cases are allowed to call their own expert witnesses and challenge the testimony of experts. Experts in legal cases are usually paid for their time (ranging from $200 to $2,000 per hour) and compensated for travel. Some experts, known as "hired guns," make over $100,000 dollars per year from providing testimony (Resnik 2007).

In several high-profile legal cases, such as the Dow Chemical breast implant case, there have been legal and political controversies about the validity of expert testimony. Many writers have argued that the courts have been far too liberal in admitting expert testimony in that they have allowed people to testify who lack legitimate qualifications, valid data, or sound theories. In a key U.S. Supreme Court case, *Daubert v. Merrell Dow Pharmaceuticals* (1993), the Court ruled that judges must be the gatekeepers for admitting expert testimony and that they can use a variety of criteria for determining who qualifies as an expert. Prior to this case, judges could admit expert testimony only if it was based on generally accepted ideas, theories, or methods. The practical effect of the general acceptance standard was that it was often used to exclude "junk" or "fringe" science as well as novel or untested science from the courtroom. Some commentators have argued that the pendulum has swung too far in the other direction and that scientists should reassert some control over expert testimony in the courtroom. Some have suggested that scientists could establish panels or boards of independent experts to provide testimony or that they could certify or license experts (Angell 1997b; Huber 1991). In addition to the issue of expertise in the courtroom, commentators have made similar arguments regarding the approval of new drugs, claiming that the Food and Drug Administration (FDA) should not bow to public demands to approve drugs.

Expert testimony raises at least two ethical issues. The first issue is financial conflict of interest (COI). Because experts in legal cases are paid by a particular party, they may have a financial interest in promoting the interests of that party, which could bias their testimony. Although attorneys' ethical rules forbid quid-pro-quo arrangements (i.e., an agreement to provide a particular kind of testimony for money), as well as contingency fees (i.e., payment based on the outcome of the case), financial interests can still influence how experts testify (Resnik 2007). For example, if a forensic science expert provides convincing testimony that helps prevent a defendant from being convicted in a criminal case, then other attorneys may seek the expert's assistance on their cases. The scientist could develop a reputation and a career based on his or her talent as an expert witness. Experts in medicine, product liability, automobile safety, and other areas of science and engineering could have similar motivations. Fortunately, the legal system has effective methods of dealing with COIs related to expert testimony. Attorneys can hire their own experts and cross-examine the opponent's experts. During cross-examination, an attorney can ask an expert to disclose his or her financial interests (i.e., who is paying for the testimony and how much). Thus, the legal system involves COI disclosure and management (Resnik 2007). Prohibiting experts from testifying based on their financial interests would not be a good idea, because this could interfere with the right to legal due process. Opposing parties have the right to call witnesses, including experts (Resnik 2007).

Experts testifying on government committees may also have financial interests that could bias their testimony. The FDA uses expert panels composed of scientists, physicians, pharmacists, and biostatisticians to provide recommendations concerning the approval and oversight of drugs, biologics, and medical devices. The opinions of these boards are nonbinding but very influential. In 1998, the FDA approved a rotavirus vaccine manufactured by Wyeth Lederle. The company took the vaccine off the market in 1999 when researchers discovered that it caused bowel obstruction in children. A congressional investigation of COIs at the FDA found that three out of the five committee members who voted to approve the vaccine had financial ties to rotavirus vaccine manufacturers. One committee member had $33,800 worth of stock from Merck, and another shared a patent on a rotavirus vaccine developed by Merck (Krimsky 2003). The congressional investigation of 177 FDA committee meetings found that in 88 meetings (49.7%) half of the committee members had a financial interest related to the topic being addressed.

Fortunately, the FDA has enacted what appear to be stringent rules concerning financial COIs on expert panels in response to criticism from Congress and others. FDA panel members and consultants must disclose their financial relationships and are not allowed to have financial interests related to the particular matter in question, unless they have been granted a waiver. Members may not participate on the panel if their total financial interests are $50,000 or more for the previous 12 months. The FDA may grant a waiver if "the need for the individual's services outweighs the potential for a conflict of interest" (Food and Drug Administration 2013). A waiver may be granted based on several factors, including the nature of the person's financial interest (e.g., stock or consulting arrangements and the amount of money involved) and the importance of their participation on the committee. Some commentators have criticized the use of waivers to include individuals on panels with COIs. Wood and Mador (2013) describe the effect of waivers on the FDA's advisory panel's decision and its threat to the integrity of FDA decisions. They cite a 2009 Institute of Medicine report stating that COIs on FDA advisory boards threaten the integrity of science.

The second issue is nonfinancial COIs. An expert may have a personal, professional, or political interest in the outcome of a court case or committee hearing. For example, a medical expert for the prosecution in a rape case, who is the mother of a daughter who was raped, would be strongly tempted to bias her testimony in favor of the prosecution. An ecologist, who is also a member of an organization that seeks to preserve wilderness, might bias his testimony in a committee hearing concerning the environmental impact of building a new electric power plant. While it may be difficult for scientists to set aside their personal, professional, or political interests when offering expert testimony, they have an obligation to do so, because the public expects that scientists will strive for objectivity when testifying in court or on government committees. Scientists who intentionally bias their testimony to promote their personal, professional, or political interests violate the public's trust. Scientists should disclose relevant personal, political, or professional interests when offering testimony and should be aware of how those interests may impact their thinking at a conscious or subconscious level.

Some might argue that, while they should not intentionally bias their testimony, scientists should be free to offer their personal or political opinions when they testify because complete objectivity is unattainable (Pielke 2007). Everyone is influenced by political, religious, economic, or other biases in some way. A scientist who claims to provide an objective presentation of the facts may actually present testimony that has been impacted by subconscious biases. For example, a scientist may omit some important evidence that impacts his conclusions, or he may use a method of data analysis that skews the results in a particular direction. While it is true that no one is perfectly objective, this is not a good reason for injecting personal or political opinions into expert testimony. Scientists who provide expert testimony should refrain from rendering opinions unless they are specifically asked to do so (Resnik 2004c).

PARTICIPATION IN POLICY DEBATES

Scientists, as informed experts and concerned citizens, can make important contributions to public policy debates on issues ranging from nuclear energy to environmental regulation to gun control. After World War II, Robert Oppenheimer and other scientists involved in the Manhattan Project sought to stop the proliferation of nuclear weapons and promoted peaceful uses of nuclear energy (Monk 2013). The pediatrician and child psychiatrist Herbert Needleman, who conducted important research demonstrating the adverse impacts of lead on human development in the 1970s, informed the public about the dangers of lead and pushed for regulations to ban lead as an ingredient in household paint and gasoline. As noted earlier, Rachel Carson advocated for additional pesticide regulations (Resnik 2012b).

There are several different ways in which scientists may participate in public policy debates (Pielke 2007; Resnik 2009a):

- Conducting research relevant to policy debates and publishing results in the open literature
- Educating the public about the relevance of their research for policy debates
- Advocating for regulations, policies, or political viewpoints

The first two ways of participating in public policy debates reinforce the image of the scientist as objective and impartial: The scientist conducts research and describes and explains facts. The third way, however, has the potential to impact the scientist's objectivity. As we have stressed several times in this book, objectivity is one of science's most important values. The public's trust in science is based, in part, on the expectation that scientists will strive to be objective. People look to scientists to provide objective information and facts. When people want opinions, they turn to political leaders, interest groups, religious organizations, newspaper columnists, bloggers, and so on (Resnik 2009a). Scientists who advocate for particular policy positions risk compromising their own objectivity and losing the public's trust. However, scientists have a right and a duty to express their opinions and participate in the political process, especially since they often have well-informed perspectives on policy issues. Because the public can benefit greatly from having scientists take an active role in policy debates, scientists who refuse to participate in policy debates in order to safeguard their objectivity may be neglecting their social responsibilities. It is worthy to note that scientists are citizens first and scientists second. To avoid compromising their objectivity or creating the impression in the public's mind that they are biased, scientists should exercise prudence and good judgment when participating in policy debates. A scientist who writes an opinion piece for a newspaper by definition is expressing his or her opinion. For example, a scientist should carefully distinguish between facts and opinions in his or her analysis.

MILITARY RESEARCH

Since ancient times, scientists have assisted with military efforts. Archimedes (287–212 B.C.E.) developed weapons to help the Greeks defend against Roman invasions, including a giant crane that could drop heavy weights on ships. The English physicist Isaac Newton (1642–1727) did research on ballistics that helped the military improve its aiming of cannons. The German chemist Fritz Haber (1868–1934), who won the Nobel Prize in 1918 for synthesizing ammonia, developed chemical weapons that were used in World War I. The American physicist Robert Oppenheimer (1904–1967) oversaw scientific research for the Manhattan Project. Other notable physicists, such as Enrico Fermi (1901–1954) and Richard Feynman (1918–1988), also worked on the project. The computer scientist Alan Turing (1912–1954) helped the British military break Germany's codes during World War II (Forge 2013).

Today, the U.S. Department of Defense (DOD) spends billions of dollars per year on military research and employs thousands of scientists. Although most people equate military research with research on weapons, strategies, and tactics, military research encompasses many different fields of science, including medicine, physiology, chemistry, physics, electronics, engineering, aeronautics, computer science, and psychology. Some of the world's most important inventions, including radar, satellites, computers, and the global positioning system, have their origins in military research (Resnik 2009a).

The primary ethical issue concerning military research is whether scientists should do it at all. Many people oppose the military on philosophical or religious grounds. Some are pacifists and oppose the use of violence for any reason. Others accept the limited use of violence (or the threat of violence) for police purposes but object to the use of violence for military goals. Still others accept the necessity of having a military but oppose specific military actions, such as the Vietnam War. Also, many people are deeply skeptical of the confluence of political and economic interests that influences the military, or what President Eisenhower referred to as the military–industrial complex. Those who have substantial qualms about the military will naturally object to military research (Forge 2013).

The justification for military research hinges on the rationale for having a military. The argument for having a military is that nations need to be able to defend themselves against threats from other nations as well as terrorism. In a utopia, there would be no need for a military because nations would coexist in peace. The real world, however, is a dangerous place. Hence, having a military is a necessary evil (Resnik 1998a). If having a military can be justified, then military research can be justified on the grounds that it is necessary for the military to achieve its goals.

While this argument for military research has considerable merit, it is important to be mindful of its limitations. The argument only shows that military research, in general, can be justified. It does not show that all types of military research are justified. One could coherently maintain that many types of military research, such as research on biological weapons or using torture as an interrogation technique, are unethical, while maintaining that other types, such as research on bulletproof vests or treatments for traumatic brain injuries resulting from battle, are ethical. Questions concerning the ethics of different types of military research are beyond the scope of this book and will not be explored here.

A secondary ethical issue concerning military research is whether it should be conducted on academic campuses. Some military research is kept secret (or classified) to protect national security interests. Access to classified information is granted on a need-to-know basis. To obtain access to classified information, one must undergo a thorough background check. There are different categories of classified information, including "top secret" (the most restricted), "secret," and "confidential" (the least restricted). For a research project to be classified, it must be funded by a government agency, such as the Department of Defense, the National Security Agency, the Department of Homeland Security, the Department of Energy, the Department of Health and Human Services, or the Federal Bureau of Investigation, that has the authority to classify research. Research that has not been explicitly classified remains open, except research on nuclear weapons, which is automatically classified (Resnik 2009a).

Some object to conducting classified military research on university or college campuses because it violates the ethical principle of openness, which is essential to academic research. Professors, students, and staff who work on classified projects must keep their work secret and not discuss it with their peers. They may also need to establish secure workspaces to prevent unauthorized access to data or materials. Although the sharing of information and ideas is vital to the academic ethos and scientific progress, military research is not the only type of secret research conducted on college or university campuses. Many academic institutions conduct research for private corporations, such as pharmaceutical, biotechnology, or computer technology companies, which treat the research they sponsor as confidential and proprietary information. If conducting secret research for private companies on campus is acceptable, then conducting secret military research should also be acceptable. Of course, one might object to all types of secret research conducted on academic campuses. However, it would be logically inconsistent to reject secret military research without rejecting secret corporate research.

DUAL USE RESEARCH

Scientific research conducted with the goal of benefiting society may yield results that can be misused by others (such as criminals or terrorists) to cause significant harm to national security, public health, society, the economy, or the environment. For example, knowledge of chemical explosives can be used to excavate land or to make bombs. Studies about the genetic makeup of human populations may be used to understand diseases or to perpetuate racist ideologies or to create a deadly gene-specific virus. The term "dual use research" was coined at the beginning of the 21st century to refer to research that may be used for either good or bad purposes (National Research Council 2004). Since 2001, the dual use research that has generated the most controversy has involved experiments involving dangerous pathogens and toxins. Some of these published studies include the following:

- Research that could be used to develop smallpox viruses that can overcome the human immune system's defenses (Rosengard et al 2002)
- A paper describing how to infect the U.S. milk supply with botulinum toxin (Wein and Liu 2005)
- A study demonstrating how to reconstruct the extinct 1918 Spanish influenza virus, which caused over 50 million deaths worldwide, from published sequence data (Tumpey et al. 2005)
- Research on genetically engineering the H5N1 avian flu virus so that it can be transmissible by air between mammals, including humans (Imai et al. 2012; Russell et al. 2012) (H5N1 has an estimated 60% mortality rate; fortunately, humans can only contract the virus by direct contact with infected birds [Resnik 2013])

In 2004, the U.S. government created the National Science Advisory Board for Biosecurity (NSABB) to provide government and institutional officials, journal editors, and scientists with advice on how to handle the findings from dual use research (Resnik 2013). The NSABB focused its attention on experiments of concern involving dangerous biological pathogens and toxins, known as select agents and toxins. Some select agents include the avian influenza virus, the 1918 Spanish influenza virus, the Marburg virus, the Ebola virus, variola viruses (animal and human pox viruses), botulinum neurotoxins, ricin, and saxitoxin (Health and Human Services and U.S. Department of Agriculture 2013). The U.S. government adopted a policy in 2012 that requires risk mitigation for government-funded experiments of concern involving select agents and toxins, including studies that

a. Enhance the harmful consequences of the agent or toxin;
b. Disrupt immunity or the effectiveness of an immunization against the agent or toxin without clinical or agricultural justification;
c. Confer to the agent or toxin resistance to clinically or agriculturally useful prophylactic or therapeutic interventions against that agent or toxin or facilitates their ability to evade detection methodologies;
d. Increase the stability, transmissibility, or the ability to disseminate the agent or toxin;
e. Alter the host range or tropism of the agent or toxin;
f. Enhance the susceptibility of a host population to the agent or toxin; or
g. Generate or reconstitute an eradicated or extinct agent or toxin. (U.S. Government 2012)

Risk mitigation could include modifying experimental protocols to reduce the risks of accidental contamination or misuse of results; enhancing biosafety measures; regularly reviewing experiments; and reviewing evidence of medical countermeasures for agents or toxins (such as treatments or vaccines). If risks cannot be adequately mitigated, options include not providing or terminating funding; redacting key information from publications and communications; or seeking classification of the research (U.S. Government 2012).

Some scientific journals have also adopted policies for reviewing dual use research. These policies involve additional review of submitted manuscripts identified by reviewers or editors as raising dual use issues. Additional review may involve gathering more information about the benefits and risks of the research (Resnik 2012c). *Science* and *Nature* conducted a dual use review of articles reporting the results of experiments that modified the H5N1 virus (Imai et al. 2012; Russell et al. 2012). The NSABB also reviewed this research. The NSABB initially concluded in December 2011 that one of the papers (Russell et al. 2012) should be published in redacted form, but it later decided in March 2012 that both papers should be published in full, after it received more information about the benefits and risks of the research. The journals published the papers shortly after the NSABB made its final determination (Resnik 2013).

Dual use research raises difficult ethical issues for scientists, funding agencies, journal editors, and society. On the one hand, the principles of openness and freedom favor no restrictions on publication or funding. Additionally, the results of research often have the potential to benefit society. For example, one of the objectives of the controversial H5N1 experiments was to determine whether this virus was capable of mutating in the wild so that it would be transmissible between mammals via respiratory water droplets. If the virus were to acquire this capacity, it could cause a global pandemic because human beings have no natural immunity to the virus. Information about potentially dangerous mutations of the virus could be useful to public health officials monitoring bird populations. If public health officials are able to detect forms of the virus with these dangerous mutations in the wild, they could take appropriate steps to try to stop the spread of the pathogen (Resnik 2013). On the other hand, social responsibility may favor restrictions on funding, publication, or both, if the results of research could be used to cause significant harm. Many scientists were concerned that terrorists, or other people with nefarious motives, could use the information produced by the controversial H5N1 studies to produce a bioweapon that could cause a global pandemic if deployed. Scientists were also concerned about the public health threats of accidental contamination of researchers working with the virus.

Dual use research can be difficult to evaluate not only because fundamental values may be at stake but also because there is usually a great deal of uncertainty concerning the risks of the research (Resnik 2013). While it may be possible to identify the risks of research, it may not be possible to quantify these risks (i.e., assign them an objective probability, such as 0.01, 0.10, 0.50, etc.). Traditional risk/benefit assessment performed by regulatory agencies, such as the FDA or the Environmental Protection Agency, usually involves weighing and comparing quantitative risks and benefits. For example, when the FDA approves a new drug, it bases its decision on scientific evidence concerning the likely effects of the drug on health outcomes in the population, such as morbidity and mortality. Traditional approaches to risk/benefit assessment may not apply to decisions concerning dual use research, due to lack of scientific evidence concerning risks. When traditional risk/benefit approaches to decision making break down, another strategy, known as the precautionary principle (PP), may apply. According to one version of the PP, one should take reasonable measures to prevent, minimize, or mitigate risks that are plausible and significant (Resnik 2012c, 2013). A measure is "reasonable" if it is effective and balances competing values appropriately. In the H5N1 example, competing values include openness, freedom, and social responsibility (i.e., the obligation to maximize benefits and minimize harms).

Publishing the H5N1 papers in full did little to prevent, minimize, or mitigate the risks of the research. Enhancing biosafety pertaining to H5N1 genetic engineering research, which was recommended by the NSABB, helped to mitigate risks, but biosafety enhancements would have been indicated even if the research had not been published. One could argue that a reasonable measure in the H5N1 case would have been to publish the research in redacted form, because this would balance competing values fairly. Although this option would limit scientific openness and freedom, it still would have alerted scientists and public health officials to H5N1's potential to mutate dangerously. Moreover, some responsible researchers working in the area could have been granted access to the full papers, with the understanding that the full papers would not be distributed. This option would also have helped to prevent or minimize potential harm to society. One problem with redacted publication, however, is that it might not be very effective, because the Freedom of Information Act (FOIA) allows the public to obtain access to nonclassified research supported by the federal government. If the research had been published in redacted form, someone probably could have gotten the result through an FOIA request and distributed them widely. Scientists would need to develop a system for making full copies of redacted papers available to responsible scientists. Scientists who receive these papers would need to undergo a background check to verify their trustworthiness and would need to agree to keep information confidential. The option of classifying the research would not have balanced competing values fairly because this would significantly restrict openness and freedom and would not alert scientists and public health officials to H5N1's potential threat (Resnik 2013).

QUESTIONS FOR DISCUSSION

1. What does it mean for a scientist to be socially responsible?
2. Why is social responsibility important in science?
3. What are some of scientists' social responsibilities?

4. Do you think scientists should conduct research sponsored by the military? Why or why not?
5. What is dual use research?
6. Can you think of any examples of dual use research from your discipline?
7. Do you think restrictions on scientific publication are warranted in some circumstances? Why or why not?
8. Should government funding organizations judge research proposals according to their potential to contribute to society? Why or why not?
9. Is it important to fund research projects that may have any practical applications?
10. Why is it important for scientists to communicate with the public and the media?
11. Should scientists take any steps to ensure that their research is not misunderstood or misinterpreted when communicating with the public or the media?
12. How should scientists participate in public policy debates? Should they offer opinions? Should they advocate for particular positions?
13. Are scientists inherently biased? How should they deal with their own biases when conducting research or communication with the media or the public?

CASES FOR DISCUSSION

CASE 1

The National Security Agency (NSA) has negotiated a $20 million contract with a large, public university to establish a research center on campus. The research conducted at the center would help the NSA mine data from emails, websites, and phone records for patterns that may indicate terrorist activity. The NSA would not access the content of particular emails or phone calls but will collect data on the locations of senders and recipients. The center would conduct basic research on statistical and analytical methods and will not access any data from emails or phone calls. The center would employ faculty, graduate students, postdoctoral students, and research staff. All of the research would be classified. A group of faculty and students who have learned about the negotiations with the NSA have begun protesting. They strongly object to the NSA's monitoring of electronic communications, which they regard as an invasion of privacy. They also object to conducting classified research on campus. They want the university to reject the contract. What should the university do? How should the university respond to the protesters?

CASE 2

A group of researchers have studied the vulnerability of the U.S. milk supply to attacks. They have identified weak (unsecure) points in the milk supply and have developed a mathematical model that predicts how many people will be killed when different amounts of the toxin are dumped into the supply at different points. They have submitted their work for publication in a top-tier journal. The National Institutes of Health (NIH), which funded the research, has contacted the editors and asked them to stop the publication. The agency is concerned that the publication will provide information that terrorists can use for an attack. The editors of the journal want to go ahead with publishing the article, because they feel that the benefits of the research will outweigh the risks. The editors believe that publishing the research will alert milk suppliers and public health officials to the significance of the problem and motivate them to take effective action to secure the milk supply. The editors and officials from NIH have a meeting to discuss these issues. Should this research be published in full, in redacted form, or not published at all? Was it appropriate for the NIH officials to inform the journal about their concerns with this research?

CASE 3

Marci Poirot, a doctoral student at a French university, has discovered a new species of truffle growing in a location near the Alps. This is an important discovery that will help biologists have a better understanding of the evolution, genetics, and ecology of this species and related ones. This discovery is important to her as well, because she will get to name the new species. Her dissertation will focus on a description of this new species. The new species is very rare, however, and could become extinct if people harvest the truffle. Truffles are a much sought-after delicacy, and truffle suppliers are always looking for new sources. Ms. Poirot is concerned that if she names the exact location of the new species that it could become extinct. Should she publish her finding in full or in redacted form?

CASE 4

Brent Barry is an anthropology professor who has studied a Native American community in Canada for several years. Dr. Barry has developed a good working relationship with members of the community and they trust him. The community is having a dispute with the Canadian government concerning ownership of some land. Tribal leaders claim that the land belongs to the tribe, based on their historical connection to the land. They claim that they have been occupying the land for more than a thousand years and should be granted ownership. Dr. Barry has learned through interviews with members of the tribe that ownership claims made by the tribal leaders cannot be substantiated. According to these members, the tribe has no historical connection to the land and has only been occupying it for a few decades. Dr. Barry is preparing to publish a paper on the tribe's history and customs. Should he mention anything about occupation of the land in the paper? Should he present evidence in the paper that contradicts the claims made by the tribal leaders? If the Canadian government asks him to testify about this issue in court, should he comply?

CASE 5

Doreen Wilkins has studied the physical and mental health of a community affected by Hurricane Katrina. She is attempting to understand how the community has been affected by the disaster and how it is recovering. She has worked closely with community leaders from the beginning of her project. A community advisory board has provided valuable input into the project and has helped with recruitment. Dr. Wilkins has given the board regular updates about the progress of her study and has shared her findings with the board prior to publication. Dr. Wilkins discovered that the community has significantly higher rates of human immunodeficiency virus (HIV) infection, hepatitis C, and drug and alcohol abuse, compared to the rest of the U.S. population. She shares this information with the board. The board asks her to not publish these results, because they are concerned that it could result in discrimination and bias against the community. What should Dr. Wilkins do? How could this predicament have been avoided?

CASE 6

Jack Johnson, a criminologist at a private university in Chicago, has been an advocate for gun control ever since his father was shot and killed 10 years ago when a person suffering from mental illness fired an assault rifle randomly into a crowded street. Six other people died in the incident. Dr. Johnson's research has focused on the effectiveness of gun control legislation. He has examined the effects of gun control laws in different nations and states. Dr. Johnson has been asked to give testimony about his research to a congressional committee considering gun control legislation, which will meet in two weeks. He has also been asked to write an opinion piece about gun control for a prominent Chicago newspaper. A student political group at his university has asked him to sign and help circulate a petition in favor of increased gun control. They have also invited him to speak at a downtown rally against gun violence. How should Dr. Johnson manage his social responsibilities related to gun control? Should he testify before the committee? How should he testify? Should he let the committee know about his personal connection to this issue? Should he write an opinion piece, circulate the petition, and speak at the rally?

CASE 7

Sophie Seymour is a pharmacologist at a medical school associated with a large university and hospital. She has conducted research on interactions between hypertension drugs and antidepressants. She has discovered a potentially dangerous interaction between a common hypertension drug and a new antidepressant medication. The interaction can lead to itching, a generalized rash, swelling, nausea, respiratory failure, and death. One person has died and several have been hospitalized. Individuals with asthma or other respiratory diseases are most at risk. The evidence she has for this interaction is based on her analysis of 82 medical records kept at the hospital during the past year for patients who have been treated for possible adverse drug reactions. Dr. Seymour has already informed the FDA about the interaction, but she believes that lives can be saved if she also warns the public immediately about this drug interaction, and she wants to call a press conference to announce her findings. Her research has not yet been submitted for peer review. Should she hold a press conference or wait until her research is published in a peer-reviewed journal? Would holding a press conference prevent her from publishing in a peer-reviewed journal?

CASE 8

Dr. Peter Protkin is a cancer epidemiologist who has studied a possible link between cell phone use and brain cancer. Several published studies have demonstrated no connection between cell phone use and brain cancer, but the studies were not very large and did distinguish between different types of phones used or methods of use (e.g., handheld, headset, etc.). Dr. Protkin's study collects data on patients with one of three types of brain cancer—glioma, meningioma, or acoustic neuroma—and compares the cases to a control group. Cases and controls are both asked questions about their cell phone use. Dr. Protkin has found evidence that the use of a particular type of cell phone that is no longer in use increases the risk of acoustic neuroma by 24%. However, the P-value for this study is 0.059, just above the accepted threshold for statistical significance (0.05). Dr. Protkin is therefore not very confident about this result, but he thinks it is interesting and warrants further study. Dr. Protkin publishes his findings in a public health journal. Shortly after his results are published, a reporter from the *Daily Planet*, a popular online publication managed by an environmental and public health interest group with over one million followers, wants to interview Dr. Protkin. During the interview, Dr. Protkin stresses that this study does not prove anything and that any possible relationship between cell phone use and brain cancer needs further study. The reporter asks Dr. Protkin if he uses a cell phone. He tells the reporter that he does, but he says he tries to minimize his use and he does not hold his phone near his head. He has the reporter's assurance that these comments are "off the record." The next day Dr. Protkin becomes very angry when he reads a story posted on the *Daily Planet*'s website. The headline says "Study Links Cell Phone Use to Brain Cancer." The article includes several other inaccuracies and Dr. Protkin's off-the-record comments. How should Dr. Protkin respond to the reporter's misrepresentation of his research? How could he have avoided this problem?

CHAPTER 13
Conclusion

In this final chapter of our book, we recommend some steps that researchers, institutional officials, government agencies, and scientific organizations can take to promote ethical conduct in scientific research, such as ethical leadership, education, and mentoring in responsible conduct of research, policy development, compliance and oversight, and international cooperation.

In this book, we discussed many different aspects of the responsible conduct of research (RCR), ranging from foundational topics like ethical theories and decision making to applied ones like conflicts of interest and research misconduct. We hope that students, trainees, investigators, and administrators will find our book to be a valuable source of information and guidance. In our final chapter, we would like to make some suggestions for putting RCR into practice. We will discuss some steps that researchers, institutional officials, government agencies, and scientific organizations can take to promote ethical conduct in scientific research. We will group these recommendations into five areas: leadership, education and mentoring, policy development, compliance and oversight, and international cooperation.

LEADERSHIP

There's a saying in business that "it all begins at the top." What this means is that for a business to be successful, it needs ethical leadership. One need not look very far for examples of how bad corporate leadership leads to poor decisions, unethical and illegal conduct, and business failures.

The Enron scandal is a perfect illustration of the consequences of bad leadership for a corporation's employees and stockholders, and the general public. Enron was an energy trading corporation led by its chief executive officer, Kenneth Lay. In 2000, the company had more than 22,000 employees and claimed more than $100 billion in revenues. In 2001, the company came crashing down when it was learned that its financial success was an illusion sustained by systematic and creatively planned accounting fraud (Fox 2003; McLean and Elkind 2003). Even before the Enron scandal broke, successful businesses understood the importance of a commitment to ethics and integrity, and many had adopted corporate ethics statements and instituted corporate ethics programs (Murphy 1998).

Ethical leadership is also important for success in scientific research. Unethical leadership at research institutions can lead to corruption and abuse, mismanagement of funds, scandals, legal liability, inefficient operations, a bad reputation, and low employee morale. Without ethical leadership, a research institution not only will fail to produce the tangible products of research, such as publications, patents, contracts, and grants, but also will fail to live up to standards of quality, ethics, and integrity. Individuals with leadership positions at academic institutions include laboratory directors, department or center heads, deans, vice presidents, presidents, and members of the board of trustees. Leadership is an important aspect of mentoring, collaboration, laboratory management, research administration, and other research activities.

Ethical leaders motivate people to work together to achieve common goals (Vroom and Jago 2007). Ethical leaders set an example for other people in the organization through their conduct, demeanor, and attitudes. Ethical leaders stress the importance of ethics in their speeches, public statements, budgets, and priorities. They do good work, and they inspire others to do the same by embodying ethical virtues, such as honesty, courage, fairness, determination, and integrity. Ethical leaders ensure that the institution makes strong commitments of financial and human resources to ethics. This commitment may include funding for ethics courses, oversight committees (such as institutional review boards [IRBs], institutional animal care and use committees [IACUCs], and conflict-of-interest [COI] committees), faculty and staff, and officials (such as ethics or compliance officers). Ethical leadership does not imply perfection—even ethical leaders make mistakes. But ethical leaders respond to mistakes by admitting them, learning from them, and taking steps to correct them, not by denying them or covering them up.

The importance of leadership illustrates how research ethics is an institutional or organizational concern, not just an individual one (Berger and

Gert 1997; National Academy of Sciences 2002; Shamoo and Davis 1989; Shamoo and Dunigan 2000). Although most ethical theories, principles, and concepts focus on the ethical duties of individuals, institutions and organizations also have ethical and legal responsibilities (De George 1995). For example, a research institution has a duty to ensure that its members obey the laws, regulations, and policies that govern the institution. A research institution also has a duty to do good work and to avoid harming individuals, society, or the environment. While all members of the institution are responsible for helping to ensure that it lives up to its obligations and duties, institutional leaders play a key role in this endeavor, because they have a greater ability to affect institutional decisions and policies. Leaders can help institutions honor their ethical obligations by helping develop an ethical culture in the institution. In an ethical culture, ethics is not an afterthought but is essential to institutional activities. People are motivated to do the right thing for the right reason, and they consider ethical principles when making decisions. They understand the importance of ethics and are willing to report conduct that is illegal or unethical (Vasgird 2007).

EDUCATION AND MENTORING

In chapter 2, we discussed the importance of education and mentoring in preventing research misconduct, but education and mentoring are vital to all aspects of ethical research, including data management, publication, and collaboration. The main rationale for RCR education is that it is a form of preventative ethics: It is better to prevent ethical problems in research than to deal with them when they arise (Vasgird 2007). To promote ethics education and mentoring, research organizations must provide financial support for these activities and make room for them in the curriculum and work schedule. Although instruction in RCR can begin at the undergraduate level, it is probably most effective at the graduate level, when students are actively involved in research and are familiar with some of the ethical questions that may arise. RCR instruction at the postgraduate level may include refresher courses and periodic updates on specialized topics, such as human subjects, animal research, and so forth.

RCR instruction should include the topics covered in this book as well as specialized ones tailored to an institution's particular needs, such as ethical aspects of bioweapons research or nanotechnology. Institutions must provide incentives for researchers to engage in mentoring activities; otherwise, they may decide that they cannot spare any time or energy for mentoring. To help support integrated learning of ethics, institutions can encourage researchers to discuss ethics topics in their regular courses. For example, courses in statistics or research methodology could discuss ethical issues related to the analysis of data, a course on pharmacology could discuss ethical aspects of drug testing, and a course on mammalian physiology and anatomy could discuss experimentation with animals. Institutions can also support informal gatherings for ethics discussions, such as brown-bag lunch meetings, focus groups, or workshops, and they can support ethics consultations by professional ethicists or researchers with ethics knowledge. To encourage experiential learning, IRBs, IACUCs, and other committees that deal with ethical issues should invite students and researchers to observe their meetings, provided that confidential information is protected. Although we have focused on the educational activities of universities, we would like to mention that other institutions or organizations involved in research, such as four-year colleges, pharmaceutical companies, government laboratories, journals, nonprofit research foundations, contract research organizations, and independent (for-profit) IRBs, should also support educational and training activities to promote an ethical culture.

As mentioned in chapter 2, research on the effectiveness of RCR education and mentoring is inconclusive. While some studies have shown that education and mentoring have a beneficial impact on ethical knowledge, awareness, and reasoning, others have suggested that education and mentoring may have little impact on behavior. Clearly, more research is needed on the effectiveness of RCR education and mentoring, as well as the effectiveness of different formats (lectures, workshops, integrated learning, etc.). We support efforts by individuals and institutions to learn more about RCR education and mentoring.

POLICY DEVELOPMENT

To help support education and mentoring activities and to establish standards of conduct and behavior, institutions should develop policies and procedures pertaining to RCR. Topics for policy development should include the following:

• Data management (acquisition, storage, analysis, sharing, etc.)
• Research misconduct (definition, procedures for investigation and adjudication)
• Conflicts of interest

- Intellectual property
- Technology transfer
- Authorship
- Publication
- Peer review
- Mentoring
- Collaboration
- Fairness in employment (e.g., discrimination, harassment)
- Human subjects
- Animal subjects
- Radiation safety, biological safety, and laboratory safety

Many university policies are already mandated by government funding agencies, such as the National Institutes of Health (NIH) or the National Science Foundation (NSF). For policy development to be meaningful and useful, it should include input from all of the key stakeholders in research (i.e., junior and senior investigators and staff), not just input from research administrators and attorneys. Researchers should perceive policies as serving important needs, not as useless red tape that caters to bureaucratic whims. All policies that are developed should also be well publicized. Copies of policies should be distributed to faculty and staff and should be available on institutional websites. Policies should be discussed and reviewed during educational or training sessions. Additionally, knowledgeable people should be available to answer questions about the interpretation and application of these policies. For example, an IRB chair or administrator could answer questions about human subjects' policies, and a technology transfer officer could answer questions about technology transfer, and so on. A person who specializes in research ethics could answer questions about various different policies, including data management, authorship, conflicts of interest, and research misconduct (de Melo-Martín et al. 2007).

Scientific journals, granting agencies, professional associations, and other organizations should also continue to develop policies. Many journals have created policies for a variety of topics, including authorship, duplicate publication, disclosure of financial interests, data sharing, human subjects' protections, clinical trial registration, and peer review (Cooper et al. 2006; Krimsky and Rothenberg 2001). The International Committee of Medical Journal Editors (2013) and the Committee on Publication Ethics (2013) have developed ethical guidelines for authors, reviewers, and editors. As mentioned in chapter 1, many different professional associations have developed ethics standards.

Because research ethics is an evolving field, policies should be updated, when needed, to reflect changes in technology, the research environment, and other areas. For example, institutions and funding agencies have revised policies pertaining to protecting the confidentiality of data in human subjects research (discussed in chapter 11) in response to developments in statistics and information technology. Scientific journals and funding agencies have formed policies pertaining to dual use (discussed in chapter 12) in response to the threat of bioterrorism. Journal policies pertaining to digital image manipulation reflect recent advances in imaging software.

Policy development and revision should be informed by empirical research pertaining to RCR. For example, surveys of what human participants want to know about studies, how much they understand, and what they are concerned about can provide useful guidance for informed consent policy development (Flory et al. 2011). Studies of the effectiveness of different forms of peer review (i.e., single blind, double blind, open) can help guide journal peer-review policies (Resnik 2011). Studies of laboratory animals' mental abilities, such as the capacity to feel pain or suffer, can provide important information for the development of policies for animal experimentation (LaFollette and Shanks 1996).

COMPLIANCE AND OVERSIGHT

Compliance and oversight activities must also be a part of any institutional ethics program. These activities include various efforts to enforce ethical and legal rules and policies at the research institution. Whereas education focuses on the prevention of ethical and legal transgressions, compliance focuses on detecting and investigating misbehaviors and implementing punishments (Vasgird 2007). Compliance is like police work. Some important compliance activities include the following:

- Establishing mechanisms for reporting, investigating, and adjudicating violations of institutional policies and laws or regulations, including protections for whistleblowers and accused parties;
- Establishing and staffing committees that deal with ethics issues in the institution, such as IRBs (human subjects), ACUCs (animals), and conflict-of-interest and biosafety committees;
- Developing mechanisms for conducting for cause and random audits of research records, including data, time and effort sheets, informed consent documents, human subjects or animal protocols, and standard operating procedures (Shamoo 1988, 1989);

- Developing mechanisms for monitoring occupational and laboratory safety and research with human and animal subjects; and
- Providing counseling and advice to researchers concerning compliance with various policies, laws, and regulations.

Other types of research organizations (journals, funding agencies, etc.) should also engage in compliance activities, where appropriate. The Korean stem cell fraud scandal discussed in chapter 2 has prompted many journals to reconsider how they should deal with misconduct and other problems (Check and Cyranoski 2005; Resnik et al. 2006). Many journals now use computers to audit articles that are submitted. Computer programs can detect improper digital image manipulation and suspected plagiarism (Butler 2007). Journals should follow up on allegations of misconduct (or other ethical problems, such as violations of human or animal protections) that they receive. Although journals do not have the power to investigate misconduct allegations, they can notify the accused's institution and retract papers if they confirm that misconduct has occurred (see the discussion of retractions in chapter 2).

As noted in chapter 2, most funding agencies have compliance and oversight offices. The Office of Research Integrity (ORI) oversees the integrity of Public Health Services (PHS)–funded research, including NIH research. Although the ORI requires institutions to conduct misconduct investigations within their jurisdiction, it retains the authority to conduct its own investigations, if appropriate. While the ORI's mission has been broadened to include RCR education and research, it maintains a strong commitment to investigation and oversight to protect the integrity of PHS research. Federal human subjects research offices, such as the Office for Human Research Protections and the Food and Drug Administration (FDA), have the authority to conduct audits for cause and on a random basis. OHRP publishes its determination letters when it finds that an institution has not complied with the federal regulations. OHRP has suspended particular studies due to compliance issues, and in some rare cases it has halted Department of Health and Human Services (DHHS)–funded research at entire institutions (Marshall 1999b; Savulescu and Spriggs 2002,).

INTERNATIONAL COOPERATION

Finally, although this chapter has focused on promoting RCR at the institutional and national level, international efforts aimed at fostering RCR should also be addressed. As discussed in chapter 5, many different aspects of research involve international collaboration. Because science has become increasingly global in scope, international cooperation on ethical and policy issues is crucial for promoting scientific progress and ensuring the public's trust of research. The Korean stem cell scandal illustrates the need for international cooperation regarding research ethics. This scandal involved researchers in two different countries and had global implications. However, the two main countries involved in the scandal, South Korea and the United States, did not have common ethical rules or guidelines pertaining to some of the important questions concerning the research, such as manipulation of digital images and authorship on scientific papers.

Because different countries may have their own laws and policies pertaining to scientific research, the development of international codes of ethics, such as the Singapore Statement on Research Integrity (mentioned in chapter 1), is an important step toward international cooperation on RCR. It is also important for international organizations, such as the United Nations Educational, Scientific, and Cultural Organization (UNESCO), and professional scientific societies, to support the development of transnational ethics codes. International conferences on research ethics and integrity can also help promote global cooperation.

REFERENCES

References that we also suggest for further reading are marked with an asterisk (*).

AAMC-AUP, Report on Managing Conflict of Interest, 2008. Protecting Patients, Preserving, Integrity, Advancing Health: Accelerating the Implementation of COI, Policies in Human Subjects Research.

AAUP, Report on Research on Human Subjects: Academic Freedom and the Institutional Review Board, 2008. Available at http://www.aaup.org/report/research-human-subjects-academic-freedom-and-institutional-review-board. Accessed on 7/2/2014.

Abbott, A. 2012. Plagiarism Charge for Romanian Minister. *Nature*. Available at http://www.nature.com/news/plagiarism-charge-for-romanian-minister-1.10646. Accessed on 10/29/2013.

Abby, M., et al. 1994. Peer Review Is an Effective Screening Process to Evaluate Medical Manuscripts. *Journal of the American Medical Association* 272: 105–107.

Aburto N. J., Ziolkovska, A., Hooper, L., Elliott, P., Cappuccio, F. P., and Meerpohl, J. J. 2013. Effect of Lower Sodium Intake on Health: Systematic Review and Meta-analyses. *British Medical Journal* 346: f1326.

Academic Freedom and the Institutional Review Board. 2006. Available at http://www.aaup.org/AAUP/About/committees/committee+repts/CommA/ResearchonHumanSubjects.htm. Accessed on February 28, 2006.

Adler, R. G. 1993. Choosing the Form of Legal Protection. In *Understanding Biotechnology Law*, Gale R. Peterson (ed.). Marcel Deckker, New York, 63–86.

Advisory Committee on Human Radiation Experiments (ACHRE). 1995. Final Report. Stock No. 061-000-00-848-9. Superintendent of Documents, U.S. Government Printing Office, Washington, DC.

Agnew, B. 1999a. NIH Eyes Sweeping Reform of Peer Review. *Science* 286: 1074–1076.

Agnew, B. 1999b. NIH Invites Activists into the Inner Sanctum. *Science* 283: 1999–2001.

Agnew, B. 2000. Financial Conflicts Get More Scrutiny at Clinical Trials. *Science* 289: 1266–1267.

Akhabue, E., and Lautenbach, E. 2010. "Equal" Contributions and Credit: An Emerging Trend in the Characterization of Authorship. *Annals of Epidemiology* 20(11): 868–871.

Alessandrini, M., Asfaha, S., Dodgen, T. M., Warnich, L., and Pepper, M. S. 2013. Cytochrome P450 Pharmacogenetics in African Populations. *Drug Metabolism Review* 45(2): 253–275.

Al-Khalili, J. 2012. *The House of Wisdom: How Arab Science Saved Ancient Knowledge and Gave us the Renaissance*. Penguin, New York.

Allen, M., and Dowell, R. 2013. Retrospective Reflections of a Whistleblower: Opinions on Misconduct Responses. *Accountability in Research* 20(5–6): 339–348.

Aller, R., and Aller, C. 1997. An Institutional Response to Patient/Family Complaints. In *Ethics in Neurobiological Research with Human Subjects*, A. E. Shamoo (ed.). Gordon and Breach, Amsterdam, 155–1172.

Altman, L. 1995. Promises of Miracles: News Releases Go Where Journals Fear to Tread. *New York Times*, January 10, C2–C3.

Altman, L. K. 1997. Experts See Bias in Drug Data. *New York Times*, April 29, C1–C8.

American Anthropological Association. 2012. Principles of Professional Responsibility. Available at http://www.aaanet.org/profdev/ethics/upload/Statement-on-Ethics-Principles-of-Professional-Responsibility.pdf. Accessed on October 2, 2013.

American Association for the Advancement of Science. 2013. R & D Budget and Policy Program. Available at http://www.aaas.org/spp/rd/guihist.shtml. Accessed on October 21, 2013.

American Association for the Advancement of Science (AAAS)–American Bar Association (ABA). 1988. Project on Scientific Fraud and Misconduct. National Conference of Lawyers and Scientists, Report on Workshop No. 1, AAAS, Washington, DC.

American Association of University Professors (AAUP). 2006. Research on Human Subjects.

American Physical Society. 2002. Guidelines for Professional Conduct. Available at http://www.aps.org/policy/statements/02_2.cfm. Accessed on October 2, 2013.

American Psychological Association. 1992. Ethical Principles of Psychologists and Code of Conduct. *American Psychologist* 47: 1597–1611.

American Society for Microbiology. 2005. Code of Ethics. Available at http://www.asm.org/index.php/governance/code-of-ethics. Accessed on October 2, 2013.

American Statistical Association. 1999. Ethical Guidelines for Statistical Practice. Available at http://www.amstat.org/about/ethicalguidelines.cfm. Accessed on October 2, 2013.

Anderson, M. S., et al. 2007. What Do Mentoring and Training in the Responsible Conduct of Research Have to Do with Scientific Misbehavior? Findings from a National Survey of NIH-Funded Scientists. *Academic Medicine* 82(9): 853–860.

Anderson, M. S, and Steneck, N. H. (Eds.). 2012. *International Research Collaborations: Much to Be Gained, Many Ways to Get in Trouble*. Routledge, New York.

Angell, M. 1997a. The Ethics of Clinical Research in the Third World. *New England Journal of Medicine* 337: 847–849.

Angell, M. 1997b. *Science on Trial*. W. W. Norton, New York.

Angell, M. 2001. Medicine in the Noise Age: What Can We Believe? *Accountability in Research* 8: 189–196.

Angel, M. 2004. *The Truth about Drug Companies—How They Deceive Us and What to Do about It*. Random House, New York.

Angell, M., and Kassirer, J. P. 1994. Setting the Record Straight in the Breast Cancer Trials. *New England Journal of Medicine* 330(20): 1448–1450.

Animal Welfare Act. 1966. Title 7 U.S. Code, 2131–2156.

Anonymous. 1993. Toxicity Tests in Animals: Extrapolating to Human Risks. *Environmental Health Perspective* 101: 396–401.

Antes, A. L., Murphy, S. T., Waples, E. P., Mumford, M. D., Brown, R. P., Connelly, S., and Devenport, L. D. 2009. A Meta-analysis of Ethics Instruction Effectiveness in the Sciences. *Ethics and Behavior* 19: 379–402.

Antes, A. L., Wang, X., Mumford, M. D., Brown, R. P., Connelly, S., and Devenport, L. D. 2010. Evaluating the Effects That Existing Instruction on Responsible Conduct of Research Has on Ethical Decision Making. *Academic Medicine* 85: 519–526.

Applebaum, P., et al. 1987. False Hopes and Best Data: Consent to Research and the Therapeutic Misconception. *Hastings Center Report* 17(2): 20–24.

Aristotle. 330 B.C. [1984]. Nichomachean Ethics. In *Complete Works of Aristotle*, J. Barnes (ed.). Princeton University Press, Princeton, NJ.

Armstrong, D., 2005. How a Famed Hospital Invests in Device It Uses and Promotes. *Wall Street Journal*, December 12. Available at http://online.wsj.com/article_print/SB113435097142119825.html. Accessed on January 12, 2006.

Armstrong, D., 2006. Cleveland Clinic to Tighten Its Disclosure Policies, February 9. Section A, p.3. Available at http://online.wsj.com/article_emaul/SB1139457922539699290-IMyQ... Accessed on February 9, 2006.

Armstrong, J. 1997. Peer Review for Journals: Evidence of Quality Control, Fairness, and Innovation. *Science and Engineering Ethics* 3(1): 63–84.

Associated Press. 1997. Test of AIDS Vaccine Sought. *Denver Post*, September 22, A3.

Association for the Assessment and Accreditation of Laboratory Animal Care (AAALAC). 2007. About AAALAC. Available at http://www.aaalac.org/. Accessed on October 21, 2007.

Association for Molecular Pathology et al v. Myriad Genetics, Inc., et al. 2013. 569 U.S. 12–398.

Association of Academic Health Centers (AAHC). 1994. *Conflict of Interest in Institutional Decision-Making.* AAHC, Washington, DC.

Association of Academic Health Centers (AAHC). 2001. Task Force on Financial Conflict of Interest in Clinical Research, Protecting Subjects, Preserving Trust, Promoting Progress II, Principles and Recommendations for Oversight of Individual Financial Interests in Human Subjects Research. AAHC, Washington, DC.

Association of Academic Health Centers (AAHC). 2002. Task Force on Financial Conflict of Interest in Clinical Research, Protecting Subjects, Principles and Recommendations for Oversight of an Institution's Financial Interests in Human Subjects Research, Preserving Trust, Promoting Progress II. AAHC, Washington, DC.

Austin, C., Battey, J., et al. 2004. The Knockout Mouse Project. *Nature Genetics* 36: 921–924.

Bacon, F. 2000 [1620]. *The New Organon.* Cambridge University Press, Cambridge.

Bailar, J. 1986. Science, Statistics, and Deception. *Annals of Internal Medicine* 105: 259–260.

Baldessarini, R. J., and Viguera, A. C. 1995. Neuroleptic Withdrawal in Schizophrenic Patients. *Archives of General Psychology* 52: 189–191.

Ball, M. P., Thakuria, J. V., et al. 2012. A Public Resource Facilitating Clinical Use of Genomes. *Proceedings of the National Academy of Sciences USA* 109(30): 11920–11927.

Ballantyne, A. 2005. HIV International Clinical Research: Exploitation and Risk. *Bioethics* 19: 476–491.

Baltimore, D. 1991. Baltimore Declares O'Toole Mistaken. *Nature* 351: 341–343.

Banoub-Baddour, S., and Gien, L. T. 1991. Student-Faculty Joint-Authorship: Mentorship in Publication. *Canadian Journal of Nursing Research* 23: 5–14.

Barbash, F. 1996. Piltdown Meltdown: A Hoaxer Revealed. *Washington Post*, May 24, A1, A34.

Barber, B. 1961. Resistance by Scientists to Scientific Discovery. *Science* 134: 596–602.

Barinaga, M. 2000. Soft Money's Hard Realities. *Science* 289: 2024–2028.

Barnard, N., and Kaufman, S. 1997. Animal Research Is Wasteful and Misleading. *Scientific American* 276(2): 80–82.

Bayles, M. 1988. *Professional Ethics*. 2nd ed. Wadsworth, Belmont, CA.

Bean, W. B. 1977. Walter Reed and the Ordeal of Human Experiments. *Bulletin of the History of Medicine* 51: 75–92.

Beardsley, T. 1994. Big-Time Biology. *Scientific American* 271(5): 90–97.

Beauchamp, T. L. 1996. Looking Back and Judging Our Predecessors. *Kennedy Institute of Ethics Journal* 6: 251–270.

Beauchamp, T. L., and Childress, J. F., 2001. *Principles of Biomedical Ethics*. 5th ed. Oxford University Press, New York.

Beaudette, C. G. 2000. *Excess Heat—Why Cold Fusion Research Prevailed*. Oak Grove Press, South Bristol, ME.

Beecher, H. 1966. Ethics and Clinical Research. *New England Journal of Medicine* 274: 1354–1360.

Bekelman, J. E., Li, Y., and Gross, G. P. 2003. Scope and Impact of Financial Conflicts of Interest in Biomedical Research, *Journal of the American Medical Association* 289: 454–465.

Bennett, T. 1994. Regulations and Requirements. In *Essentials for Animals Research*, T. Bennett, et al. (eds.). National Agricultural Library, Beltsville, MD.

Bentham, J. 1789 [1988]. *Introduction to Principles of Morals and Legislation*. Penguin, New York.

Berg, J., Applebaum, P., Parker, L., and Lidz, C. 2001. *Informed Consent: Legal Theory and Clinical Practice*. Oxford University Press, New York.

Berger, E., and Gert, B. 1997. Institutional Responsibility. In *Research Ethics: A Reader*, D. Elliot and J. Stern (eds.). University Press of New England, Hanover, NH, 197–212.

Berman, F., and Cerf, V. 2013. Who Will Pay for Public Access to Research Data? *Science Magazine*, August 9, 616–617.

Bero, L. A., et al. 1994. Publication Bias and Public Health on Environmental Tobacco Smoke. *Journal of the American Medical Association* 272: 133–136.

Beskow, L. and Burke, W. 2010. Offering Individual Genetic Research Results: Context Matters. *Science Translational Medicine* 2(38): 38cm20.

Beskow, L., Fullerton, S. M., Namey, E. E., Nelson, D. K., Davis, A. M., Wilford, B. S. 2012. Recommendations for Ethical Approaches to Genotype-Driven Research Recruitment. *Human Genetics* 131: 1423–1431.

Bingham, C. 2000. Peer Review and the Ethics of Internet Publishing. In *Ethical Issues in Biomedical Publication*, A. Jones and F. McLellan (eds.). Johns Hopkins University Press, Baltimore, 85–112.

Blinderman, C. 1986. *The Piltdown Inquest*. Prometheus, Buffalo, NY.

Blumenthal, D. 1995. Academic-Industry Relationships in the 1990s: Continuity and Change. Paper presented at the symposium "Ethical Issues in Research Relationships between Universities and Industry," Baltimore, MD, November 3–5.

*Blumenthal, D. 1997. Withholding Research Results in Academic Life Science: Evidence from a National Survey of Faculty. *Journal of the American Medical Association* 277: 1224–1228.

Blumenthal, D., et al. 1986. University-Industry Research Relationships in Biotechnology: Implications for the University. *Science* 232: 1361–1366.

Blumenthal, D., et al. 1996a. Participation of Life-Science Faculty in Relationships with Industry. *New England Journal of Medicine* 335: 1734–1739.

Blumenthal, D., et al. 1997. Withholding Research Results in Academic Life Science: Evidence from a National Survey of Faculty. *Journal of the American Medical Association* 287(4): 473–480.

Blumenthal D., et al. 2006. Data Withholding in Genetics and the Other Life Sciences: Prevalences and Predictors. *Academic Medicine* 81: 137–145.

Bok, D. 2003. *Universities in the Marketplace—The Commercialization of Higher Education*. Princeton University Press, Princeton, NJ.

Bonham, V., and Moreno, J. 2011. Research with Captive Populations: Prisoners, Students, and Soldiers. In *The Oxford Textbook of Clinical Research Ethics*, Emanuel, E. et al (eds.). Oxford University Press, New York, 461–474.

Bonner, J. 1980. *The Evolution of Culture in Animals*. Princeton University Press, Princeton, NJ.

Borenstein, J. 2011. Responsible Authorship in Engineering Fields: An Overview of Current Ethical Challenges. *Science and Engineering Ethics* 17: 355–364.

Borry, P., Schotsmans, P., and Dierickx, K. 2006. Author, Contributor or Just a Signer? A Quantitative Analysis of Authorship Trends in the Field of Bioethics. *Bioethics* 20: 213–220.

Bosch, X., Hernández, C., Pericas, J. M., Doti, P., and Marušić, A. 2012. Misconduct Policies in High-impact Biomedical Journals. *PLoS One* 7(12): e51928.

Botkin, J. 2001. Protecting the Privacy of Family Members in Survey and Pedigree Research. *Journal of the American Medical Association* 285: 207–211.

Botting, J., and Morrison, A. 1997. Animal Research Is Vital to Medicine. *Scientific American* 276(2): 83–85.

Bower, B. 1991. Peer Review under Fire. *Science News* 139: 394–395.

Bowie, N. 1994. *University-Business Partnerships: An Assessment*. Rowman and Littlefield, Lanham, MD.

Bradley, G. 2000. Managing Conflicting Interests. In *Scientific Integrity*, Francis Macrina (ed.). American Society for Microbiology Press, Washington, DC, 131–156.

Broad, W. J. 1981. The Publishing Game: Getting More for Less. *Science* 211: 1137–1139.

*Broad, W., and Wade, N. 1982 [1993]. *Betrayers of the Truth: Fraud and Deceit in the Halls of Science*. Simon and Schuster, New York.

Bronowski, J. 1956. *Science and Human Values*. Harper and Row, New York.

Brown, J. 2000. Privatizing the University—the New Tragedy of the Commons. *Science* 290: 1701–1702.

Bulger, R. 1987. Use of Animals in Experimental Research: A Scientist's Perspective. *Anatomical Record* 219: 215–220.

Burke, J. 1995. *The Day the Universe Changed*. Little, Brown, Boston.

Burnham, J. C. 1990. The Evolution of Editorial Peer Review. *Journal of the American Medical Association* 263: 1323–1329.

Butler, D. 1999a. The Writing Is on the Web for Science Journals in Print. *Nature* 397: 195–199.

Butler, D. 2007. Copycat Trap. *Nature* 448: 633.

Butler, D. 2010. Journals Step Up Plagiarism Policing. *Nature* 466: 167.

Buzzelli, D. 1993. NSF's Approach to Misconduct in Science. *Accountability in Research* 3: 215–222.

Callahan, S. 1998. The Ethical Challenge of the New Reproductive Technology. In *Health Care Ethics—Critical Issues for the 21st Century*, J. Monagle and D. Thomasma (eds.). Aspen Publishers, Boulder, CO, 45–55.

Campbell, E., Clarridge, B., Gokhale, M., Birenbaum, L., Hilgartner, S., Holtzman, N., and Blumenthal, D. 2002. Data Withholding in Academic Genetics: Evidence from a National Survey. *Journal of the American Medical Association* 287(4): 473–480.

Caplan, A. 1983. Beastly Conduct: Ethical Issues in Animal Experimentation. *Annals of the NY Academy of Science* 406: 159–169.

*Capron, A. M. 1989. Human Experimentation. In *Medical Ethics*, R. M. Veatch (ed.). Jones and Bartlett, Boston, 125–172.

Capron, A. M. 2011. Legal and Regulatory Standards of Informed Consent in Research. In *The Oxford Textbook of Clinical Research Ethics*, Emanuel, E., Grady, C., and Crouch, R., et al. (eds). Oxford University Press, New York, 613–632.

Carey, J., et al. 1997. The Biotech Century. *Business Week*, March 10, 79–88.

Carruthers, P. 1992. *The Animals Issue*. Cambridge University Press, Cambridge.

Carson, R. 1962. *Silent Spring*. Houghton Mifflin, Boston.

Cassell, E. 1991. *The Nature of Suffering*. Oxford University Press, New York.

Cech, T., and Leonard, J. 2001. Conflicts of Interest: Moving beyond Disclosure. *Science* 291: 989.

Centers for Disease Control and Prevention. 2013. *Salt*. Available at http://www.cdc.gov/salt/. Accessed on September 27, 2013.

Chalmers, T. C., et al. 1990. Minimizing the Three Stages of Publication Bias. *Journal of the American Medical Association* 263: 1392–1395.

Chapman, A. (ed.). 1999. *Perspectives on Genetic Patenting*. AAAS, Washington, DC.

Check, E., and Cyranoski, D. 2005. Korean Scandal Will Have Global Fallout. *Nature* 438: 1056–1057.

*Cheny, D. (Ed.). 1993. *Ethical Issues in Research*. University Publishing Group, Inc., Frederick, MD.

Chickering, R. B., and Hartman, S. 1980. *How to Register a Copyright and Protect Your Creative Work*. Charles Scribner's Sons, New York.

Cho, M., et al. 2000. Policies on Faculty Conflicts of Interest at US Universities. *Journal of the American Medical Association* 284: 2203–2208.

Cho, M. K. 1997. Letters to the Editor, Disclosing Conflicts of Interest. *Lancet* 350: 72–73.

Cho, M. K. 1998. Fundamental Conflict of Interest. *HMS Beagle: The BioMedNet Magazine*, issue 24. Available at http://biomednet.com/hms beagle/1998/24/people/op-ed.htm.

Cho, M. K., and Bero, L. A. 1996. The Quality of Drug Studies Published in Symposium Proceedings. *Annals of Internal Medicine* 124: 485–489.

Chubb, S. 2000. Introduction to the Series of Papers in Accountability in Research Dealing with "Cold Fusion." *Accountability in Research* 8: 1–18.

Chubin, D., and Hackett, E. 1990. *Peerless Science*. State University of New York Press, Albany.

Cohen, C. 1986. The Case for the Use of Animals in Biomedical Research. *New England Journal of Medicine* 315: 865–870.

Cohen, J. 1991. What Next in the Gallo Case? *Science* 254: 944–949.

Cohen, L., and Hahn, R. 1999. A Solution to Concerns over Public Access to Scientific Data. *Science* 285: 535–536.

Cohen, S. 1995. Human Relevance of Animal Carcinogenicity Studies. *Regulatory Toxicology and Pharmacology* 21: 75–80.

Cole, S., et al. 1978. *Peer Review in the NSF: Phase One*. National Academy of Sciences, Washington, DC.

Cole, S., and Cole, J. R. 1981. *Peer Review in the NSF: Phase Two*. National Academy of Sciences, Washington, DC.

The Committee on Publication Ethics. 2013. Guidelines on Good Publication and the Code of Conduct. Available at http://publicationethics.org/about. Accessed on March 13, 2014.

Committee on Science, Engineering, and Public Policy, National Academy of Sciences, National Academy of Engineering, and Institute of Medicine. 2009. *On Being a Scientist: A Guide to Responsible Conduct in Research*. 3rd ed. National Academies Press, Washington, DC.

Cooper, R., Gupta, M., Wilkes, M., and Hoffman, J. 2006. Conflict of Interest Disclosure Policies and Practices in Peer-reviewed Biomedical Journals. *Journal of Internal Medicine* 21(12): 1248–1252.

Corbie-Smith, G., Thomas, S. B., and St George, D. M. 2002. Distrust, Race, and Research. *Archives of Internal Medicine* 162(21): 2458–2463.

Corbie-Smith, G., Thomas, S. B., Williams, M. V., and Moody-Ayers, S. 1999. Attitudes and Beliefs of African Americans toward Participation in Medical Research. *Journal of General Internal Medicine* 14(9): 537–546.

Cottrell, C. 2013. University Revokes German Official's Doctorate. Available at http://www.nytimes.com/2013/02/06/world/europe/german-university-revokes-minister-annette-schavans-doctorate.html?_r=0. Accessed on October 29, 2013.

Council for the Organizations of Medical Sciences. 2002. International Ethical Guidelines for Biomedical Research Involving Human Subjects. Available at http://www.cioms.ch/publications/layout_guide2002.pdf. Accessed on November 12, 2013.

Couzin, J. 2006. Truth and Consequences. *Science* 313: 1222–1226.

Crossen, C. 1994. *Tainted Truth*. Simon and Schuster, New York.

Crow, T. J., MacMillian, J. F., Johnson, A. L., and Johnstone, B. C. 1986. A Randomised Controlled Trial of Prophylatic Neuroleptic Treatment. *British Journal of Psychiatry* 148: 120–127.

Culliton, J. 1977. Harvard and Monsanto: The $23 Million Alliance. *Science* 195: 759–763.

Culliton, B. J. 1990. Gallo Inquiry Takes Puzzling Turn. *Science* 250: 202–203.

Cummings, M. 2002. Informed Consent and Investigational New Drug Abuses in the U.S. Military. *Accountability in Research* 9: 93–103.

Dalton, R. 2001. Peers under Pressure. *Nature* 413: 102–104.

Daubert v. Merrell Dow Pharmaceutical. 1993. 113 S CT 2768: 92–102.

Davidoff, F. 1998. Masking, Blinding, and Peer Review: The Blind Leading the Blinded. *Annals of Internal Medicine* 128: 66–68.

Davidson, R. 1986. Source of Funding and Outcome of Clinical Trials. *Journal of General Internal Medicine* 1: 155–158.

Davis, J. 2003. Self-Experimentation. *Accountability in Research* 10: 175–187.

Davis, M. 1982. Conflict of Interest. *Business and Professional Ethics Journal* 1(4): 17–27.

Davis, M. 1991. University Research and the Wages of Commerce. *Journal of College and University Law* 18: 29–39.

Davis, M. 1995a. A Preface to Accountability in the Professions. *Accountability in Research* 4: 81–90.

Davis, M. 1995b. Panel discussion at the symposium "Ethical Issues in Research Relationships between Universities and Industry," Baltimore, MD.

De Cock, K., Fowler, M., Mercier, E., de Vincenzi, I., Saba, J., Hoff, E., Alnwick, D., Rogers, M., and Shaffer N. 2000. Prevention of Mother-to-Child HIV Transmission in Resource-poor Countries: Translating Research into Policy and Practice. *Journal of the American Medical Association* 283: 1175–1182.

Deer, B. 2011. How the Case against the MMR Vaccine Was Fixed. *British Medical Journal* 342: c5347.

De George, R. 1995. *Business Ethics.* 4th ed. Prentice-Hall, Englewood Cliffs, NJ.

DeGrazia, D. 1991. The Moral Status of Animals and their Use in Research. *Kennedy Institute of Ethics Journal* 1: 48–70.

de Melo-Martín, I., Palmer, L., and Fins, J. 2007. Viewpoint: Developing a Research Ethics Consultation Service to Foster Responsive and Responsible Clinical Research. *Academic Medicine* 82: 900–904.

DeMets, D. 1999. Statistics and Ethics in Medical Research. *Science and Engineering Ethics* 5: 97–117.

Deming, N. et al. 2007. Incorporating Principles and Practical Wisdom in Research Ethics Education: A Preliminary Study. *Academic Medicine* 82: 18–23.

Department of Health and Human Services. 2011. Responsibility of Applicants for Promoting Objectivity in Research for Which Public Health Service Funding Is Sought and Responsible Prospective Contractors; Final Rule. *Federal Register* 76(165): 53256–53293.

Department of Health and Human Services. 2013. Summary of the HIPAA Privacy Rule. Available at http://www.hhs.gov/ocr/privacy/hipaa/understanding/ summary/. Accessed on November 19, 2013.

Descartes, R. 1970. *Descartes: Philosophical Letters.* A. Kenny (trans. and ed.). Oxford University Press, Oxford.

de Waal, F. 1996. *Good Natured: The Origins of Right and Wrong in Humans and Other Animals.* Harvard University Press, Cambridge, MA.

de Waal, F. 2009. *Primates and Philosophers: How Morality Evolved.* Princeton University Press, Princeton, NJ.

Deyo, R. A., et al. 1997. The Messenger under Attack—Intimidation of Research by Special-Interest Groups. *New England Journal of Medicine* 336: 1176–1180.

Diamond v. Chakrabarty. 1980. 447 US 303–310.

Dickert, N., and Grady, C. C. 2011. Incentives for Research Participants. In *The Oxford Textbook of Clinical Research Ethics*, Emanuel, E. et al (eds.). Oxford University Press, New York, 386–396.

Dickson, D. 1988. *The New Politics of Science.* University of Chicago Press, Chicago.

Dickson, D. 1995. *Between Politics and Science.* Cambridge University Press, Cambridge.

Diguisto, E. 1994. Equity in Authorship: A Strategy for Assigning Credit When Publishing. *Social Science and Medicine* 38: 55–58.

Djerassi, C. 1999. Who Will Mentor the Mentors? *Nature* 397: 291.

Doucet, M. S., et al. 1994. An Application of Stratified Sampling Techniques for Research Data. *Accountability in Research* 3: 237–247.

Drenth, J. 1996. Proliferation of Authors on Research Reports in Medicine. *Science and Engineering Ethics* 2: 469–480.

Dresser, R. 2001. *When Science Offers Salvation.* Oxford University Press, New York.

Dreyfuss, R. 2000. Collaborative Research: Conflicts on Authorship, Ownership, and Accountability. *Vanderbilt Law Review* 53: 1161–1232.

Ducor, P. 2000. Coauthorship and Coinventorship. *Science* 289: 873–875.

Duft, B. J. 1993. Preparing Patent Application. In *Understanding Biotechnology Law*, Gale R. Peterson (ed.). Marcel Dekker, New York, 87–186.

Duke University. Duke Policies, Regulations, and Committees. 2013. Available at https://gradschool.duke.edu/academics/degree_reqs/rcr/policies.php. Accessed on October 10, 2013.

Dustira, A. K. 1992. The Funding of Basic and Clinical Biomedical Research. In *Biomedical Research: Collaboration and Conflict of Interest*, R. J. Porter and T. E. Malone (eds.). Johns Hopkins University Press, Baltimore.

The Economist. 2013. Unreliable Research, Trouble at the Lab—Scientists Like to Think of Science as Self-correcting. To an Alarming Degree, It Is Not. Available at http://www.economist.com/news/briefing/21588057-scientists-think-science-self-correcting-alarming-degree-it-not-trouble. Accessed on 10/29/2013.

Egilman, D., et al. 1998a. Ethical Aerobics: ACHREs Flight from Responsibility. *Accountability in Research* 6: 15–62.

Egilman, D., et al. 1998b. A Little Too Much of the Buchenwald Touch? Military Radiation Research at the University of Cincinnati, 1960–1972. *Accountability in Research* 6: 63–102.

Ehringhause, S. H., et al. 2008. Responses of Medical Schools to Institutional Conflicts of Interest. *Journal of the American Medical Association* 299: 665–671.

Eisen, H. N. 1991. Origins of MIT Inquiry. *Nature* 351: 343–344.

Eisenberg, R. 1995. Patenting Organisms. In *Encyclopedia of Bioethics*, rev. ed. Simon and Schuster, New York, 1911–1914.

Elliott, K. C. 2006. An Ethics of Expertise Based on Informed Consent. *Science and Engineering Ethics* 12(4): 637–661.

Elliott, K. C. 2008. Scientific Judgment and the Limits of Conflict-of-Interest Policies. *Accountability in Research*, 15(1): 1–29.

Emanuel E., and Miller, F. 2003. The Ethics of Placebo-Controlled Trials – A Middle Ground. *The New England Journal of Medicine* 345: 915–919.

Emanuel, E., et al. 2000. What Makes Clinical Research Ethical? *Journal of the American Medical Association* 283: 2701–2711.

Emanuel, E. J., Crouch, R. A., Arras, J. D., Moreno, J. D., and Grady, C. C. (Eds.). 2003. *Ethical and Regulatory Aspects of Clinical Research: Readings and Commentary.* Johns Hopkins University Press, Baltimore.

Emanuel, E. J., Grady, C. C., Crouch, R. A., Lie, R. K., Miller, F. G., and Wendler, D. D. (Eds.). 2011. *Oxford Textbook of Clinical Research Ethics.* Oxford University Press, New York.

Enriquez, J. 1998. Genomics and the World's Economy. *Science* 281: 925–926.

Etkowitz, H., et al. 1994. The Paradox of Critical Mass for Women in Science. *Science* 266: 51–54.

Faden, R. R., and Beauchamp, T. L. 1986. *A History of Informed Consent*. Oxford University Press, New York.

Fanelli, D. 2009. How Many Scientists Fabricate and Falsify Research? A Systematic Review and Meta-analysis of Survey Data. *PLoS One* 4(5): e5738.

Fang, F. C., Steen, R. G., and Casadevall, A. 2012. Misconduct Accounts for the Majority of Retracted Scientific Publications. *Proceedings of National Academy of Science USA* 109(42): 17028–17033.

Federal Policy for the Protection of Human Subjects ('Common Rule'). Available at http://www.hhs.gov/ohrp/humansubjects/commonrule/. Accessed on 7/2/2014.

Feinberg, J. 1973. *Social Philosophy*. Prentice-Hall, Englewood Cliffs, NJ.

Ferber, D. 2002. HHS Intervenes in Choice of Study Section Members. *Science* 298: 1323–1323.

Fields, K. L., and Price, A. R. 1993. Problems in Research Integrity Arising from Misconceptions about the Ownership of Research. *Academe Medicine Supplement* 3: S60–S64.

Flanagin, A., et al. 1998. Prevalence of Articles with Honorary and Ghost Authors in Peer-Reviewed Medical Journals. *Journal of the American Medical Association* 280: 222–224.

Fleischmann, M. 2000. Reflections on the Sociology of Science and Social Responsibility in Science, in Relationship to Cold Fusion. *Accountability in Research* 8: 19–54.

Fletcher, R., and Fletcher, S. 1997. Evidence for the Effectiveness of Peer Review. *Science and Engineering Ethics* 3(1): 35–50.

Fletcher, S.W., and Fletcher, R.H. 1999. Medical Editors, Journal Owners, and the Sacking of George Lundberg. *Journal of General Internal Medicine* 14(3): 200–202.

Flory, J., Wendler, D., and Emanuel, E. 2011. Empirical Issues in Informed Consent for Research. In *The Oxford Textbook of Clinical Research Ethics*, E. Emanuel, et al. (eds.). Oxford University Press, New York, 645–660.

Food and Drug Administration (FDA). 2002. Best Pharmaceutical for Children Act. Available at http://www.fda.gov/opacom/laws/pharmkids/pharmkids.html. Accessed on December 19, 2007.

Food and Drug Administration. 2013. Policies and Procedures for Handling Conflicts of Interest with FDA Advisory Committee Members, Consultants, and Experts. Available at http://www.fda.gov/oc/advisory/conflictofinterest/policies.html. Accessed on September 27, 2013.

Forge, J. 2008. *The Responsible Scientist: A Philosophical Inquiry*. University of Pittsburgh Press, Pittsburgh, PA.

Forge, J. 2013. *Designed to Kill: The Case against Weapons Research*. Springer, New York.

Foster, F., and Shook, R. 1993. *Patents, Copyrights, and Trademarks*. 2nd ed. John Wiley, New York.

Fox, L. 2003. *Enron—The Rise and Fall*. John Wiley and Sons, New York.

Fox, R., and DeMarco, J. 1990. *Moral Reasoning*. Holt, Rinehart, and Winston, Chicago.

Frankena, W. 1973. *Ethics*. 2nd ed. Prentice-Hall, Englewood Cliffs, NJ.

Freedom of Information Act (FOIA). 2002. 5 U.S.C. 552.

Frey, R. 1980. *Interests and Rights: The Case against Animals.* Oxford University Press, New York.

Frey, R. 1994. The Ethics of the Search for Benefits: Experimentation in Medicine. In *Principles of Health Care Ethics*, R. Gillon (ed.). John Wiley, Chichester, 1067–1075.

Friedberg, M., Saffran, B., Stinson, T., Nelson, W., and Bennett, C. 1999. Evaluation of Conflict of Interest in New Drugs Used in Oncology. *Journal of the American Medical Association* 282: 1453–1457.

Friedly, J. 1996a. How Congressional Pressure Shaped the Baltimore Case. *Science* 273: 873–875.

Friedly, J. 1996b. After 9 Years, a Tangled Case Lurches toward a Close. *Science* 272: 947–948.

Friedman Ross, L. 2006. *Children in Medical Research: Access vs. Protection.* Oxford University Press, New York.

Funk, Carolyn L., Barrett, Kirsten A., and Macrina, Francis L. 2007. Authorship and Publication Practices: Evaluation of the Effect of Responsible Conduct of Research Instruction to Postdoctoral Trainees. *Accountability in Research* 14(4): 269–305.

Garfield, E. 1987. The Anomie-Deviant Behavior Connection: The Theories of Durkheim, Merton, and Srole. *Current Contents*, September 28, 39: 3–12.

*Garfield, E. 1990. The Impact of Fraudulent Research on the Scientific Literature—the Stephen Breuning Case. *Journal of the American Medical Association* 263: 1424–1426.

Garfunkel, J. M., et al. 1994. Effect of Institutional Prestige on Reviewer's Recommendations and Editorial Decisions. *Journal of the American Medical Association* 272: 137–138.

Garner, B. A. (Ed.). 1999. *Black's Law Dictionary.* 7th ed. West Group, St. Paul, MN.

Garrett, J. (ed.). 2012. *The Ethics of Animal Research: Exploring the Controversy.* MIT Press, Cambridge, MA.

Geison, G. L. 1978. Pasteur's Work on Rabies: Reexamining the Ethical Issues. *Hastings Center Report* 8: 26–33.

Geison, G. L. 1995. *The Private Science of Louis Pasteur.* Princeton University Press, Princeton, NJ.

Gelsinger, P., and Shamoo, A. E. 2008. Eight Years after Jesse's Death, Are Human Research Subjects Any Safer? *Hastings Center Report* 38(2): 25–27.

Gert, B. 2007. *Common Morality: Deciding What to Do.* Oxford University Press, New York.

Gibbard, A. 1992. *Wise Choices, Apt Feelings.* Harvard University Press, Cambridge, MA.

Gibbs, W. 1996. The Price of Silence: Does Profit-Minded Secrecy Retard Scientific Progress? *Scientific American* 275(5): 15–16.

Giere, R. 1991. *Understanding Scientific Reasoning.* 3rd ed. Holt, Rinehart and Winston, Chicago.

Gilbert, P. L., et al., 1995. Neuroleptic Withdrawal in Schizophrenic Patients: A Review of the Literature. *Archives of General Psychiatry* 52: 173–188.

Glantz, S. A., and Bero, L. A. 1994. Inappropriate and Appropriate Selection of "Peers" in Grant Review. *Journal of the American Medical Association* 272: 114–116.

Glick, J. L. 1992. Scientific Data Audit—a Key Management Tool. *Accountability in Research* 2: 153–168.

Glick, J. L. 1993. Perceptions Concerning Research Integrity and the Practice of Data Audit in the Biotechnology Industry. *Accountability in Research* 3: 187–195.

Glick, J. L., and Shamoo, A. E. 1991. Auditing Biochemical Research Data: A Case Study. *Accountability in Research* 1: 223–243.

Godlee, F. 2000. The Ethics of Peer Review. In *Ethical Issues in Biomedical Publication*, A. Jones, and F. McLellan (eds.). Johns Hopkins University Press, Baltimore, 59–84.

Godlee, F. 2002. Making Reviewers Visible—Openness, Accountability, and Credit. *Journal of the American Medical Association* 287: 2762–2765.

Godlee, F., Gale, C. R., and Martyn, C. N. 1998. Effect on the Quality of Peer Review of Blinding Reviewers and Asking Them to Sign Their Reports: A Randomized Controlled Trial. *Journal of the American Medical Association* 280(3): 237–240.

Godlee, F., Smith, J., and Marcovitch H. 2011. Wakefield's Article Linking MMR Vaccine and Autism Was Fraudulent. *British Medical Journal* 342: c7452.

Goh, K. P. 2004. Management of Hyponatremia. *American Family Physician* 69(10): 2387–2394.

*Goode, S. 1993. Trying to Declaw the Campus Copycats. *Insight Magazine*, April 18, 10–29.

Goodman, S. 1994. Manuscript Quality before and after Peer Review and Editing at the Annals of Internal Medicine. *Annals of Internal Medicine* 121: 11–21.

Gøtzsche, P. C., et al. 2007. Available at http://www.plosmedicine.org/article/info%3Adoi%2F10.1371%2Fjournal.pmed.0040019. Accessed on 7/1/2014.

Graham, G. 1999. *The Internet: A Philosophical Inquiry*. Routledge, London.

Graudal, N. A., Galløe, A. M., and Garred, P. 1998. Effects of Sodium Restriction on Blood Pressure, Renin, Aldosterone, Catecholamines, Cholesterols, and Triglyceride: A Meta-analysis. *Journal of the American Medical Association* 279(17): 1383–1391.

Griffin, P. 1992. *Animal Minds*. University of Chicago Press, Chicago.

Grimlund, R. A., and Doucet, M. S. 1992. Statistical Auditing Techniques for Research Data: Financial Auditing Parallels and New Requirements. *Accountability in Research* 2: 25–53.

Grinnell, F. 1992. *The Scientific Attitude*. 2nd ed. Guilford Press, New York.

Gross, C., et al. 1999. The Relation between Funding at the National Institutes of Health and the Burden of Disease. *New England Journal of Medicine* 340: 1881–1887.

Grossman, R. 1997. In Academe, the Serfs Are Toppling the Lords. *Chicago Tribune*, August 24, A1.

Guston, D. 2000. *Between Politics and Science*. Cambridge University Press, Cambridge.

Guttman, D. 1998. Disclosure and Consent: Through the Cold War Prism. *Accountability in Research* 6: 1–14.

Haack, S. 2003. *Defending Science within Reason*. Prometheus, New York.

Haidt, J. 2007. The New Synthesis in Moral Psychology. *Science* 316: 998–1002.

Hambruger, P. 2005. The New Censorship: Institutional Review Boards, The Law School, The University of Chicago. Available at http://www.law.uchicago.edu/academics/publiclaw/95-ph-censorship.pdf. Accessed on March 15, 2007.

Hamilton, D. P. 1991. NIH Finds Fraud in Cell Paper. *Science* 25: 1552–1554.

Harman, G. 1977. *The Nature of Morality*. Oxford University Press, New York.

Hauser, M. 2006. *Moral Minds: How Nature Designed Our Universal Sense of Right and Wrong*. HarperCollins, New York.

Health and Human Services and U.S. Department of Agriculture. 2013. Select Agents and Toxins. Available at http://www.selectagents.gov/resources/List_of_Select_Agents_and_Toxins_2013-2009-10.pdf. Accessed on September 23, 2013.

Hempel, C. 1965. *Philosophy of Natural Science*. Prentice-Hall, Englewood Cliffs, NJ.

Hilts, P. 1994. Philip Morris Blocked '83 Paper Showing Tobacco Is Addictive, Panel Finds. *New York Times*, April 1, A1.

Hinman, L. 2002. *Ethics: A Pluralistic Approach to Moral Theory*. Wadsworth, Belmont, CA.

Hixson, J. 1976. *The Patchwork Mouse*. Doubleday, Garden City, NJ.

Holden, C. 2000. NSF Searches for Right Way to Help Women. *Science* 289: 379–381.

Holden, C. 2007. Prominent Researchers Join the Attack on Stem Cell Patents. *Science* 317: 187.

Hollander, R., et al. 1996. Why Teach Ethics in Science and Engineering? *Science and Engineering Ethics* 1: 83–87.

Holton, G. 1978. Subelectrons, Presuppositions, and the Millikan-Ehrenhaft Dispute. *Historical Studies in the Physical Sciences* 9: 166–224.

Homer, N., Szelinger, S., Redman, M., Duggan, D., Tembe, W., Muehling, J., Pearson, J., Stephan, D., Nelson, S., and Craig, D. 2008. Resolving Individuals Contributing Trace Amounts of DNA to Highly Complex Mixtures Using High-density SNP Genotyping Microarrays. *PLoS Genetics* 4(8): e1000167.

Hoppe, S. K. 1996. Institutional Review Boards and Research on Individuals with Mental Disorders. *Accountability in Research* 4: 187–196.

*Hornblum, A. M. 1998. *Acres of Skin*. Routledge, New York.

Huber, P. 1991. *Galileo's Revenge: Science in the Courtroom*. Basic Books, New York.

Hull, D. 1988. *Science as a Process*. University of Chicago Press, Chicago.

Hurt, R., and Robertson, C. 1998. Prying Open the Door to the Tobacco Industry's Secrets about Nicotine. *JAMA* 280: 1173–1181.

Huth, E. 2000. Repetitive and Divided Publication. In *Ethical Issues in Biomedical Publication*, A. Jones and F. McLellan (eds.). Johns Hopkins University Press, Baltimore, 112–136.

Hwang, W., Roh, S., et al. 2005. Patient-specific Embryonic Stem Cells Derived from Human SCNT Blastocysts. *Science* 308: 1777–1783 (RETRACTED).

Hwang, W., Ryu, Y., et al. 2004. Evidence of a Pluripotent Human Embryonic Stem Cell Line Derived from a Cloned Blastocyst. *Science* 303: 1669–1674 (RETRACTED).

Hyder, A. A., and Wali, S. A. 2006. Informed Consent and Collaborative Research: Perspectives from the Developing World. *Developing World Bioethics*. 6: 33–40.

Iltis, A. 2000. Bioethics as Methodological Case Resolution: Specification, Specified Principlism and Casuistry. *Journal of Medicine and Philosophy* 25: 271–284.

Imai, M., Watanabe, T., et al. 2012. Experimental Adaptation of an Influenza H5 HA Confers Respiratory Droplet Transmission to a Reassortant H5 HA/H1N1 Virus in Ferrets. *Nature* 486(7403): 420–428.

Imanishi-Kari, T. 1991. OSI's Conclusions Wrong. *Nature* 351: 344–345.

Institute of Medicine (IOM). 2002. *Integrity in Scientific Research: Creating an Environment That Promotes Responsible Conduct*, National Academy Press, Washington, DC.

Institute of Medicine (IOM). 2004. *Intentional Human Dosing Studies for EPA Regulatory Purposes: Scientific and Ethical Issues*. National Academies Press, Washington, DC.

Institute of Medicine (IOM). 2009. Dietary Reference Intakes for Water, Potassium, Sodium, Chloride, and Sulfate, 2004. Available at http://www.nap.edu/openbook.php?isbn=0309091691. Accessed on September 27, 2013.

International Committee of Medical Journal Editors. 2013. Defining the Roles of Authors and Contributors. Available at http://www.icmje.org/roles_a.html. Accessed on October 29, 2013.

International Council on Harmonization (ICH). 1996. Guidance for Industry: Good Clinical Practice. Available at http://www.fda.gov/cder/guidance/959fnl.pdf. Accessed on November 12, 2006.

Irving, D. N., and Shamoo, A. E. 1993. Which Ethics for Science and Public Policy. *Accountability in Research* 3: 77–100.

Isaacson, W. 2007. *Einstein: His Life and Universe*. Simon and Schuster, New York.

Jaffe, A. 1996. Trends and Patterns in Research and Development Expenditures in the United States. *Proceedings of the National Academy of Sciences of the USA* 93: 12658–12663.

Jasanoff, S. 1990. *The Fifth Branch: Science Advisors as Policy Makers*. Harvard University Press, Cambridge, MA.

Johnsen, A., and Toulmin S. 1988. *The Abuse of Casuistry A History of Moral Reasoning*. University of California Press, Berkeley.

Johnson, H. 1993. The Life of a Black Scientist. *Scientific American* 268 1: 160.

Jones, A. 2000. Changing Traditions of Authorship. In *Ethical Issues in Biomedical Publication*, A. Jones and F. McLellan (eds.). Johns Hopkins University Press, Baltimore, pp.3 –29.

Jones, J. H. 1981. *Bad Blood*. Free Press, London.

Journal of Cell Biology. 2007. Image Manipulation. Available at http://www.jcb.org/misc/ifora.shtml#image_aquisition. Accessed on November 26, 2007.

Justice, A., et al. 1998. Does Masking the Author Identity Improve Peer Review Quality? *Journal of the American Medical Association* 280: 240–242.

Kaiser, J. 2004. Scientific Publishing. Seeking Advice on 'open access,' NIH Gets an Earful. *Science* 305(5685):764.

Kaiser, J. 2005. NIH Chief Clamps Down on Consulting and Stock Ownership. *Science* 307:824–825.

Kaiser, J. 2006. Court Decides Tissue Samples Belong to University, Not Patients. *Science* 312: 346. http://www.sciencemag.org/content/312/5772/346.full, Accessed 8/19/2014.

Kaiser, K. 2009. Protecting Respondent Confidentiality in Qualitative Research. *Qualitative Health Research* 19(11): 1632–1641.

Kant, I. 1753 [1981]. *Grounding for the Metaphysics of Morals*. J. Ellington (transl.). Hackett, Indianapolis.

Karlawish, J. 2011. Emergency Research. In *The Oxford Textbook of Clinical Research Ethics*, E. Emanuel et al (eds.). Oxford University Press, New York, 280–289.

Kass, N. E., Faden, R. R., Goodman, S. N., Pronovost, P., Tunis, S., and Beauchamp, T. L. 2013. The Research-treatment Distinction: A Problematic Approach for Determining Which Activities Should Have Ethical Oversight. Ethical Oversight of Learning Health Care Systems, *Hastings Center Report Special Report* 43, no. 1: S4–S15.

Katz, D., Caplan, A., and Merz, J. 2003. All Gifts Large and Small: Toward an Understanding of the Ethics of Pharmaceutical Industry Gift-giving. *American Journal of Bioethics* 3(3): 39–46.

Katz, J. 1972. *Experimentation with Human Beings*. Russell Sage Foundation, New York.

*Katz, J. 1993. Human Experimentation and Human Rights. *Saint Louis University Law Journal* 38: 7–54.

Katz, J. 1996. Ethics in Neurobiological Research with Human Subjects—Final Reflections. *Accountability in Research* 4: 277–283.

Kayton, I. 1995. *Patent Practice*, vol. 1. Patent Resources Institute, Charlottesville, VA.

Kempner, J. 2008. The Chilling Effect: How Do Researchers React to Controversy? *PLoS Medicine* 5(11): e222.

Kennedy, D. 2006. Responding to Fraud. *Science* 316: 1353.

Kesselheim, A. S., Cook-Deegan, R. M., Winickoff, D. E., Mello, M. M. 2013. Gene Patenting—the Supreme Court Finally Speaks. *New England Journal of Medicine* 369(9): 869–875.

Kesselheim, A. S., Cook-Deegan, R. M., Winickoff, D. E., and Mello, M. M. 2013. Gene Patenting—the Supreme Court Finally Speaks. *New England Journal of Medicine* 369(9): 869–875.

Kesselheim, A. S., and Karlawish, J. 2012. Biomarkers Unbound—the Supreme Court's Ruling on Diagnostic-test Patents. *New England Journal of Medicine* 366(25): 2338–2340.

Kevles, D. J. 1996. The Assault on David Baltimore. *New Yorker*, May 27, 94–109.

King, N. 1995. Experimental Treatment: Oxymoron or Aspiration? *Hastings Center Report* 25(4): 6–15.

Kirk, R. 1995. *Experimental Design*. 3rd ed. Brooks/Cole, New York.

Kitcher, P. 1993. *The Advancement of Science*. Oxford University Press, New York.

Kitcher, P. 2001. *Science, Truth, and Democracy*. Oxford University Press, New York.

Knoll, E. 1990. The Communities of Scientists and Journal Peer Review. *Journal of the American Medical Association* 263: 1330–1332.

Koenig, R. 1999. European Researchers Grapple with Animal Rights. *Science* 284: 1604–1606.

Koenig, R. 2001. Scientific Misconduct: Wellcome Rules Widen the Net. *Science* 293: 1411–1412.

Kolata, G. 2013. No Benefit Seen in Sharp Limits on Salt in Diet. *New York Times*, May 14, A1.

*Kong, D., and Whitaker, R. 1998. Doing Harm: Research on the Mentally Ill. *Boston Globe*, November 15, A1.

Koocher, G. P., 2005, Chapter 10, see Kodish, E. (ed.) 2005. *Ethics and Research with Children – A Case-Based Approach*, Oxford University Press.

Kopelman, L. 2000a. Moral Problems in Assessing Research Risk. *IRB: A Review of Human Subjects Research* 22(5): 7–10.

Kopelman, L. 2000b. Children as Research Subjects: A Dilemma. *Journal of Medicine and Philosophy* 25: 745–764.

Koppelman-White, E. 2006. Research Misconduct and the Scientific Process: Continuing Quality Improvement. *Accountability in Research* 13: 325–346.

Korsgaard, C. 1996. *The Sources of Normativity*. Cambridge University Press, Cambridge.

Kravitz, R. L., Franks, P., Feldman, M. D., Gerrity, M., Byrne, C., and Tierney, W. M. 2010. Editorial Peer Reviewers' Recommendations at a General Medical Journal: Are They Reliable and Do Editors Care? *PLoS One* 5(4): e10072.

Krimsky, S. 1996. Financial Interest of Authors in Scientific Journals: A Pilot Study of 14 Publications. *Science and Engineering Ethics* 2(4): 1–13.

Krimsky, S. 2003. *Science in the Private Interest—Has the Lure of Profits Corrupted Biomedical Research?* Rowman and Littlefield, Lanham, MD.

Krimsky, S. 2007. *Defining Scientific Misconduct When Conflict-of-Interest Is a Factor in Scientific Misconduct. Medicine and Law* 26: 447–463.

Krimsky, S., and Rothenberg, L. 2001. Conflict of Interest Policies in Science and Medical Journals: Editorial Practices and Author Disclosures. *Science and Engineering Ethics* 7: 205–218.

Krimsky, S., and Simocelli, T. 2007. Testing Pesticides in Humans—Of Mice and Men Divided by Ten. *Journal of the American Medical Association* 297: 2405–2407.

Krimsky, S., et al. 1996. Financial Interests of Authors in Scientific Publications. *Science and Engineering Ethics* 2(4): 396–410..

Kronic, D. A., 1990. Peer Review in 18th-Century Scientific Journalism. *Journal of the American Medical Association* 263: 1321–1322.

Kuflik, A. 1989. Moral Foundations of Intellectual Property Rights. In *Owning Scientific and Technical Information*, V. Weil and Snapper, J. (eds.). Rutgers University Press, Brunswick, NJ, 29–39.

Kuhn, T. 1970. *The Structure of Scientific Revolutions*. 2nd ed. University of Chicago Press, Chicago.

Kuznik, F. 1991. Fraud Buster. *Washington Post Magazine*, April 14, 22–26, 31–33.

Laband, D. N., and Piette, M. J. 1994. A Citation Analysis of the Impact of Blinded Peer Review. *Journal of the American Medical Association* 272: 147–149.

*LaFollette, H., and Shanks, S. 1996. *Brute Science*. Routledge, New York.

*LaFollette, M. C., 1992. *Stealing into Print—Fraud, Plagiarism, and Misconduct in Scientific Publishing*. University of California Press, Berkeley.

LaFollette, M. C. 1994a. The Pathology of Research Fraud: The History and Politics of the US Experience. *Journal of Internal Medicine* 235: 129–135.

LaFollette, M. 1994b. Measuring Equity—the U.S. General Accounting Office Study of Peer Review. *Science Communication* 6: 211–220.

LaFollette, M. C. 2000. The Evaluation of the "Scientific Misconduct" Issues: An Historical Overview. *Proceedings for the Society for Experimental Biology and Medicine* 224: 211–215.

Laine, C., De Angelis, C., et al. Clinical Trial Registration: Looking Back and Moving Ahead. 2007. *Annals of Internal Medicine* 147: 275–277.

Lawler, A. 2000. Silent No Longer: A "Model Minority" Mobilizes. *Science* 290: 1072–1077.

Lawrence, P. 2003. The Politics of Publication. *Nature* 422: 259–261.

Lederer, S. 1995. *Subjected to Science: Human Experimentation in America before the Second World War*. Johns Hopkins University Press, Baltimore.

Lenzer, J. 2011. Pfizer Settles with Victims of Nigerian Drug Trial. *British Medical Journal* 343: d5268.

Levine, R. J. 1988. *Ethics and Regulation of Clinical Research*. 2nd ed. Yale University Press, New Haven, CT.

Lin, Z., Owen, A., and Altman, R. 2004. Genomic Research and Human Subject Privacy. *Science* 305: 183.

Lo, B., and Garan, N. 2011. Research with Ethnic and Minority Populations. In *The Oxford Textbook of Clinical Research Ethics*, E. Emanuel et al. (eds.). Oxford University Press, New York, 423–430.

Lock, S. 1991. *A Difficult Balance: Editorial Peer Review in Medicine*. BMJ Publishing, London.

Lock, S. 1993. Research Misconduct: A Resume of Recent Events. In *Fraud and Misconduct in Medical Research*, S. Lock and F. Wells (eds.). BMJ Publishing, London, 5–24.

Locke, J. 1764 [1980]. Second Treatise of Government, C. Macpherson (ed.). Hackett, Indianapolis, IN.

Loeb, S. E., and Shamoo, A. E. 1989. Data Audit: Its Place in Auditing. *Accountability in Research* 1: 23–32.

London, A. 2001. Equipoise and International Human-subjects Research. *Bioethics* 15: 312–332.

Lowrance, W. W., and Collins, F. S. 2007. Identifiability in Genomic Research. *Science* 317: 600–602.

Lucky, R. 2000. The Quickening Pace of Science Communication. *Science* 289: 259–264.

Lurie, P., and Wolfe, S. 1997. Unethical Trials of Interventions to Reduce Perinatal Transmission of the Human Immunodeficiency Virus in Developing Countries. *New England Journal of Medicine* 337: 853–856.

Macilwain, C. 1999. Scientists Fight for the Right to Withhold Data. *Nature* 397: 459.

Macklin R. 2003. Bioethics, Vulnerability, and Protection. *Bioethics* 17: 472–486.

MacQueen, K., and Buehler, J. 2004. Ethics, Practice, and Research in Public Health. *American Journal of Public Health* 94: 928–931.

Macrina, F (Ed.). 2013. *Scientific Integrity*. 4th ed. American Society for Microbiology Press, Washington, DC.

Madey v. Duke University. 2002. 307 F. 3d 1351 (Fed. Cir. 2002).

Malakoff, D. 2000. Researchers Fight Plan to Regulate Mice, Birds. *Science* 290: 23.

Malek, J. 2010. To Tell or Not to Tell? The Ethical Dilemma of the Would-be Whistleblower. *Accountability in Research* 17(3): 115–129.

Manning, K. 1998. Science and Opportunity. *Science* 282: 1037–1038.

Marshall, E. 1997a. NIH Plans Peer Review Overhaul. *Science* 276: 888–889.

Marshall, E. 1998. Embargoes: Good, Bad, or "Necessary Evil"? *Science* 282: 860–865.

Marshall, E. 1999b. Duke Told to Stop Clinical Trials. *Science News*, May 12. Available at http://news.sciencemag.org/1999/05/duke-told-stop-clinical-trials. Accessed on November 26, 2013.

Martinson, B. C., Anderson, M. S., and de Vries, R. 2005. Scientists Behaving Badly. *Nature* 435: 737–738.

Mastroianni, A., and Kahn, J. 2001. Swinging on the Pendulum. Shifting Views of Justice in Human Subjects Research. *Hastings Center Report* 31(3): 21–28.

May, D. R., and Luth, M. T. 2013. The Effectiveness of Ethics Education: A Quasi-experimental Field Study. *Science and Engineering Ethics* 19: 545–568.

McCrary, V. S., et al. 2000. A National Survey of Policies on Disclosure of Conflicts of Interest in Biomedical Research. *New England Journal of Medicine* 343: 1621–1626.

McGuire, A., and Gibbs R. 2006. No Longer De-identified. *Science* 312: 370–371.

McKeon, R. (Ed.). 1947. *Modern Library*. Introduction to Aristotle. New York.

McLean, B., and Elkind, P. 2003. *The Smartest Guys in the Room: The Amazing Rise and Scandalous Fall of Enron*. Penguin, New York.

McLellin, F. 1995. Authorship in Biomedical Publications: How Many People Can Wield One Pen? *American Medical Writers Association* 10: 11.

McNutt, R., et al. 1990. The Effects of Blinding on the Quality of Peer Review: A Randomized Trial. *JAMA* 263: 1371–1376.

Meadows, J. 1992. *The Great Scientists*. Oxford University Press, New York.

Merton, R. 1973. *The Sociology of Science*. University of Chicago Press, Chicago.

Mervis, J. 1999. Efforts to Boost Diversity Face Persistent Problems. *Science* 284: 1757–1758.

Mervis, J. 2002. Science with an Agenda: NSF Expands Centers Program. *Science* 297: 506–507.

Milgram, S. 1974. Obedience to Authority. Harper and Rowe, New York.

Miller, A., and Davis, M. 2011. *Intellectual Property*. 4th ed. Thompson West, St. Paul, MN.

Miller, F., and Brody, H. 2002. What makes placebo-controlled trials unethical? *American Journal of Bioethics* 2(2): 3–9.

Miller, F. G., and Fins, J. J. 1999. Protecting Vulnerable Research Subjects without Unduly Constraining Neuropsychiatric Research, *Archives of General Psychiatry* 56: 701–702.

Miller, F. G., and Wertheimer, A. 2007. Facing up to Paternalism in Research Ethics. *Hastings Center Report* 37(3): 24–34.

Miller, G. 2008. Neurobiology. The Roots of Morality. *Science* 320(5877): 734–737.

Miller, L., and Bloom, F. 1998. Publishing Controversial Research. *Science* 282: 1045.

Millum, J. 2011. Post-trial Access to Antiretrovirals: Who Owes What to Whom? *Bioethics* 25(3): 145–154.

Monk, R. 2013. *Robert Oppenheimer: His Life and Mind*. Random House, New York.

Monson, N. 1991. How the Scientific Community Protects Its Black Sheep at the Expense of the Whistleblowers and the Public. *Health Watch*, July/August: 25–33.

Moore v. Regents of the University of California. 1990. 51 Cal 3d 120 134–147.

Moreno, J., and Hynes, R. 2005. Guidelines for Human Embryonic Stem Cell Research. *Nature Biotechnology*. 23(7): 793–794.

Moreno, J. D. 2000. *Undue Risk—Secret State Experiments on Humans*. W. H. Freeman and Company, New York.

Morreim, E. 2005. The Clinical Investigator as Fiduciary: Discarding a Misguided Idea. *Journal of Law Medicine and Ethics* 33: 586–598.

Moses, H., and Martin, B. 2001. Academic Relationships with Industry: A New Model for Biomedical Research. *Journal of the American Medical Association* 285: 933–935.

Mosimann, J. E., et al. 1995. Data Fabrication: Can People Generate Random Digits? *Accountability in Research* 4: 31–56.

Müller-Hill, B. 1992. Eugenics: The Science and Religion of the Nazis. In *When Medicine Went Mad*, A. Caplan (ed.). Humana Press, Totowa, NJ, 43–53.

Mulligan, A. 2005. Is Peer Review in Crisis? *Oral Oncology* 41: 135–141.

Munson, R. 1992. *Intervention and Reflection*. 4th ed. Wadsworth, Belmont, CA.

Murphy, P. 1998. *80 Exemplary Ethics Statements*. University of Notre Dame Press, Notre Dame, IN.

National Academy of Science (NAS). 1992. *Responsible Science—Ensuring the Integrity of the Research Process*, vol. 1. Panel on Scientific Responsibility and the Conduct of Research, NAS, Washington, DC.

National Academy of Sciences (NAS). 1994. *On Being a Scientist*. NAS, Washington, DC.

*National Academy of Science (NAS). 1997. *Advisor, Teacher, Role Model, Friend: On Being a Mentor to Students in Science and Engineering*. NAS, Washington, DC.

National Academy of Science (NAS). 2002. *Integrity in Scientific Research: Creating an Environment That Promotes Responsible Conduct.* NAS, Washington, DC.

National Academy of Sciences. 2011. Examining Core Elements of International Research Collaboration. Available at http://www.nap.edu/catalog. php?record_id=13192. Accessed on 7/1/2014.

*National Bioethics Advisory Commission (NBAC). 1998. *Research Involving Persons with Mental Disorders That May Affect Decisionmaking Capacity,* vol. 1, Report and Recommendations. NBAC, Rockville, MD.

*National Bioethics Advisory Commission (NBAC). 1999. Report on Ethical Issues in Human Stem Cell Research, vol. 1. NBAC, Rockville, MD.

National Commission for the Protection of Human Subjects of Biomedical and Behavioral Research. 1979. *The Belmont Report.* Department of Health, Education, and Welfare, Washington, DC. Available at http://ohsr.od.nih.gov/ guidelines/belmont.html. Accessed on November 21, 2013.

National Institutes of Health (NIH). 1998. Report of the National Institute of Health Working Group on Research Tools. Available at http://www.nih.gov/ news/researchtools/index.htm.

National Institutes of Health (NIH). 2002. A Guide to Mentoring and Training in the Intramural Program at NIH. National Institutes of Health, Bethesda, MD. Available at http://sourcebook.od.nih.gov/ethic-conduct/ TrainingMentoringGuide_7.3.02.pdf. Accessed on February 12, 2014.

National Institutes of Health (NIH). 2003. NIH Data Sharing and Policy Implementation Guidance. Available at http://grants.nih.gov/grants/policy/ data_sharing/data_sharing_guidance.htm. Accessed on October 15, 2007.

National Institutes of Health (NIH). 2007a. Guidelines for the Conduct of Research at the Intramural Program of the NIH. Available at http://www1.od.nih.gov/ oir/sourcebook/ethic-conduct/Conduct%20Research%206-211-07.pdf.

National Institutes of Health (NIH). 2007b. Award Data. Available at http://grants. nih.gov/grants/award/success/Success_ByIC.cfm. Accessed on December 26, 2007.

National Institutes of Health. 2007c. Genome-Wide Association Studies: Frequently Asked Questions. Available at http://grants.nih.gov/grants/gwas/GWAS_faq. htm. Accessed on April 30, 2008.

National Institutes of Health (NIH). 2007d. Guidelines for the Conduct of Research at the Intramural Program of the NIH. Available at http://www1.od.nih.gov/ oir/sourcebook/ethic-conduct/Conduct%20Research%206-211-07.pdf.

National Institutes of Health (NIH). 2008a. NIH Policy Manual, 3/10/2008. Available at http://oma1.od.nih.gov/manualchapters/management/1184/. Accessed on February 11, 2014.

National Institutes of Health (NIH). 2008b. Scientists Isolate a Toxic Key to Alzheimer's Disease in Human Brains. Available at http://www.nih.gov/ news/health/jun2008/nia-22.htm. Accessed on Februrary 24, 2014.

National Institutes of Health (NIH). 2009a. Update on the Requirement for Instruction in Responsible Conduct of Research. Available at http://grants1. nih.gov/grants/guide/notice-files/NOT-OD-10-019.html. Accessed on October 10, 2013.

National Institutes of Health (NIH). 2009b. *Guidelines for the Conduct of Research in the Intramural Program at NIH.* National Institutes of Health, Bethesda, MD.

National Institutes of Health (NIH). 2009c. Genomic Data Sharing. Available at http://gds.nih.gov/03policy2.html. Accessed on July 1, 2014.

National Institutes of Health (NIH). 2013. Available at http://news.sciencemag.org/funding/2013/09/sequester-cuts-may-have-driven-nih-grant-success-rates-down-14-2013. Accessed on November 8, 2013.

National Research Council (NRC). 1996. *Guide for the Care and Use of Laboratory Animals*. National Academy Press, Washington, DC.

National Research Council (NRC). 2004. *Biotechnology in the Age of Terrorism*. National Academies Press, Washington, DC.

National Science Foundation (NSF). 1997. Scientists and Engineers Statistical Data System. Science Resources Studies Division, SESTAT, NSF, Washington, DC.

National Science Foundation (NSF). 2009. Responsible Conduct of Research. Available at http://www.gpo.gov/fdsys/pkg/FR-2009-2008-20/html/E9-19930.htm. Accessed on January 22, 2014.

Nature. 1999. Policy on Papers' Contributors. *Nature* 399: 393.

Newton, I. 1687 [1995]. *The Principia*. A. Motte (trans.). Prometheus Books, Amherst, NY.*New York Times*. 2013. We Paid for the Research, So Let's See It. February 25. Available at http://www.nytimes.com/2013/02/26/opinion/we-paid-for-the-scientific-research-so-lets-see-it.html?_r=0. Accessed on October 31, 2013.

Nuffield Council. 2002. *The Ethics of Patenting DNA*. Nuffield Council, London.

Obama, B. 2009. Executive Order 13505, March 9. Available at http://edocket.access.gpo.gov/2009/pdf/E9-5441.pdf. Accessed on October 14, 2013.

Office of Human Research Protections. 2011. Advanced Notice of Proposed Rulemaking. Available at http://www.hhs.gov/ohrp/humansubjects/index.html. Accessed on November 12, 2013.

Office of Human Research Protections. 2013. 2013 Edition of the International Compilation of Human Research Standards. Available at http://www.hhs.gov/ohrp/international/intlcompilation/intlcomp2013.pdf. Accessed on November 12, 2013.

Office of Research Integrity (ORI). 2003. Survey of Research Measures Utilized in Biomedical Research Laboratories. Final Report—Executive Summary. Available at http://ori.dhhs.gov/documents/research/intergity_measures_final_report_11_07_03.pdf. Accessed on October 23, 2007.

Office of Research Integrity (ORI). 2005a. UV Press Release Poehlman. Available at http://ori.hhs.gov/misconduct/cases/press_release_poehlman.shtml. Accessed on October 23, 2007.

Office of Research Integrity (ORI). 2007a. About ORI. ORI, Rockville, MD. Available at http://ori.dhhs.gov/about/index.shtml. Accessed on October 23, 2007.

Office of Research Integrity (ORI). 2007b. Forensic Tools. Available at http://ori.hhs.gov/tools/index.shtml.

Office of Research Integrity (ORI). 2011. Historical Background. Available at http://ori.dhhs.gov/historical-background. Accessed on October 11, 2013.

Office of Research Integrity (ORI). 2012. Case Summary: Marc Hauser. Available at http://ori.hhs.gov/content/case-summary-hauser-marc. Accessed on October 7, 2013.

Office of Science and Technology Policy. 2000. Federal Research Misconduct Policy. *Federal Register* 65(235): 76260–76264.

Office of Technology Assessment (OTA). 1986. *Alternatives to Animal Use in Research, Testing, and Education*. OTA, Washington, DC.

Office of Technology Assessment (OTA). 1990. *New Developments in Biotechnology—Patenting Life*. Dekker, New York.

Oliver, D. T. 1999. *Animal Rights—the Inhumane Crusade*. Capital Research Center, Merril Press, Washington, DC.

Ollove, M. 2001. The Lessons of Lynchburg. *Baltimore Sun*, May 6, 7F.

Orlans, F, Beauchamp, T., Dresser, R., Morton, D., and Gluck, J. 1998. *The Human Use of Animals*. Oxford University Press, New York.

Oxman, A., et al. 1991. Agreement among Reviewers of Review Articles. *Journal of Clinical Epidemiology* 44: 91–98.

Participants in the 2001 Conference on Ethical Aspects of Research in Developing Countries. 2004. Moral Standards for Research in Developing Countries: From "Reasonable Availability" to "Fair Benefits." *Hastings Center Report* 34(3): 17–27.

Pellegrino, E. 1992. Character and Ethical Conduct of Research. *Accountability in Research* 2: 1–2.

Pence, G. 1995. Animal Subjects. In *Classic Cases in Medical Ethics*. McGraw-Hill, New York, 203–224.

Pence, G. 1996. *Classic Cases in Medical Ethics*. 2nd ed. McGraw-Hill, New York.

Penslar, R. 1995. *Research Ethics: Cases and Materials*. Indiana University Press, Bloomington.

Peters, D., and Ceci, S. 1982. Peer-Review Practices of Psychological Journals: The Fate of Published Articles, Submitted Again. *Behavioral and Brain Sciences* 5: 187–195.

Pfund, C., Maidl Pribbenow, C., Branchaw, J., Miller Lauffer, S., and Handelsman, J. 2006. Professional Skills. The Merits of Training Mentors. *Science* 311(5760): 473–474.

Pielke, R. 2007. *The Honest Broker: Making Sense of Science in Policy and Politics*. Cambridge University Press, Cambridge.

Plemmons, D. K., Brody, S. A., and Kalichman, M. W. 2006. Student Perceptions of the Effectiveness of Education in the Responsible Conduct of Research. *Science and Engineering Ethics* 12: 571–582.

Plous, S., and Herzog, H. 2000. Poll Shows Researchers Favor Animal Lab Protection. *Science* 290: 711.

Pojman, J. 1995. *Ethics*. Wadsworth, Belmont, CA.

Popper, K. 1959. *The Logic of Scientific Discovery*. Routledge, London.

*Porter, D. 1993. Science, Scientific Motivation, and Conflict of Interest in Research. In *Ethical Issues in Research*, D. Cheny (ed.). University Publishing Group, Frederick, MD, 114–125.

Porter, R. 1997. *The Greatest Benefit to Mankind*. W. W. Norton, New York.

Powell, S., Allison, M., and Kalichman, M. 2007. Effectiveness of a Responsible Conduct of Research Course: A Preliminary Study. *Science and Engineering Ethics* 13: 249–264.

President's Commission for the Study of Ethical Problems in Medicine and Biomedical and Behavioral Research. 1983a. Summing Up. U.S. Government Printing Office, Washington, DC.

President's Commission for the Study of Ethical Problems in Medicine and Biomedical and Behavioral Research. 1983b. Splicing Life: A Report on the Social and Ethical Issues of Genetic Engineering with Human Beings, U.S. Government Printing Office, Washington.

Press, E., and Washburn, J. 2000. The Kept University. *Atlantic Monthly* 285(3): 39–54.

Price, A. R., and Hallum, J. V. 1992. The Office of Scientific Integrity Investigations: The Importance of Data Analysis. *Accountability in Research* 2: 133–137.

Proctor, R. 1988. *Radical Hygiene—Medicine under the Nazis*. Harvard University Press, Cambridge, MA.

Proctor, R. 1999. *The Nazi War on Cancer*. Princeton University Press, Princeton, NJ.

Rajakumar, K., Thomas, S. B., Musa, D., Almario, D., and Garza, M. A. 2009. Racial Differences in Parents' Distrust of Medicine and Research. *Archives of Pediatric Adolescent Medicine* 163(2): 108–114.

Ravitsky, V., and Wilfond, B. 2006. Disclosing Individual Results to Research Participants. *American Journal of Bioethics* 6(6): 8–17.

Rawls, J. 1971. *A Theory of Justice*. Harvard University Press, Cambridge, MA.

Ready, T. 1999. Science for Sale. *Boston Phoenix*, April 29, 60–62.

Redman, B., and Merz, J. 2006. Research Misconduct Policies of Highest Impact Biomedical Journals. *Accountability in Research* 13: 247–258.

Regaldo, A. 1995. Multiauthor Papers on the Rise. *Science* 268: 25–27.

Regan, T. 1983. *The Case for Animal Rights*. University of California Press, Berkeley.

Regan, T., and Singer, P. (Eds.). 1989. *Animal Rights and Human Obligations*. 2nd ed. Prentice-Hall, Englewood Cliffs, NJ.

Reich, E. S. 2009. *Plastic Fantastic: How the Biggest Fraud in Physics Shook the World*. Palgrave Macmillan, New York.

Rennie, D. 1989a. How Much Fraud? Let's Do an Experimental Audit. *AAAS Observer*, 3(3): 4.

Rennie, D. 1989b. Editors and Auditors. *Journal of the American Medical Association*, 261: 2543–2545.

Rennie, D., et al. 1997. When Authorship Fails: A Proposal to Make Contributors Accountable. *Journal of the American Medical Association* 278: 579–585.

Rescher, N. 1965. The Ethical Dimension of Scientific Research. In *Beyond the Edge of Certainty: Essays on Contemporary Science and Philosophy*, N. Rescher (ed.). Prentice-Hall, Englewood Cliffs, NJ, 261–276.

Resnik, D. 1994. Methodological Conservatism and Social Epistemology. *International Studies in the Philosophy of Science* 8: 247–264.

Resnik, D. 1997. A Proposal for a New System of Credit Allocation in Science. *Science and Engineering Ethics* 3: 237–243.

Resnik, D. 1998a. *The Ethics of Science*. Routledge, New York.

*Resnik, D. 1998b. Conflicts of Interest in Science. *Perspectives on Science* 6(4): 381–408.

Resnik, D. 1998c. The Ethics of HIV Research in Developing Nations. *Bioethics* 12(4): 285–306.

Resnik, D. 2000. Statistics, Ethics, and Research: An Agenda for Education and Reform. *Accountability in Research* 8: 163–188.

*Resnik, D. 2001a. DNA Patents and Scientific Discovery and Innovation: Assessing Benefits and Risks. *Science and Engineering Ethics* 7(1): 29–62.

*Resnik, D. 2001b. Financial Interests and Research Bias. *Perspectives on Science* 8(3): 255–285.

Resnik, D. 2001c. Ethical Dilemmas in Communicating Medical Information to the Public. *Health Policy* 55: 129–149.

Resnik D. 2003a. Exploitation in Biomedical Research. *Theoretical Medicine and Bioethics* 24: 233–259.

Resnik, D. 2003b. From Baltimore to Bell Labs: Reflections on Two Decades of Debate about Scientific Misconduct. *Accountability in Research* 10: 123–135.

Resnik, D. 2004a. *Owning the Genome: A Moral Analysis of DNA Patenting*. SUNY Press, Albany.

Resnik, D. 2004b. Disclosing Conflicts of Interest to Research Subjects: An Ethical and Legal Analysis. *Accountability in Research* 11: 141–159.

Resnik, D. B. 2004c. Punishing Medical Experts for Unethical Testimony: A Step in the Right Direction or a Step Too Far? *Journal of Philosophy, Science, and Law* 4. Available at http://www6.miami.edu/ethics/jpsl/archives/all/punishing. pdf. Accessed on September 27, 2013.

Resnik, D. 2005. Affirmative Action in Science and Engineering. *Science & Education* 14: 75–93.

Resnik, D. 2006. A Survey of Research Practices at the National Institutes of Environmental Health Sciences. Proceedings from 2006 ORI Conference on Research on Research Integrity, Potomac, MD.

Resnik, D. 2007. *The Price of Truth: How Money Affects the Norms of Science.* Oxford University Press, New York.

Resnik, D. B. 2008. COI Issues in Research Misconduct Investigations and Inquiries. *ORI Newsletter* 16(4): 1, 4.

Resnik, D. B. 2009a. *Playing Politics with Science: Balancing Scientific Independence and Government Oversight.* Oxford University Press, New York.

Resnik, D. B. 2009b. The Investigator-Subject Relationship: A Contextual Approach. *Journal of Philosophy, Ethics, Humanities in Medicine* 4: 16.

Resnik, D. B. 2010. Genomic Research Data: Open vs. Restricted Access. *IRB* 32(1): 1–6.

Resnik, D. B. 2011. Scientific Research and the Public Trust. *Science and Engineering Ethics* 17(3): 399–409.

Resnik, D. B. 2012a. Ethical Virtues in Scientific Research. *Accountability in Research* 19(6): 329–343.

Resnik, D. B. 2012b. Ethical Issues Concerning Transgenic Animals in Biomedical Research. In: J. Garrett (ed.), The Ethics of Animal Research: Exploring the Controversy. MIT Press, Cambridge, MA: 169–179.

Resnik, D. B. 2012c. *Environmental Health Ethics.* Cambridge University Press, Cambridge.

Resnik, D. B. 2013. H5N1 Avian Flu Research and the Ethics of Knowledge. *Hastings Center Report* 43(2): 22–33.

Resnik, D. B., Barner, D. D., and Dinse, G. E. 2012. Dual-use Review Policies of Biomedical Research Journals. *Biosecurity and Bioterrorism* 9(1): 49–54.

Resnik, D. B., and Dinse, G. E. 2012a. Scientific Retractions and Corrections Related to Misconduct Findings. *Journal of Medical Ethics* 39: 46–50.

Resnik, D. B., and Dinse, G. E. 2012b. Do U.S. Research Institutions Meet or Exceed Federal Mandates for Instruction in Responsible Conduct of Research? A National Survey. Academic Medicine 87(9): 1237–1242.

Resnik, D. B., and Elliott, K. C. 2013. Taking Financial Relationships into Account When Assessing Research. *Accountability in Research* 20(3): 184–205.

Resnik, D. B., and Master, Z. 2013a. Policies and Initiatives Aimed at Addressing Research Misconduct in High-income Countries. *PLoS Medicine* 10(3): e1001406.

Resnik, D. B., and Master, Z. 2013b. Authorship Policies of Bioethics Journals. Journal of Medical Ethics 2011; 37:424–428. doi:10.1136/jme.2010.040675. Accessed on 7/1/2014.

Resnik, D. B., Neal, T., Raymond, A., and Kissling, G. E. 2014. Research Misconduct Definitions Adopted by U.S. Research Institutions. *Accountability in Research* 22(1): 14–21.

Resnik, D. B., Patrone, D., Peddada, S. 2010. Research Misconduct Policies of Social Science Journals and Impact Factor. *Accountability in Research* 17(2):79–84.

Resnik, D. B., Peddada, S., and Ford, C. 2008. Perceptions of Ethical Problems with Scientific Journal Peer Review: An Exploratory Study. *Science and Engineering Ethics* 14: 305–310.

Resnik, D., and Portier, C. 2005. Pesticide Testing on Human Subjects: Weighing Benefits and Risks. *Environmental Health Perspectives* 113: 813–817.

Resnik, D., and Shamoo, A. E. 2002. Conflict of Interest and the University. *Accountability in Research* 9: 45–64.

Resnik, D. B., and Shamoo, A. E. 2011. The Singapore Statement on Research Integrity. *Accountability in Research* 18(2): 71–75.

Resnik, D., Shamoo, A., and Krimsky, S. 2006. Fraudulent Human Embryonic Stem Cell Research in South Korea: Lesson Learned. *Accountability in Research* 13: 101–109.

Resnik, D. B., and Sharp, R. R. 2006. Protecting Third Parties in Human Subjects Research. *IRB* 28(4): 1–7.

Resnik, D. B., and Stewart, C. N. Jr. 2012. Misconduct versus Honest Error and Scientific Disagreement. *Accountability in Research* 19(1): 56–63.

Rial-Sebbag, E., and Cambon-Thomsen, A. 2012. The Emergence of Biobanks in the Legal Landscape: Towards a New Model of Governance. *Journal of Law and Society* 39(1): 113–130.

Richardson, H. 2000. Specifying, Balancing, and Interpreting Bioethical Principles. *Journal of Medicine and Philosophy*. 25: 285–307.

Richardson, H. S., and Belsky, L. 2004. The Ancillary-care Responsibilities of Medical Researchers. An Ethical Framework for Thinking about the Clinical Care That Researchers Owe Their Subjects. *Hastings Center Report* 34(1): 25–33.

Ridker, P. M., and Torres, J. 2006. Reported Outcomes in Major Cardiovascular Clinical Trials Funded by For-Profit and Not-Profit Organizations: 2000–2005. *Journal of the American Medical Association* 295: 2270–2274.

Robbins, L. E. 2001. *Louis Pasteur and the Hidden World of Microbes*. Oxford University Press, New York.

Robert, J. 2006. The Science and Ethics of Making Part-human Animals in Stem Cell Biology. *FASEB J* 20: 838–845.

Robert, J., and Baylis, F. 2003. Crossing Species Boundaries. *American Journal of Bioethics* 3(3): 1–13.

Robertson, H., and Gorovitz, S. 2000. Pesticide Toxicity, Human Subjects, and the Environmental Protection Agency's Dilemma. *Journal of Contemporary Health Law and Policy* 16: 427–458.

Rollin, B., 1989. *The Unheeded Cry: Animal Consciousness, Animal Pain, and Science*. Oxford University Press, New York.

Rollin, B. 1992. *Animal Rights and Human Morality*. 2nd ed. Oxford University Press, Oxford.

Ronan, C. 1982. *Science: Its History and Development among the World Cultures*. Facts on File, New York.

Rooyen, S., et al. 1998. Effect of Blinding and Unmasking on the Quality of Peer Review. *Journal of the American Medical Association* 280: 234–237.

Rose, M., and Fischer, K. 1995. Policies and Perspectives on Authorship. *Science and Engineering Ethics* 1: 361–370.

Rosenberg, S. A. 1996. Sounding Board—Secrecy in Medical Research. *New England Journal of Medicine* 334: 392–394.

Rosengard, A. M., Liu, Y., Nie, Z., and Jimenez, R. 2002. Variola Virus Immune Evasion Design: Expression of a Highly Efficient Inhibitor of Human Complement. *Proceedings of the National Academy of Sciences* 99(13): 8808–8813.

Roy, R. 1993. Science Publishing Is Urgently in Need of Reform. *The Scientist*, September 6, 11, 22.

Rule, J. T., and Shamoo, A. E. 1997. Ethical Issues in Research Relationships between Universities, and Industry. *Accountability in Research* 5: 239–250.

Russell, C. A., Fonville, J. M., et al. 2012. The Potential for Respiratory Droplet-Transmissible A/H5N1 Influenza Virus to Evolve in a Mammalian Host. *Science* 336(6088): 1541–1547.

Russell, W., and Birch, R. 1959. *Principles of Humane Animal Experimentation*. Charles C. Thomas, Springfield, IL.

Salvaterra, E., Lecchi, L., et al. 2008. *EMBO Reports* 9(4): 307–313.

Saul, S. 2005. F.D.A. Approves a Heart Drug for African-Americans. *New York Times*, June 24, 2005: A1.

Savulescu, J., and Spriggs, M. 2002. The Hexamethonium Asthma Study and the Death of a Normal Volunteer in Research. *Journal of Medical Ethics* 28: 3–4.

Scheetz, M. D. 1999. Office of Research Integrity: A Reflection of Disputes and Misunderstandings. *Croatian Medical Journal.*, September; 40(3) 321–325.

Schreier, A., Wilson, K., and Resnik, D. 2006. Academic Research Record-keeping: Best Practices for Individuals, Group Leaders, and Institutions. *Academic Medicine* 81(1): 42–47.

Schroter, S, Tite, L, and Smith, R. 2005. Perceptions of Open Access Publishing: Interviews with Journal Authors. *British Medical Journal* 330(7494):756.

Semeniuk, I., and Reverby, S. 2010. A Shocking Discovery. *Nature* 467(7316): 645.

Shah, S., et. al. 2004. How Do Institutional Review Boards Apply the Federal Risk and Benefit Standards for Pediatric Research? *Journal of the American Medical Association* 291: 476–482.

Shamoo, A. E. 1988. We Need Data Audit. *AAAS Observer November* 4: 4.

Shamoo, A. E. 1989. *Principles of Research Data Audit*. Gordon and Breach, New York.

Shamoo, A. E. 1991a. Quality Assurance. *Quality Assurance: Good Practice, Regulation, and Law* 1: 4–9.

Shamoo, A. E. 1991b. Policies and Quality Assurance in the Pharmaceutical Industry. *Accountability in Research* 1: 273–284.

*Shamoo, A. E. 1992. Role of Conflict of Interest in Scientific Objectivity—a Case of a Nobel Prize. *Accountability in Research* 2: 55–75.

Shamoo, A. E. 1993. Role of Conflict of Interest in Public Advisory Councils. In *Ethical Issues in Research*, D. Cheney (ed.). University Publishing Group, Frederick, MD, 159–174.

Shamoo, A. E. 1994a. Editors, Peer Reviews, and Ethics. *AAAS Perspectives* 14: 4–5.

Shamoo, A. E. 1994b. Our Responsibilities Toward Persons with Mental Illness as Human Subjects in Research. *Journal of the California Alliance for the Mentally Ill* 5: 14–16.

Shamoo, A. E. 1997a. Brain Disorders—Scientific Facts, Media, and Public Perception. *Accountability in Research* 5: 161–174.

Shamoo, A. E. 1997b. The Ethical Import of Creation. *Baltimore Sun*, March 2, F1, F7.

Shamoo, A. E. (Ed.). 1997c. *Ethics in Neurobiological Research with Human Subjects*. Gordon and Breach, Amsterdam.

Shamoo, A. E. 1999. Institutional Review Boards (IRBs) and Conflict of Interest. *Accountability in Research* 7: 201–212.

Shamoo, A. E. 2000. Future Challenges to Human Subject Protection. *The Scientist*, June 26, 35.

Shamoo, A. E. 2005. Debating Moral Issues in Developing Countries. *Applied Clinical Trials* 14(6): 86–96.

Shamoo, A. E. 2012. *Equal Worth—When Humanity Will Have Peace*. University Press of America, Lanham, MD.

Shamoo A. E. 2013. Data Audit as a Way to Prevent/Contain Misconduct. *Accountability in Research* 20(5–6): 369–379.

Shamoo, A. E., and Annau, Z. 1987. Ensuring Scientific Integrity [correspondence]. *Nature* 327: 550.

Shamoo, A. E., and Annau, Z. 1989. Data Audit—Historical Perspective. In *Principles of Research Data Audit*, A. E. Shamoo (ed.). Gordon and Breach, New York, 1–12.

Shamoo, A., and Davis, S. 1989. The Need for Integration of Data Audit Research and Development Operations. In *Principles of Research Data Audit*, A. Shamoo (ed.). Gordon and Breach, Amsterdam, 119–128.

*Shamoo, A., and Dunigan, C. 2000. Ethics in Research. *Proceedings of the Society for Experimental Biology and Medicine* 224: 205–210.

Shamoo, A. E., and Irving, D. N. 1993. Accountability in Research Using Persons with Mental Illness. *Accountability in Research* 3: 1–17.

*Shamoo, A. E., and Keay, T. 1996. Ethical Concerns about Relapse Studies. *Cambridge Quarterly of Health Care Ethics* 5: 373–386.

Shamoo, A. E., and O'Sullivan, J. L. 1998. The Ethics of Research on the Mentally Disabled. In *Health Care Ethics—Critical Issues for the 21st Century*, J. F. Monagle and D. C. Thomasma (eds.). Aspen Publishers, Gaithersburg, MD, 239–250.

Shamoo, A. E., and Resnik, D. B. 2006a. Ethical Issues for Clinical Research Managers. *Drug Information Journal* 40: 371–383.

Shamoo, A. E., and Resnik, D. B. 2006b. Strategies to Minimize Risks and Exploitation in Phase One Trials on Healthy Subjects. *American Journal of Bioethics* 6(3): W1–13.

Shamoo, A. E., and Teaf, R. 1990. Data Ownership. *CBE Views* 13: 112–114.

Shamoo, A. E., and Woeckner, E. 2007. Ethical Flaws in the TeGenero Trial. *American Journal of Bioethics* 7(2): 90–92.

Sharav, V. H., and Shamoo, A. E. 2000. Are Experiments That Chemically Induce Psychosis in Patients Ethical? *BioLaw* 2(1): S1–S36.

Shenk, D. 1999. Money & Science = Ethics Problems on Campus. *The Nation*, May 22, 11–18.

Shrader-Frechette, K. 1994. *Ethics of Scientific Research*. Rowman and Littlefield, Boston.

Sigma Xi. 1986. *Honor in Science*. Sigma Xi, Research Triangle Park, NC.

Singapore Statement. 2010. Available at http://www.singaporestatement.org/. Accessed on October 4, 2013.

*Singer, P. 1975 [1990]. *Animal Liberation*. 2nd ed. Random House, New York.

Singer, P. 1985. *In Defense of Animals*. Harper and Row, New York.

Sismondo, S. 2008. Pharmaceutical Company Funding and Its Consequences: A Qualitative Systematic Review. *Contemporary Clinical Trials* 29: 109–113.

Smith, R. 2006a. Research Misconduct: The Poisoning of the Well. Journal of the Royal Society of Medicine 99: 232–237.

Smith, R. 2006b. Peer Review: A Flawed Process at the Heart of Science and Journals. *Journal of the Royal Society of Medicine* 99: 178–182.

Snow, C. 1964. *The Two Cultures and the Scientific Revolution*. Cambridge University Press, Cambridge.

Sobel, A. 1978. Deception in Social Science Research: Is Informed Consent Possible? *Hastings Center Report* 8(5): 40–45.

Sprague, R. 1991. One Man's Saga with the University Federal System. Paper presented at the Second Conference on Research Policies and Quality Assurance, Rome, May 6–7.

Sprague, R. L. 1993. Whistblowing: A Very Unpleasant Avocation. *Ethics and Behavior* 3: 103–133.

Steen, R. G. 2011. Retractions in the Scientific Literature: Is the Incidence of Research Fraud Increasing? *Journal of Medical Ethics* 37(4): 249–253.

Steiner, J. F., et al. 2004. Assessing the Role of Influential Mentors in the Research Development of Primary Care Fellows. *Academic Medicine* 79: 865–872.

Stelfox, H.T., et al. 1998. Conflict of Interest in the Debate over Calcium-Channel Antagonists. *New England Journal of Medicine* 338: 101–106.

Steneck, N. 1999. Confronting Misconduct in Science in the 1980s and 1990s: What Has and Has Not Been Accomplished. *Science and Engineering Ethics* 5: 161–176.

*Steneck, N. 2000. Assessing the Integrity of Publicly Funded Research. In Proceedings from the ORI Conference on Research Integrity, ORI, Washington, DC, 1–16.

Steneck, N. 2006. *ORI Introduction to Responsible Conduct of Research*. Office of Research Integrity, Washington, DC.

Steneck, N., and Bulger, R. 2007. The History, Purpose, and Future of Instruction in the Responsible Conduct of Research. *Academic Medicine* 82: 829–834.

Stephens, T., and Brynner, R. 2001. *Dark Remedy: The Impact of Thalidomide and Its Revival as a Vital Medicine*. Perseus, New York.

Stewart, W. W., and Feder, N. 1987. The Integrity of the Scientific Literature. *Nature* 325: 207–214.

Stewart, W. W., and Feder, N. 1991. Analysis of a Whistle-blowing. *Nature* 351: 687–691.

Stokstad, E. 1999. Humane Science Finds Sharper and Kinder Tools. *Science* 286: 1068–1071.

Strong, C. 2000. Specified Principlism: What Is It, and Does It Really Resolve Cases Better Than Casuistry? *Journal of Medicine and Philosophy*. 25: 323–341.

Swazey, J., and Bird, S. 1997. Teaching and Learning Research Ethics. In *Research Ethics: A Reader*, D. Elliot and J. Stern (eds.). University Press of New England, Hanover, NH, 1–19.

Swazey, J. 1993. Teaching Ethics: Needs, Opportunities, and Obstacles. In *Ethics, Values, and the Promise of Science*. Sigma Xi, Research Triangle Park, NC, pp.233 –242.

Swisher, K. 1995. *What Is Sexual Harassment?* Greenhaven, San Diego.

Tagney, J. P. 1987. Fraud Will Out—or Will It? *New Scientist*, August 6, 62–63.

Tamot, R., Arsenieva, D., and Wright, D. E. 2014. The Emergence of the Responsible Conduct of Research (RCR) in PHS Policy and Practice. *Accountability in Research* 20: 349–368.

Taubes, G. 1998. The (Political) Science of Salt. *Science* 281(5379): 898–907.

*Tauer, C. A. 1999. Testing Drugs in Pediatric Populations: The FDA Mandate. *Accountability in Research* 7: 37–58.

Taylor J. 2013. IRS Audit Red Flags: The Dirty Dozen. *Kiplinger*, March. Available at http://www.kiplinger.com/article/taxes/T054-C000-S001-irs-audit-red-flags-the-dirty-dozen.html. Accessed on October 10, 2013.

Taylor, P. 1986. *Respect for Nature*. Princeton University Press, Princeton, NJ.

Teitelman, R. 1994. *The Profits of Science*. Basic Books, New York.*Thompson, D. 1993. Understanding Financial Conflict of Interest. *New England Journal of Medicine* 329: 573–576.

Titus, S. L. 2014. Evaluating U.S. Medical Schools' Researchers on Research Integrity and Research Misconduct Policies and Procedures. *Accountability in Research* 21: 9–25.

Tsuchiya T. 2011. The imperial Japanese Experiments in China. In: E. Emanuel, C. C. Grady,R. A. Crouch,R. K. Lie,F. G. Miller,D. D. Wendler (eds.). *Oxford Textbook of Clinical Research Ethics*, pp. 31–45, Oxford University Press, New York.

Tumpey, T. M., Basler, C. F., et al. 2005. Characterization of the Reconstructed 1918 Spanish Influenza Pandemic Virus. *Science* 310(5745): 77–80.

U.S. Congress, Committee on Government Operations. 1990. Are Scientific Misconduct and Conflict of Interests Hazardous to Our Health? Report 101–688, U.S. Government Printing Office, Washington, DC.

U.S. Department of Health, Education, and Welfare (DHEW). 1973. Final Report of the Tuskegee Syphilis Study Ad Hoc Advisory Panel. DHEW, Washington, DC.

U.S. Department of Justice. 2007. Strategic Plan. Available at http://www.google.com/url?sa=t&rct=j&q=&esrc=s&frm=1&source=web&cd=2&ved=0CCwQFjAB&url=http%3A%2F%2Fwww.justice.gov%2Farchive%2Fmps%2Fstrategic2007-2012%2Fstrategic_plan20072012.pdf&ei=SGb6UtGgNcLI0QGYk4DYCw&usg=AFQjCNEFExPHDcdYDnNam4QV_g7Xef3ycA. Accessed on February 11, 2014.

U.S. General Accounting Office (GAO). 1994. Peer Review—Reforms Needed to Ensure Fairness in Federal Agency Grant Selection. GAO/PEMD-94-1. GAO, Washington, DC.

U.S. Government. 2012. Policy for Overseeing Life Sciences Dual Use Research of Concern. Available at http://oba.od.nih.gov/oba/biosecurity/PDF/United_States_Government_Policy_for_Oversight_of_DURC_FINAL_version_032812.pdf. Accessed on September 23, 2013.

U.S. Public Health Service (PHS). 2000. *Policy on the Humane Care and Use of Laboratory Animals*. PHS, Bethesda, MD.

U.S. Public Health Service Policies on Research Misconduct. 2005 Final Rule. Available at http://ori.dhhs.gov/documents/42_cfr_parts_50_and_93_2005.pdf. Accessed on October 22.

Van Noorden, R. 2013. Open Access: The True Cost of Science Publishing. *Nature* 495: 426–429.

Varmus, H., and Satcher, D. 1997. Ethical Complexities of Conducting Research in Developing Countries. *New England Journal of Medicine* 337: 1000–1005.

Vroom, V. H., and Jago, A. G. 2007. The Role of the Situation in Leadership. *American Psychologist* 62: 17–24.

Vasgird D. 2007. Prevention over Cure: The Administrative Rationale for Education in the Responsible Conduct of Research. *Academic Medicine* 82(9):835–837.

Wade, N. 1981. The Rise and Fall of a Scientific Superstar. *New Scientist* 91: 781–782.

Wade, N. 2010. Harvard Finds Scientist Guilty of Misconduct. *New York Times*, August 20, A1.

Wadman, M. 1996. Drug Company Suppressed Publication of Research. *Nature* 381: 4.

Wager, E., Parkin, E. C., and Tamber, P. S. 2006. Are Reviewers Suggested by Authors as Good as Those Suggested by Editors? Results of a Rater-blinded,

Retrospective Study. *BMC Medicine* 4: 13. Available at http://www.
biomedcentral.com/1741-7015/4/13.

Wahlberg, A., et. al. 2013. From Global Bioethics to Ethical Governance of
Biomedical Research Collaborations, *Social Science and Medicine* 98:
293–300.

Wakefield, A. J., Murch, S. H., et al. 1998. Ileal-lymphoid-nodular Hyperplasia,
Non-specific Colitis, and Pervasive Developmental Disorder in Children.
Lancet 351(9103): 637–641.

Walsh. et al. 2000. Open Peer Review: A Randomized Controlled Trial. *British
Journal of Psychiatry*, 176:47–51.

Washburn, J. 2006. *University, Inc.: The Corporate Corruption of American Higher
Education*. Basic Books, New York.

Washington, H. A. 2006. *Medical Apartheid—The Dark History of Medical Experimentation
on Black Americans from Colonial Times to the Present*. Doubleday, New York.

Weaver, D., et al. 1986. Altered Repertoire of Endogenous Immunoglobulin Gene
Expression in Transgenic Mice Containing a Rearranged mu Heavy Chain
Gene. *Cell* 45: 247–59.

Wecker, M. 2012. 10 High-Profile People Whose Degrees Were Revoked. Available at
http://www.usnews.com/education/top-world-universities/articles/2012/
05/02/10-high-profile-people-whose-degrees-were-revoked. Accessed on
October 29, 2013.

Weed, D. L., and McKeown, R. E. 2003. Science and Social Responsibility in Public
Health. *Environmental Health Perspectives* 111(14): 1804–1808.

Weijer, C., and Emanuel, E. E. 2000. Protecting Communities in Biomedical
Research. *Science* 289: 1142–1144.

Weil, V. 1993. Teaching Ethics in Science. In *Ethics, Values, and the Promise of Science*,
Sigma Xi, Research Triangle Park, NC, 242–248.

Weil, V., and Arzbaecher, R. 1997. Relationships in Laboratories and Research
Communities. In *Research Ethics: A Reader*, D. Elliott and J. Stern (eds.).
University of New England Press, Hanover, NH, 69–90.

Wein, L., and Liu, Y. 2005. Analyzing a Bioterror Attack on the Food Supply: The
Case of Botulinum Toxin in Milk. *Proceedings of the National Academy of
Sciences* 102: 9984–9989.

Weiss, R. 1997. Thyroid Drug Study Reveals Tug of War over Privately Financed
Research. Washington Post, April 16, A3.

Welsome, E. 1999. *The Plutonium File*. Dial Press, New York. Wendler, D. 2006. Three
Steps to Protecting Pediatric Research Participants from Excessive Risks.
PloS Clinical Trials 1(5): e25. doi:10.1371/journal.pctr.

Wendler, D. 2013. Do U.S. Regulations Allow More Than a Minor Increase over
Minimal Risk Pediatric Research? Should They? *IRB and Human Research*,
November-December.

Wendler, D., and Miller F. G. 2011a. Deception in Clinical Research. In *The Oxford
Textbook of Clinical Research Ethics*, E. Emanuel et al (eds.). Oxford University
Press, New York, 315–324.

Wendler, D., and Miller, F. G. 2011b. Risk-Benefit Analysis and the Net Risks Test.
In *The Oxford Textbook of Clinical Research Ethics*, E. Emanuel et al (eds.).
Oxford University Press, New York, 503–513.

Wendler, D. et. al. 2005. Quantifying the Federal Minimal Risk Standard—
Implications for Pediatric Research without a Prospect of Direct Benefit,
Journal of the American Medical Association 29: 826–832.

Whitbeck, C. 1996. Ethics as Design. Doing Justice to Moral Problems. *Hastings Center Report* 26(3): 9–16.

Whitbeck, C. 1998. *Ethics in Engineering Practice and Research*. Cambridge University Press, Cambridge.

White, M. 2007. A Right to Benefit from International Research: A New Approach to Capacity Building in Less-developed Countries. *Accountability in Research* 14: 73–92.

Whon, D., and Normile D. 2006. Hwang Indicted for Fraud, Embezzlement. *ScienceNow*, May 12.

Wilcox, B. L. 1992. Fraud in Scientific Research: The Prosecuters Approach. *Accountability in Research* 2: 139–151.

Wilcox, L. 1998. Authorship: The Coin of the Realm, The Source of Complaints. *Journal of the American Medical Association* 280: 216–217.

Williams, T. 1987. *The History of Invention*. Facts on File, New York.

Williams, R., Flaherty, L., and Threadgill, D. 2003. The Math of Making Mutant Mice. *Genes, Brain, and Behavior* 2: 191–200.

Willman, D. 2005. NIH Inquiry Shows Widespread Ethical Lapses, Lawmaker Says. *Los Angeles Times*, July 14.

Wilmut, I. 1997. Cloning for Medicine. *Scientific American* 279(6): 58–63.

Wilson, K., Schreier, A., Griffin, A., and Resnik, D. 2007. Research Records and the Resolution of Misconduct Allegations at Research Universities. *Accountability in Research* 14: 57–71.

Wislar, J. S., Flanagin, A., Fontanarosa, P. B., and Deangelis, C. D. 2011. Honorary and Ghost Authorship in High Impact Biomedical Journals: A Cross Sectional Survey. *British Medical Journal* 343: d6128.

Wolf, S., Lawrenz, F., et al. 2008. Managing Incidental Findings in Human Subjects Research: Analysis and Recommendations. *Journal of Law, Medicine and Ethics* 36: 219–248.

Wood, S. F., and Mador, J. K. 2013. Uncapping Conflict of Interest? *Science* 340: 1172–1173.

World Medical Association. 2013. Declaration of Helsinki—Ethical Principles for Medical Research Involving Human Subjects. Available at http://www.wma.net/en/30publications/10policies/b3/. Accessed on November 12, 2013.

World Trade Organization (WTO). 2007. TRIPS. Available at http://www.wto.org/english/tratop_e/trips_e/t_agm2_e.htm. Accessed on November 17, 2007..

Wyatt, R. J. 1986. Risks of Withdrawing Antipsychotic Medication. *Archives of General Psychiatry* 52: 205–208.

Wyatt, R. J., et al., 1999. The Long-term Effects of Placebo in Patients with Chronic Schizophrenia. *Biological Psychiatry* 46: 1092–1105.

Zeng, W., and Resnik, D. 2010. Research Integrity in China: Problems and Prospects. *Developing World Bioethics* 10(3): 164–171.

Ziman, J. 1984. *Introduction to Science Studies*. Cambridge University Press, Cambridge.

Zolla-Parker, S. 1994. The Professor, the University, and Industry. *Scientific American* 270(3): 120.

Zuckerman, H. 1977a. Deviance Behavior and Social Control in Science. In *Deviance and Social Change*, E. Sagrin (ed.). Sage, Beverly Hills, CA, 87–138.

Zuckerman, H. 1977b. *Scientific Elite: Nobel Laureates in the United States*. Free Press, New York.

Zurer, P. 1993. NIH Peer Reviewers to Watch for High-Risk, High-Payoff Proposals. *Chemical and Engineering News*, June 7, 25–26.

INDEX

Locators in **bold** indicate major concepts

Broad, William, 28, 29, 46, 65, 71, 98, 123
Buxton, Peter, 244

Capron, Alexander Morgan, 236, 237, 241, 251, 252, 264
career, 1, 5, 24, 30, 48, 77, 79, 87, 93, 117, 154, 166, 169, 198, 289
carefulness, 18
Carson, Rachel, 285, 291
categorical imperative, 13
Chalmers, Thomas, 147
children, 6, 15, 27, 30, 35, 112, 215, 218–20, 234, **242–5**, 248, 252, 253, 262, 268–71, 277, 289
citation, 22, 39, 123, 124, 126
citation amnesia, 126
clinical research, 3, 63, 66, 73, 115, 158
clinical trials, 56, 61, 97, 98, 112, 113, 124, 128, 190, 191, 249, 256, 259, 270, 277, 278
cloning, 10, 33, 160, 265, 275
coauthors, 31, 33, 44, 45, 88, 124
Cobbe, Francis Powers, 215
code of medical ethics, 237
codes of conduct, 6, 36
codes of ethics, 4, 19, 310
cold fusion, 163
collaboration, 2, 33, 41, 49, 59, 74, **96–121**, 122, 172, 191, 304, 305, 307, 310
  with industry, **96–121**, 172
Common Rule, **253–5**, 263, 268–70
conflict of interest, 35, 36, 43, 50, 96, 100, 152, 156, 165, **194–212**, 288
  individual, 197, 273, 288, 289, 304, 308
  institutional, 56, 203
  policies, 195
consequentialism, 13
cooperation, 3, 74, 303, 309, **310**
Copernicus, Nicholas, 61, 138
copyright, 18, 67, 99, 126, 134, 161, 171–3, **178**, 179, 181, 183, 184, 188, 193
credit, 8, 18, 38, 39, 47, 63, 76, 88, 94, 118, 125, 126, 131, 133, 136, 166, 172, 279

Dalton, 29, 155
Darsee, John, 30, 31
Darwin, Charles, 76, 122
data, viii, 1, 2, 5, 10, 18, 19, 21, 22, 24, **29**, **37**, 39, 42, 44, 45, 47, 48, 50, 54–6, 61, 64–6, 69, 72–4, 78, 107, 114, 126, 128, 129, 144, 148, 171, 254
  analysis, 5, 18, 62, 66, 69, **70**, 114, 128
  archives, 77
  fabrication, 4, 6, 17, 20, **29–37**, 39, 42, 44, 47, 56, 114, 149
  interpretation, 18, **72**, 73
  management, **60**, 67, 96–9, 117, 306, 307
  misrepresentation, 18
  ownership, 60, 68, **180**
  raw, 67
  sharing, 3, 6, 19, **74–6**, 79, 108, 110, 199, 265, 266, 307
data audit, **51**, **52**, 54
Daubert v. Merrell Dow Pharmaceuticals, 288
Declaration of Helsinki, 251, 257, 268
deontological, 13
Department of Defense, 103, 104, 274, 292, 293
Department of Energy (DOE), 140
Descartes, Rene, 139, 214
Diamond v. Chakrbarty, 176, 185
Dong, Betty, 109
do no harm, 4, 237
dual use research, 294–6, 298
Durkheim, Emile, 48

Edison, Thomas, 173
editorial independence, 137, **159**
editors, 33, 34, **44**, 46, 57, 66, 72, 127, 130, 145, 147, 148–50, 153–8, 160, 162, 166, 211, 295, 296, 299, 307
education
  ethics, 155–8
  science, 33, 34, 127, 128, 130
Egyptians, 137
Einstein, Albert, 148, 285
enlightenment, 12
ethical, vii, viii, **1–12**, 14–17, 19, 25, 26, 28, 37, 45, 49–51, 60, 61, 70,

National Science Foundation (NSF), vii, 38, 42, 49, 75, 96, 101, 140, 143, 151, 200, 307
natural law, 187
Nazi, 236, 241, 246, 261
Newkirk, Ingrid, 215
Newton, Isaac, 5, 28, 96, 122, 139, 292
Nobel Prize, 31, 70, 72, 292
nonobviousness, 177
novelty, 177
Nuremberg Code, 236, 243, 246, 251, 263

objectivity, 3, 12, 60, 64, 70, 85, 87, 108, 141, 146, 152, **194–9**, 201, 202, 205, 290, 291
in ethics, 12, 18
Office of Human Research Protections (OHRP), 252, 254, 309
Office of Research Integrity (ORI), vii, 34–6, 42, 45, 49, 53, 123, 309
Olivieri, Nancy, 109, 110
openness, 18, 19, 20, 74, 77, 85, 108, 110, 111, 154, 161, 266, 283, 285, 293, 296, 297
Oppenheimer, Robert, 291
Origin of Species, 122
Osler, William, 239, 243

Pacheco, Alex, 215
Pasteur, Louis, 29, 31, 238, 239, 285
patents, 18, 67, 74, 76, 78, 105–7, 116, 125, 146, 171–3, **175–9**, 304
DNA, 177, **185–8**, 195
peer review, 3, 5, 18, 25, 34, 37, 38, 49, 60, 97, **137–70**, 252, 307, 308
blinding, 153
fair, 154, 156
People for the Ethical Treatment of Animals (PETA), 212, 215, 232
pharmaceutical companies, 74, 112–14, 124, 177, 185, 188, 208, 270, 306
pharmacogenomics, vii
phase I studies, 260
Phinney, Carolyn, 89
Piltdown man, 29
placebo, 111, 247, 249, 250, 256, 257
plagiarism, 22, 36–9, 44–7, 51, 63, 97, 123, 125–7, 146, 149, 158, 309
Plato, 12, 85, 137

Poehlman, Eric, 34, 35, 38, 40, 198
Pons, Stanley, 163
principal investigator, 63, 88, 129, 143, 194, 232
printing press, 5, 138–40, 172, 173
prisoners, 215, 236, 242, 246, 251, 252, 264, 268, 269, 272, 275
privacy, 66, 77, 236, 253, **265, 266**, 268, 275
private foundations, 141, 143, 204
publication, 3, 4, 18, 22, 32, 44–6, 49, 50, 52, 55, 71–6, 96, 100, 104, 109–11, 113, 117, 122–5, 128–31, **137–70**, 177, 181, 282, 296, 297, 305, 307
electronic, 46, 137, **160–2**
quality control, 76, 137, 139–41, 148, 154, 162
public policy, 73, 157, 283, 290, 291
public trust, 3
publish or perish, 123

quality assurance, 67, 69
quality control, 76, 137, 139–41, 148, 154, 162

radiation experiments, 236, 240, 245, 251, 253
raw data, 52, 67, 68
record keeping, 39, 50, 66–9
redundancy, 226
Reed, Walter, 239, 240
Regan, Tom, 212, 216, 219–21
reliability, 149, 258
religion, 9, 10, 18, 25, 284
repeatability, 146
replacement, 212, 225, 227
replication, 45, 74
research, **1–310**
as a career, 5
collaboration, 33, 41, 49, 59, 74, 96, 122, 172, 304, 305, 307, 310
dissemination, 74, 110, 143
hypothesis, 56, 60, 61–**3**, 64, 129, 148, 238, 239, 286
interdisciplinary, 122, 147
protocol, 63, 65, 226, 231, 247–50
record, 37, 39, 42, 44, 50, 62, 65–9, 80, 86, 122, 129, 137, 145, 174